Gender in the Middle Ages

Volume 11

MEDICINE, RELIGION AND GENDER IN MEDIEVAL CULTURE

Gender in the Middle Ages

ISSN 1742-870X

This series investigates the representation and construction of masculinity and femininity in the Middle Ages from a variety of disciplinary and interdisciplinary perspectives. It aims in particular to explore the diversity of medieval genders, and such interrelated contexts and issues as sexuality, social class, race and ethnicity, and orthodoxy and heterodoxy.

Proposals or queries should be sent in the first instance to the editors or to the publisher, at the addresses given below; all submissions will receive prompt and informed consideration.

Professor Jacqueline Murray, College of Arts, University of Guelph, Guelph, Ontario, N1G 2W1, Canada

Professor Diane Watt, School of English and Languages, University of Surrey, Guildford, Surrey GU5 7XH, UK

Boydell & Brewer Limited, PO Box 9, Woodbridge, Suffolk IP12 3DF, UK

Previously published volumes in the series are listed at the end of this book.

MEDICINE, RELIGION AND GENDER IN MEDIEVAL CULTURE

Edited by

Naoë Kukita Yoshikawa

D. S. BREWER

First published 2015
D. S. Brewer, Cambridge

ISBN 978 1 84384 401 3

D. S. Brewer is an imprint of Boydell & Brewer Ltd
PO Box 9, Woodbridge, Suffolk IP12 3DF, UK
and of Boydell & Brewer Inc.
668 Mt Hope Avenue, Rochester, NY 14620–2731, USA
website: www.boydellandbrewer.co.uk

A CIP catalogue record for this book is available
from the British Library

In memoriam

Masako Yoshikawa

1928–2012

CONTENTS

CONTRIBUTORS

Diane Watt is Professor of English and Head of the School of English and Languages at the University of Surrey. She works on medieval and early modern English Literature, women's writing and gender and sexuality. Her most recent publications include *The History of British Women's Writing, 700–1500*, co-edited with Liz Herbert McAvoy (Basingstoke: Palgrave Macmillan, 2012), *The Lesbian Premodern*, co-edited with Noreen Giffney and Michelle M. Sauer (Basingstoke: Palgrave Macmillan, 2011) and *Medieval Women's Writing* (Cambridge: Polity, 2007).

Roberta Magnani is Lecturer in Medieval English Literature at Swansea University, where she teaches medieval and early modern literature as well as gender theory. Interested in the works of Geoffrey Chaucer and, more broadly, in the intersection between manuscript studies and queer theory, she is currently completing a monograph, *Chaucer's Queer Textualities: Manuscripts and the Challenging of Authority*, New Middle Ages series (Basingstoke: Palgrave Macmillan, forthcoming 2016). Her research interests also lie in medieval medicine, spirituality and gendered spaces such as the *hortus conclusus*.

Naoë Kukita Yoshikawa is Professor of English in the Faculty of Humanities and Social Sciences at Shizuoka University. She has widely published on late medieval devotional texts, including *Margery Kempe's Meditations: The Context of Medieval Devotional Literature, Liturgy and Iconography* (Cardiff: University of Wales Press, 2007). Her research also focuses on late medieval medicine and religion. Her recent publications include 'Holy Medicine and Diseases of the Soul: Henry of Lancaster and *Le Livre de Seyntz Medicines*', *Medical History* 53, 3 (2009) and 'The Translation of the *Regimen Sanitatis* into a Handbook for the Devout Laity: a New Look at the *Kalender of Shepherds* and Its Context', in *Medieval Translator XV: In Principio Fuit Interpres*, ed. Alessandra Petrina (Turnhout: Brepols, 2013).

Liz Herbert McAvoy is Professor of Medieval Literature at the Centre for Medieval and Early-Modern Studies, Swansea University. She has published widely in the area of gender and medieval women's literature. Her recent publications include *Medieval Anchoritisms: Gender, Space and the Solitary Life* (Cambridge: D. S. Brewer, 2011) and the edited collection *A Companion to Julian of Norwich* (Cambridge: D. S. Brewer, 2008).

Juliette Vuille is currently a Fonds National Suisse de la Recherche Scientifique (FNS) Early Postdoctoral Mobility Fellow at the University of Oxford. She holds a doctorate from the University of Lausanne and a Master of Studies (honors) degree from the University of Oxford. She has published articles on topics ranging from late medieval female mystics in England to medieval translations of the Bible, by way of palaeography. Connected to her contribution in this present volume are 'The Magdalene as an Authorizing Tool in the Book of Margery Kempe', in *Mary Magdalene in Medieval Culture: Conflicted Roles*, ed. Peter Loewen and Robin Waugh (London: Routledge, 2014) and '"Towche Me Not": Uneasiness in the Translation of the Noli Me Tangere Episode in the Late Medieval English Period', in *Medieval Translator XV: In Principio Fuit Interpres*, ed. Alessandra Petrina (Turnhout: Brepols, 2013).

Takami Matsuda is Professor of English at the Department of English and American Literature, Faculty of Letters, Keio University. He works on medieval English literature, early printed books and digitisation of medieval and early modern manuscripts. His publications include *Death and Purgatory in Middle English Didactic Poetry* (Cambridge: D. S. Brewer, 1997), *The Medieval Book and a Modern Collector: Essays in Honour of Toshiyuki Takamiya*, co-edited with Richard A. Linenthal and John Scahill (Cambridge: D. S. Brewer/ Tokyo: Yushodo, Press, 2004) and the edited collection, *Codices Keionenses: Essays on Western Manuscripts and Early Printed Books in Keio University Library* (Tokyo: Keio University Press, 2005).

Louise M. Bishop is Associate Professor of literature at Clark Honors College, University of Oregon. She specialises in fourteenth-century Middle English poetry and prose, and has written on medieval medicine in her book *Words, Stones and Herbs: The Healing Word in Medieval and Early Modern England* (Syracuse, NY: Syracuse University Press, 2007) as well as on the poetry of William Langland and Geoffrey Chaucer, most recently in *Icons of the Middle Ages*, ed. Lister Matheson (Westport, CT: Greenwood, 2011). Other work includes an essay on the myth of the flat earth for *Misconceptions about the Middle Ages* (London: Routledge, 2008) and on Shakespeare's *Winter's Tale* in *Medieval Shakespeare in Performance* (Jefferson, NC: MacFarland, 2009).

Irina Metzler holds a Wellcome Trust University Award at Swansea University. She is a leading expert on cultural, religious and social aspects of physical and mental disability in the European Middle Ages. Books on these topics include *Disability in Medieval Europe* (London and New York: Routledge, 2006, 2010), *A Social History of Disability in the Middle Ages* (London and New York: Routledge, 2013), as well as the forthcoming *Fools and Idiots? Intellectual Disability in the Middle Ages* (2015). Her wider research interests revolve around perceptions of the natural world and historical anthropology in the Middle Ages, with essays such as heretical cats and animal symbolism in *Medium Aevum Quotidianum* 59 (2009), and the article, 'Perceptions of Hot Climate in Cosmography and Travel Literature', in *The Medieval Ethnographies: European Perceptions of the World Beyond*, ed. Joan-Pau Rubiés (Farnham: Ashgate, 2009).

Patricia Skinner is Reader in Medieval History at the University of Winchester. Her research interests focus on the social and cultural history of medieval Italy, gender and the Jewish communities of medieval Europe. Her most recent publication in gender history is *Medieval Writings on Secular Women*, co-edited with Elisabeth van Houts (London: Penguin, 2011). She is currently completing a monograph for Palgrave Macmillan on facial mutilation in the Middle Ages

Joy Hawkins is a Tutor in History in the Faculty of Arts and Humanities, University of East Anglia. She completed her Ph.D. on 'The Blind in Later Medieval England: Medical, Social and Religious Responses' under the supervision of Professor Carole Rawcliffe. Her publications include 'Seeing the Light? Blindness and Sanctity in Later Medieval England', *Studies in Church History* 47 (2011) and *On Light*, Medium Aevum monograph, ed. K. P. Clarke and S. Baccianti (2013), exploring the role of vision in health during the Middle Ages. She is currently researching several aspects of medieval medical history, including the interactions of the visually impaired with the law.

Elma Brenner is Specialist, Medieval and Early Modern Medicine, at the Wellcome Library, London. Her research examines medicine and religious culture in medieval France and England, particularly responses to leprosy and mental illness in the duchy of Normandy. Her most recent publications are 'Leprosy and Public Health in Late Medieval Rouen', in *The Fifteenth Century XII: Society in an Age of Plague*, ed. Linda Clark and Carole Rawcliffe (Woodbridge: Boydell, 2013), and 'The Leprous Body in Twelfth- and Thirteenth-Century Rouen: Perceptions and Responses', in *The Ends of the Body: Identity and Community in Medieval Culture*, ed. Suzanne Conklin Akbari and Jill Ross (Toronto: University of Toronto Press, 2013). Her recent publications also include *Memory and Commemoration in Medieval Culture*, co-edited with Meredith Cohen and Mary Franklin-Brown (Aldershot: Ashgate, 2013) and *Society and Culture in Medieval Rouen, 911–1300*, co-edited with Leonie V. Hicks (Turnhout: Brepols, 2013). Her monograph, *Leprosy and Charity in Medieval Rouen*, is forthcoming in 2015/2016.

Denis Renevey is Professor of Medieval English Language and Literature at the University of Lausanne. He is the author of several articles and book chapters on vernacular theology. His recent book publications include *The Doctrine of the Hert: A Critical Edition with Introduction and Commentary*, co-edited with Christiania Whitehead and Anne Mouron (Exeter: University of Exeter Press, 2010), *A Companion to the Doctrine of the Hert: The Middle English Translations and its Latin and European Contexts*, co-edited with Christiania Whitehead (Exeter: University of Exeter Press, 2010); *Poetica* 72, Special Issue, *Convergence/Divergence: The Politics of Late Medieval English Devotional and Medical Discourses*, co-edited with Naoë Kukita Yoshikawa (Tokyo: Yushodo Press, 2009). His most recent book, *Medieval and Early Modern Literature, Science and Medicine*, co-edited with Rachel Falconer (Tübingen: Gunter Narr, 2013), explores the meeting of the literary and scientific spheres of knowledge in medieval and early modern England.

ACKNOWLEDGEMENTS

It is a pleasure to acknowledge the abundant support I have received in producing this collection. My thanks are due first and foremost to the contributors for collaborating with me during its production and entrusting me with editing and proofreading. Many colleagues and friends generously shared their time, intelligence and expertise with me.

I would especially like to thank Professor Carole Rawcliffe, who introduced me to the history of medieval medicine through her work and provided me with her profound knowledge and expertise during my research leave at the University of East Anglia in the autumn semester of 2006. I would also like to thank my former UEA colleagues: Dr Christopher Bonfield, Professor Stephen Church, Dr Joy Hawkins, Dr Carole Hill, Mr David King, Mrs Elizabeth Rutledge and Dr Sarah Salih. Their interest in my work and their friendship always encouraged me to explore this interdisciplinary area. I should extend my thanks to Professor Monica Green, who generously shared her work in progress with me and inspired me to a variety of ideas through The Medieval Medicine listserv run by her, to Professor Elizabeth Robertson and Professor Tess Tavormina, who gave me discerning comments on this project, and to Dr Julie Orlemanski and Dr Katie Walter, who have shared with me a recent article and a summary of a PhD thesis, respectively. I would also like to thank Dr Juliette Vuille, who produced a very fine essay in a short space of time, following the withdrawal of two of the original contributors, and Professor Denis Renevey, for contributing an astute Afterword to this collection.

Special thanks go to Professor Liz Herbert McAvoy, who not only gave me perceptive suggestions and unflagging encouragement in most difficult circumstances but also offered to read all non-native English speakers' essays with me and supported my efforts at editing with tremendous generosity in the last stage of submission. I would also like to warmly thank Professor Catherine Innes-Parker and Dr Christiania Whitehead, who have helped me at various moments with care, generosity and thoughtfulness. Indeed, they are my sisters at heart.

Three essays in this volume were originally presented at the International Symposium on Medicine, Religion and Gender in Medieval Culture at Shizuoka University in 2012. I owe my thanks to Professor Takami Matsuda, Professor Liz Herbert McAvoy and Professor Diane Watt for participating in this event when the anxiety about occasional earthquakes and the unstable situation of the nuclear plant in the wake of the natural disaster in the spring of 2011 had repercussions, especially on the mind of foreign visitors.

I am grateful to Ms Caroline Palmer at Boydell & Brewer for her expertise and enthusiasm at all stages of the project. It has also been a pleasure to collaborate with her associates Mr Robert Kinsey and Ms Rosie Pearce for the publication of this volume. This volume benefited greatly from insightful and constructive comments from the publisher's anonymous readers, to whom I am immensely grateful. Financial support for research and the symposium was provided by the Japanese Ministry of Education (2006) and the Japan Society for the Promotion of Science (2010–13). I appreciate the generosity of these organisations.

Finally, my thanks, as ever, go to my three children, and this time, perhaps, especially to Tomoko, who trailed around medieval hospitals and churches with me over a decade and produced exciting photographical resources for my research and teaching. This collection of essays is dedicated to the memory of my mother, Masako Yoshikawa, who earned her MD and PhD in post-war Japan. Practising as a paediatrician, she was as circumscribed as any medieval female physician by society's assumptions about women's traditional roles. Yet, by the time she retired in her eighties, she was keeping company with female physicians including her granddaughter, Asako. This volume is a tribute to her and an expression of hope that the future generations of women will flourish with confidence, moral courage and compassion.

Naoë Kukita Yoshikawa
Tokyo, January 2015

ABBREVIATIONS

AA.SS.	*Acta Sanctorum*
CBA	Council for British Archaeology
EETS	Early English Text Society
e.s.	extra series
FSGA	Freiherr-vom-Stein-Gedächtnisausgabe
HMSO	Her Majesty's Stationery Office
MED	Middle English Dictionary
MGH	*Monumenta Germaniae Historica*
n.s.	new series
PL	*Patrologiae cursus completus ... Series Latina*, ed. J.-P. Migne (Paris, 1844–65)
o.s.	original series
s.s.	supplementary series
TEAMS	Consortium for the Teaching of the Middle Ages

INTRODUCTION

Naoë Kukita Yoshikawa

Preoccupations with the body in the twenty-first century have led to a growing interest in the intersections between literature, religion and the history of medicine, and, more specifically, how they converge within a given culture. In her plenary lecture delivered at the 2012 conference at Swansea University entitled 'Cure and Care: Diseases, Disabilities and Therapies',[1] Professor Monica Green, a leading historian of medieval medicine, not only emphasised the importance of a continued historical perspective but also called for active dialogue and concerted multi-disciplinary approaches in order to develop a deeply nuanced understanding of the social and cultural factors of disease, both modern and premodern. In response to such imperatives, this volume comprises a collection of essays exploring the ways in which aspects of medieval culture were predicated upon an interaction between medical and religious discourses, particularly those inflected by contemporary gendered ideologies. Indeed, during the Middle Ages there was frequently a fusion of such discourses, one that became increasingly fissured within post-Enlightenment contexts – to the extent that it has become largely lost to us today.[2] During the medieval period, however, the inseparability of bodily and spiritual concerns was paramount, as displayed in the Church's dominance over all issues concerning sickness, health, life, death and the salvation of all individual souls. This inseparability is witnessed clearly in medical and devotional texts of all types and genres during the period: such texts interrelate thematically, entering into dialogue with one another by means of powerful metaphors linked to cultural and religious norms. Medieval socio-religious culture, therefore, offers an ideal site for an investigation into such

[1] This lecture was based on Green's essay, entitled 'The Value of Historical Perspective', in *The Ashgate Research Companion to the Globalization of Health*, ed. Ted Strecker et al. (forthcoming).

[2] On medicine and the eighteenth century, see *Literature and Medicine during the Eighteenth Century*, ed. Marie Mulvey Roberts and Roy Porter (London and New York, 1993).

a close cohabitation of religious and medical discourses, along with the *mentalités* this produced.

The overarching aim of this volume is to investigate this interaction of medieval medicine and religion in the Middle Ages, taking its lead from those scholars working in the Early Modern period who have already made some inroads into examining the time immediately preceding the emergence of the stark dichotomous separation of literature and science that characterised the eighteenth century.[3] For example, in her article, 'Literature and Medicine: Traditions and Innovations', Anne Hudson Jones argues that the fields of literature and medicine share a number of common themes and foci: illness, suffering, death, healers, physician-writers, to name but a few, as well as their common depiction of literature as a healing mechanism. Indeed, as Jones argues, within these shared interests, literary and bodily hermeneutics speak cogently to one another. In her discussion of the use made of literary texts in North American medical schools, Jones argues that a training in subtle critical reading of such works can – and should – be used by doctors as a tool for improving patient diagnoses.[4] As this present volume will demonstrate, this type of practice finds its precedent in medieval medical training, which aimed to make physicians good readers of bodies by training them first to become good readers of texts. In this way, medical students are able to become better readers of their patients' bodies, obtaining a heightened sense of their individual and hermeneutic qualities. What has been all but forgotten, too, is that before the eighteenth century, the physician-writer was a common figure in the humanist landscape and someone who employed both medical and literary discourses without any sense of discontinuity or tension.[5]

As an intrinsic component of textuality, both rhetoric and metaphor have long been fundamental in shaping a specific culture's understanding of disease and illness, and, as such, also constitute another of this volume's major concerns. As medical anthropologists continue to argue, illness is and always has been shaped by a culture's normative functions: each culture provides a different set of hermeneutic tools for interpreting the experience labelled as 'disease'. Byron Good, for instance, describes illness as a 'set of words, experiences, and feelings which typically "run together" for members of a society'.[6]

3 See George S. Rousseau, *Enlightenment Borders: Pre- and Post-modern Discourses: Medical, Scientific* (Manchester and New York, 1991), especially 'The Discourses of Literature and Science', pp. 202–52.

4 See Anne Hudson Jones, 'Literature and Medicine: Traditions and Innovations', in *The Body and the Text: Comparative Essays in Literature and Medicine*, ed. Bruce Clarke and Wendell Aycock (Lubbock, TX, 1990), pp. 11–24.

5 On our preoccupations with the body and the field of literature and medicine, see George S. Rousseau, 'Bridges of Light: The Domains of Literature and Medicine', *The Aberdeen University Review* 56 (1995), 1–22.

6 Byron J. Good, *Medicine, Rationality, and Experience: An Anthropological Perspective* (Cambridge, 1994), p. 5. See further *Poetica* 72, Special Issue, *Convergence/Divergence:*

Each society, therefore, is likely to offer a different set of paradigms for the construction, authorisation and contestation of personal experiences of illness. Such a variety of interpretative practices, explored synchronically and diachronically by medical anthropologists, suggests that disease as a cultural phenomenon is subject to interpretation, becoming a site for the display and/or imposition of power and authorisation, with rhetoric also playing a significant role within this equation. Again, it is just such contingency of meaning that preoccupies many of the essays in this volume, particularly those offering a literary focus and analysis sensitive to both the metaphorical and material aspects of medieval medicine. Combined with those essays offering historical approaches, they serve to broaden the range of the developing field.

This is not to say that this type of focus is unique to this present volume: indeed, the project is indebted to a wealth of earlier scholarship examining notions of healing in late medieval culture and its texts. For example, Glending Olson's study posits a therapeutic value in the experience of reading literature as able to moderate the 'accidents of the soul'. Olson argues that the pleasure of the literary text can generate for the reader an inner harmony that promotes bodily and mental health.[7] This remains true, not just for secular literature but also – far more explicitly, perhaps – for devotional literature as a site where allusions to bodily/spiritual health are almost ubiquitous. Among those scholars who have already investigated the wide deployment of medical metaphors and discourses in medieval writing is Louise Bishop (one of the contributors to this volume), who, in her 2007 monograph, links the image of Christ in *Piers Plowman* to 'theriac', a medieval antidote to snake venom, arguing that Christ's sacrifice is the medicinal antidote for the venom of Original Sin. Grounded in the powerful connection between healing and theology that characterised medieval epistemology, Bishop reveals that 'medicine is the vehicle for epistemological, lexical, and pious analysis' of religious texts.[8]

Another critic who has identified some of the ways in which medieval medical discourses are intertwined with theology and confessional practice is Virginia Langum, drawing on the close connection between care and cure of illness with the discernment and cure of sins as predominant in penitential literature, in particular.[9] Based on an area of Augustinian theology that perceives skin as having become darkened after the Fall, Langum reveals how confessors read the surface of confessants' skin to determine the *complexio* and

The Politics and Late Medieval English Devotional and Medical Discourses, ed. Denis Renevey and Naoë Kukita Yoshikawa (Tokyo, 2009), 'Introduction'.

7 Glending Olson, *Literature as Recreation in the Middle Ages* (Ithaca, NY, 1982).

8 Louise M. Bishop, *Words, Stones, Herbs: The Healing Word in Medieval and Early Modern England* (Syracuse, NY, 2007), p. 6.

9 For a study of Penitentials in terms of therapy for sin, see George Christian Anderson, 'Medieval Medicine for Sin', *Journal of Religion and Health* 2. 2 (1963), 156–65.

the sins they committed. Langum also identifies the overlapping of knowledge and practice within the fields of surgery and confession, arguing that 'medieval beliefs about the relationship between body and soul posit a literal connection between sins and illnesses and spiritual and physical cures'.[10] Here, she joins Jeremy J. Citrome, who employs a variety of approaches to examine the type of surgical metaphors that became prominent following the Fourth Lateran Council (1215). He presents illuminating reinterpretations of Middle English literature, such as *Cleanness*, *Siege of Jerusalem* and John Audelay's poems, with an exemplary awareness of the need for a concerted interdisciplinary approach to medieval literature and the history of medicine.[11]

Alongside surgeons, university-trained, elite physicians have also provided an important focus for literary interrogation. For example, Huling E. Ussery has explored Chaucer's portrait of the Physician and his tale in *The Canterbury Tales*, examining historical and literary accounts of physicians as compared with surgeons in fourteenth-century England.[12] In his work, Ussery argues against the tendency to see the Doctour of Physik as a stock figure to be read through irony and satire, and contends that through Chaucer's realistic characterisation of the Physician he emerges as a learned man (probably a cleric) who is highly suited to the telling of a moral and erudite tale of chastity and goodness. Similarly, William Langland's portrayal of medical practice and practitioners in *Piers Plowman* has also been investigated by scholars: Rosanne Gasse, for example, argues for the inseparability of the body and the soul embedded in the text and demonstrates how Langland envisages an ideal medical practitioner as one who heals both the body and the soul.[13]

Another important area where literature and medicine converge is in the context of sensory experience. Mystical texts from the period, which often display a heightened convergence of the senses, convey the mystic's experience as accompanied by myriad sensory perceptions. Good smells, for example, prominently feature such experiences, since it was believed that a floral fragrance permeated Heaven where one may breathe eternal bliss into the soul by means of that fragrance.[14] Indeed, it is no coincidence that Christ

10 Virginia Langum, 'Discerning Skin: Complexion, Surgery, and Language in Medieval Confession', in *Reading Skin in Medieval Literature and Culture*, ed. Katie L. Walter (New York, 2013), pp. 141–60 (p. 147).

11 Jeremy J. Citrome, *The Surgeon in Medieval English Literature* (New York, 2006).

12 Huling E. Ussery, *Chaucer's Physician: Medicine and Literature in Fourteenth-Century England*, Tulane Studies in English 19 (New Orleans, LA, 1971). I would like to thank Dr Roberta Magnani for sharing her thoughts on this with me.

13 Rosanne Gasse, 'The Practice of Medicine in *Piers Plowman*', *The Chaucer Review* 39, 2 (2004), 177–97. See also Raymond St-Jacques, 'Langland's Christus Medicus Image and the Structure of *Piers Plowman*', *Yearbook of Langland Studies* 5 (1991), 111–27.

14 Conversely, Purgatory and Hell were associated with vile stench. Julian of Norwich describes the temptation by the devil as a feverish state in which Julian, in her sickbed,

appeared to Mary Magdalene as a gardener on Easter morning (John 20:15).[15] Similarly, we find in Richard Rolle (d. 1349) a comparison of Christ's body to 'a medow ful of swete flours and holsome herbes'.[16] Thus, the healing powers of floral perfume are attributed to Christ who, by extension, is conceived as Physician and Apothecary in a healthy, redeemed garden.[17] Noteworthy in this context is C. M. Woolgar's thorough study of ideas concerning the senses in later medieval England. Examining various theories of sensation produced both by a learned culture and by popular belief, Woolgar analyses sources ranging from hagiographical accounts, miracle and medical collections and sermons to royal household books, arguing ultimately that 'Christianity and devotional practice opened up a range of possibilities for sensory perception.'[18]

Such a 'range of possibility' in the context of taste and touch was the focus of Katie Walter's doctoral thesis on the human mouth, which also explores the intersection of religious and medical texts in the later medieval period.[19] Arguing that the mouth is deeply implicated in religious thinking about sin and salvation, Walter examines the anatomy, physiology and pathology of the human mouth as well as its place in religious discourses, and presents new readings of pastoral and devotional works. Especially illuminating is the nexus of oral introspection and confessional self-knowledge shown by the analogy of barber-surgeon (an agent of dentistry) and confessor, a point also discussed by Langum and Citrome.

Linked also to the hermeneutic potential of the human senses in the Middle Ages is that of the human heart. Within this context, Heather Webb has identified an all-encompassing sensory system centred on the medieval heart. By examining the image and function of the heart – both medical and literary, Webb reconstructs a 'cardiosensory' model, a model which, based on a combination of Aristotelian and Galenic models for sense perception, emerged in the thirteenth and fourteenth centuries. Ultimately, Webb argues that this model responded to 'both philosophical and medical concepts of the

smells his stench: see *A Vision Showed to a Devout Woman* (known as her short text), in *The Writings of Julian of Norwich: A Vision Showed to a Devout Woman and A Revelation of Love*, ed. Nicholas Watson and Jacqueline Jenkins, Medieval Women: Texts and Contexts 5 (Turnhout, 2006), section 23, lines 18-22.

15 See, for example, 'Resurrection of Christ', Book of Hours, France, c. 1410, Bruges, Openbare Bibliotheek, MS 321, fol. 26v.

16 *English Writings of Richard Rolle*, ed. Hope Emily Allen (Oxford, 1968), p. 36; see Carole Rawcliffe, '"Delectable Sightes and Fragrant Smelles": Gardens and Health in Late Medieval and Early Modern England', *Garden History* 36 (2008), 3–21 (pp. 7–8).

17 For the image of Christ the Apothecary, see *Chants royaux sur la Conception couronnee du Puy de Rouen*, Paris, Bibliothèque nationale de France, MS Fr. 1537, fol. 82v.

18 C. M. Woolgar, *The Senses in Late Medieval England* (New Haven, CT, 2006), p. 269.

19 Katie Walter, 'Discourses of the Human: Mouths in Late Medieval Religious Literature', unpublished doctoral thesis, University of Cambridge, 2007.

human and of corporal sensation, envisioning an intimate cohabitation of body and soul'.[20]

Clearly, then, in the types of cohabitation of body and soul being identified here, the material and the metaphorical are rendered contiguous and boundaries between spiritual and bodily ailments and healing are blurred. Indeed, the question of how clear distinctions can be drawn between medical cure and miraculous cure within medieval perceptions of holistic health is key in this capacity. Therefore, if we are to reconstruct – and understand – the sheer hybridity of knowledge embedded in medieval medical and literary texts and appreciate the nuanced plurality of interpretation, it is imperative that those religious and medical discourses be brought together, along with the texts that house them.[21] Moreover, it is now becoming anachronistic to consider medical, religious and literary discourses as working separately during the medieval period (or, in reality, in any period), for those discourses are inscribed within a far larger social and cultural context. Adding to and complementing these foundational works, then, this present volume seeks to explore the literariness of medical knowledge and the medical aspects of religious literature.

Such a task, however, would be fundamentally untenable, were it not for the wide variety of studies produced by medical historians over the decades of the twentieth and twenty-first centuries focussing on medieval medicine in its Christian context. Foremost among these are Carole Rawcliffe's authoritative investigations of medical practice in late medieval English society, along with her more focused studies on hospitals, leprosy and, more recently, on public health (although her work does not particularly foreground the medical intersection with devotional writing and theology that is central to this volume). The excellent work of Peter Biller and Joseph Ziegler, however, does illuminate our thematic concerns in part, although, in their focus upon European clerical physicians and medico-theological debates taking place in elite university centres in Italy and France, their work distinguishes itself from this volume, which places a close focus upon English textual culture.[22] Nevertheless, this Anglocentric focus can be fruitfully informed by pan-European contexts.

20 Heather Webb, 'Cardiosensory Impulses in Late Medieval Spirituality', in *Rethinking the Medieval Senses: Heritage, Fascinations, Frames*, ed. Stephen G. Nichols, Andreas Kablitz and Alison Calhoun (Baltimore, MD, 2008), pp, 265–85 (p. 266); Heather Webb, *The Medieval Heart* (New Haven, CT, 2010).

21 See *Medieval and Early Modern Literature, Science and Medicine*, ed. Rachel Falconer and Denis Renevey, Swiss Papers in English Language and Literature, 28 (Tübingen, 2013).

22 Carole Rawcliffe, *Medicine and Society in Later Medieval England* (Stroud, 1995); *Medicine for the Soul: The Life, Death and Resurrection of an English Medieval Hospital, St Giles's, Norwich, c. 1249–1550* (Stroud, 1999); *Leprosy in Medieval England* (Woodbridge, 2006); *Urban Bodies: Communal Health in Late Medieval English Towns and Cities* (Woodbridge, 2013). Joseph Ziegler, *Medicine and Religion c. 1300: The Case*

Indeed, although we are now aware that professionally-trained doctors were rarer in England than in some other countries, such as France, Italy and Spain, late medieval English society was not isolated from the advanced medicine of the continent – French physicians and surgeons, for example, were attached to English royal households from the late thirteenth century. Like Pascal of Bologna, a *medicus* who served Henry of Lancaster (c. 1310–1361) who, in turn, obtained 'several ecclesiastical benefices in England for Pascal from the pope',[23] a number of Italian medical practitioners came to England as the opportunities for commerce increased. English medical practitioners also benefited from growing opportunities to travel, leading them to integrate themselves within a much larger world of medical experience.[24] In fact, recent research has shown that English surgeons were using continental texts to inform their practice. As Peter Murray Jones has argued, John of Arderne (1307–c. 1380) acquired knowledge and practice of scholastic surgery from that which originated in the milieu of the north Italian medical schools of the thirteenth and fourteenth centuries, particularly through texts by Lanfranco of Milan and Roger of Parma.[25] Such wide socio-cultural contexts for 'English' medicine certainly justify recourse to European medical discourse to inform our work.[26] As Monica Green argues, 'even if a historian is not immediately interested in apothecaries in the south of France ... midwives in England, or sick people in any of these areas, it *is* relevant to all historians that certain patterns of literacy, gender structures, economics ... are being documented by these studies'.[27] This is also true of the literary scholarship documented above, and for the same reasons: both medical culture and practices have trans-regional manifestations as well as local idiosyncrasies. Hence, here, Irina Metzler, Patricia Skinner and Elma Brenner do not specifically concentrate on English contexts but assist in an understanding of English medical culture as it operated within a wider, pan-European context.

of Arnau de Vilanova (Oxford, 1998); *Religion and Medicine in the Middle Ages*, ed. Peter Biller and Joseph Ziegler (York, 2001).

23 Faye Getz, *Medicine in the English Middle Ages* (Princeton, 1998), p. 29.

24 Getz, *Medicine in the English Middle Ages*, ch. 2, especially pp. 24–30.

25 Peter Murray Jones, 'John of Arderne and the Mediterranean Tradition of Scholastic Surgery', in *Practical Medicine from Salerno to the Black Death*, ed. Luis García-Ballester, Roger French, Jon Arrizabalaga and Andrew Cunningham (Cambridge, 2010), pp. 289–321.

26 See Nancy Siraisi, *Medieval and Early Renaissance Medicine* (Chicago, IL, 1990); Katharine Park, 'Medicine and Society in Medieval Europe, 500–1500', in *Medicine in Society: Historical Essays*, ed. Andrew Wear (Cambridge, 1992), pp. 59–90. See also Iona McCleery, 'Medical "Emplotment" and Plotting Medicine: Health and Disease in Late Medieval Portuguese Chronicles', *Social History of Medicine* 24, 1 (2011), 125–41; John Henderson, *The Renaissance Hospital: Healing the Body and Healing the Soul* (New Haven, CT and London, 2006).

27 Monica Green, 'Integrative Medicine: Incorporating Medicine and Health into the Canon of Medieval European History', *History Compass* 7, 4 (2009), 1218–45 (p. 1230).

Additionally, this volume also probes the way the literature-medicine nexus operates within a culture deeply inflected by gender discourse – for medieval culture manifests itself as one heavily influenced by gender divisions, as a myriad of recent studies has shown[28] – and, of course, medical discourse proves to be no exception. In exploring the gender-inflected nature of the medico-literary discourse and rhetoric, this volume also seeks to uncover the type of dialogues established – both positive and negative – between the medical, the religious and the gendered in the period under scrutiny. One might add to this mix the importance of the work of Irina Metzler on late medieval perceptions of disability and the discourses it generated. In her ground-breaking book of 2006, Metzler demonstrated how modern concepts can, indeed, be used to study the past and help to make visible many of those things that might otherwise have remained invisible.[29] Following her lead, therefore, this volume will also explore how disease and disability have been represented in medieval texts and images; it will also consider the problem of social attitudes and stigma – medical, spiritual and highly gendered – that were directed toward disability and impairment during the period. As such, the volume also focuses on an area of study increasingly attracting the attention of scholars in what is now broadly called the 'medical humanities'.

*

At this point it may be useful to consider some of the more specific cultural spaces in which medical and devotional discourses converged. Firstly, there was the widespread concept of *Christus medicus*, or Christ the Physician, that

28 There are too many studies to attempt a comprehensive list, but the most significant include: Joan Cadden, *The Meanings of Sex Difference in the Middle Ages: Medicine, Science, and Culture* (Cambridge and New York, 1993); Thomas Laqueur, *Making, Sex: Body and Gender form the Greeks to Freud* (Cambridge, MA, 1990); Elizabeth Robertson, 'Medieval Medical Views of Women and Female Spirituality in the *Ancrene Wisse* and Julian of Norwich's *Showings*', in *Feminist Approaches to the Body in Medieval Literature*, ed. Linda Lomperis and Sarah Stanbury (Philadelphia, 1993), pp. 142–67; Nancy Caciola, *Discerning Spirits: Divine and Demonic Possession in the Middle Ages* (Ithaca, NY and London, 2003), ch. 3. For numerous other works, see Monica Green's 'Bibliography on Medieval Women, Gender, and Medicine, 1980–2009': http://www.sciencia.cat/biblioteca/documents/Green_CumulativeBib_Feb2010.pdf (accessed 4 January 2014). Alexandra Barratt's illuminating reading of Julian's mystical text through the lens of medieval gynaecology, for example, still gives us an insightful methodology with which to appreciate the scientific and medical context of medieval texts: see '"In the Lowest Part of Our Need": Julian and Medieval Gynecological Writing', in *Julian of Norwich: A Book of Essays*, ed. Sandra J. McEntire, Garland Medieval Casebooks 21 (New York, 1998), pp. 239–56.

29 Irina Metzler, *Disability in Medieval Europe: Thinking about Physical Impairment during the High Middle Ages, c. 1100–1400* (London and New York, 2006); *A Social History of Disability in the Middle Ages: Cultural Considerations of Physical Impairment* (London and New York, 2013).

formed a powerful discourse within the Christian faith during the Middle Ages.[30] The concept dates back to the synoptic gospels where Christ was conceived as the physician of both soul and body. The intense struggle during the second and third centuries between the cult of Asclepius, the pagan healer, and the worship of Christ stimulated the early Church fathers to describe God's salvation of mankind by using similes taken from medicine in order to reconcile perceived incompatibilities.[31]

Fundamental to the concept of Christ the Physician is the widely held belief that sin and disease are interrelated. Within pre-Cartesian society the body and soul were regarded as unified entities, as mentioned above, the one influencing the condition of the other. Within this context too, sin could well be the root of disease, and physical healing could result directly from confession by virtue of its cleansing effect. Christ offered repentant sinners a remedy for their own personal transgressions as well as the collective burden, both physical and spiritual, of Original Sin. St Augustine (c. 354–430), among others, makes frequent use of the idea of *Christus medicus*. He saw the Passion of Christ as the best medicine through which man might recover his spiritual and physical health. Following Augustine, successive generations of theologians long maintained that holy medicine derived from Christ's flesh and blood, and emphasised the therapeutic effects of the Eucharist upon souls consumed with sin.[32] Indeed, the Eucharist was believed to radiate healing power. Exposure to the miracle of transubstantiation, even without reception, might have a beneficial effect on bodily infirmities. In medieval hospitals, Mass became hugely important in the daily regimen for the sick: as Carole Rawcliffe has demonstrated, it was 'in every sense a *medicina sacramentalis*, suffused with occult power'.[33] Moreover, the location of altars in medieval hospital shows that the Mass took place in full view of the inmates lying in their beds.[34]

Such interconnection between physical and spiritual health was reinforced around the time of the Gregorian Reform, a series of reforms initiated by Pope Gregory VII (c. 1050–80) and culminating in the Fourth Lateran Council (1215). Among the decrees of the Council, Canon 21 (*Omnis utriusque sexus*) demanded annual confession and communion and thus affected medieval spiritual life more than any other ruling.[35] Although lay confession long

30 For the notion of *Christus medicus* and its history, see R. Arbesmann, 'The Concept of "*Christus medicus*" in St Augustine', *Traditio* 10 (1954), 1-28. William Flete, a mid fourteenth-century Norwich hermit, presents God as the cruel-to-be-kind physician in *De Remediis contra Temptaciones [The Remedy ayenst the troubles of temptacyons]*. See further Liz Herbert McAvoy's essay in this volume.

31 Arbesmann, 'The Concept of "*Christus medicus*"', p. 3.

32 Rawcliffe, *Medicine and Society*, p. 18.

33 Rawcliffe, *Leprosy in Medieval England*, p. 339.

34 A notable example is found in the l'Hôtel-Dieu, Beaune (mid fifteenth century).

35 See Jacques Le Goff, *La naissance du purgatoire* (Paris, 1981), pp. 288–95; R. N. Swanson, *Religion and Devotion in Europe, c. 1215–c. 1515* (Cambridge, 1995), pp. 25–30;

preceded the Council, nevertheless it is important to acknowledge that a new emphasis was placed on the sacraments of confession and the Eucharist after 1215.[36] These developments in spiritual practice had an effect on notions of physical and spiritual health especially. Although the use of medicalised terms to explicate the efficacy of the process of confession was not a new literary phenomenon, as we have seen, with Lateran IV the canon was explicitly presented by means of medical imagery:

> Sacerdos autem sit discretus et cautus, ut more periti medici superinfundat vinum et oleum vulneribus sauciati, diligenter inquirens et peccatoris circumstantias et peccati, per quas prudenter intelligat, quale illi consilium debeat exhibere et cuiusmodi remedium adhibere, diversis experimentis utendo ad sanandum aegrotum.
>
> [The priest shall be discerning and prudent, so that like a skilled doctor he may pour wine and oil over the wounds of the injured one. Let him carefully inquire about the circumstances of both the sinner and the sin, so that he may prudently discern what sort of advice he ought to give and what remedy to apply, using various means to heal the sick person.][37]

Here, the terminology reflects explicitly the inextricability between medical and spiritual discourses I have been identifying elsewhere in this Introduction. In a culture in which sin and sickness were intimately related, sickness was seen as a sign of spiritual corruption and the metaphor of sin as a wound was widely accepted. Within the confessional ideology emerging from Lateran IV, auricular confession was embraced as the cleansing of wounds of sin and the purifying of the transgressor.[38] In terms of humoral pathology, one long favoured by theologians, it was thought that confession and communion enabled a reconciliation with God and the restoration of humoral balance. William of Auvergne (d. 1247), for example, a scholastic who relates penance to the metaphor of medicine, explicates in his *Sacrament*, that confession is 'a vomiting of necessary and healthy purgation, and spiritual emptying'.[39]

Handling Sin: Confession in the Middle Ages, ed. Peter Biller and A. J. Minnis (York, 1998).

36 Sarah Hamilton, *The Practice of Penance, 900–1050* (Woodbridge, 2001), pp. 5, 7, 10. According to Citrome, private confession was explained in manuals of Celtic origin as early as the sixth century, but it had been performed only sporadically: see *The Surgeon in Medieval English Literature*, p. 3.

37 *Decrees of the Ecumenical Councils*, ed. Norman P. Tanner, 2 vols (London and Washington, DC, 1990), vol. 1, p. 245. See also McAvoy's discussion of confession in this volume.

38 For the metaphorical application of medieval surgery and a highly charged metaphor of the surgeon-confessor, see Citrome, *The Surgeon in Medieval English Literature*, pp. 3–5.

39 Lesley Smith, 'William of Auvergne and Confession', in *Handling Sin*, ed. Biller and Minnis, pp. 95–107 (p. 96).

Literature of pastoral care was quick to respond to the conciliar reforms. A popular manual of confession from the diocese of Exeter, written in 1240, makes extensive use of medical language based on humoral pathology and treatments:

> Christus ergo medicus altissimus est, et dat *dimissionem* in contritione, medicinam laxativam in confessione, dietam iniungit in observatione ieiuniorum, balneum precipit in lacrimarum effusione, flebotomiam iniungit in passionis Christi recordatione.
>
> [Christ is the best physician: he gives us relief from our pain through contrition, and through confession we receive a purgative; he recommends a healthful diet through our keeping of fasts; he orders therapeutic baths through our outpouring of tears; he prescribes blood letting through our recollection of Christ's passion.][40]

Le Livre de seyntz medicines – a long meditation on spiritual therapeutics by Henry of Lancaster, mentioned above[41] – also bears witness to a broader development of sacramental confession in the context of medicine. Before unfolding the therapeutic regimen required for his healing, Henry first confesses the circumstances of the innumerable and grievous sins committed during his life and asks God to help him cleanse his soul:[42]

> [T]resdouz Sires, eietz mercy de moy et me donetz grace qe jeo peusse ou ma lang garrir l'ord plaie de ma bouche, et nettoier de l'ordure qe y est ou ma lange, c'est a dire par regeier les ordes pecchés de ma bouche ou touz les autres par verraie confessione ou tristece de coer.
>
> [Most sweet Lord, have mercy on me and give me grace that I might with my tongue heal the foul wound of my mouth, and with my tongue clean it of the filth that is there, that is, by confessing the filthy sins of my mouth and all the others, by true confession, with heartfelt sorrow.][43]

40 The *Summula* for the synod of the diocese of Exeter (1287?), *Councils and Synods with Other Documents Relating to the English Church*, vol. 2, ed. F. M. Powicke and C. R. Cheney (Oxford, 1964), p. 1061; *Pastors and the Care of Souls in Medieval England*, ed. John Shinners and William J. Dohar (Notre Dame, IN, 1998), p. 171.

41 *Le Livre de Seyntz Medicines: The Unpublished Devotional Treatise of Henry of Lancaster*, ed. E. J. Arnould (Oxford, 1940). See Naoë Kukita Yoshikawa, 'Holy Medicine and Disease of the Soul: Henry of Lancaster and *Le Livre de Seyntz Medicines*', *Medical History* 53, 3 (2009), 397–414, which argues for the interface of the devotional self and contemporary medical knowledge in this celebrated book.

42 Apart from any spiritual benefits confession may have had, it also imparted some physical improvements due to the psychosomatic effect of relieving the mind from any burden or guilt which may have been causing stress and worry. For a discussion of the psychological state of an individual having a real effect on his or her health, see Michael R. McVaugh, 'Bedside Manners in the Middle Ages', *Bulletin of History of Medicine* 71 (1997), 201–23 (pp. 212–14).

43 *Livre de Seyntz Medicines*, p. 181. I would like to thank Dr Catherine Batt for sharing her translation in progress with me.

The subsequent meditations show how Henry's wounds are healed by Christ the Physician and the Virgin, who acts as a nurse in the service of her Son: at the end of the treatment, Henry asks the Virgin for some clean, white bandages to protect the wounds from air, dust and flies.[44]

The popularity of the idea of the Virgin as nurse is illustrated by the fact that most medical care in late medieval England was supplied by women, both at home and in hospitals. Midwives, nurses and female empirics, for instance, fed their patients in accordance with an appropriate regimen, cleansing and comforting them, all of which demanded exhausting amounts of labour and courage. The image of St Elizabeth of Hungary, who tends the lepers by bathing them and feeding them with chicken, conveys the caring nature of such women – and holy women, in particular.[45] It is, therefore, fitting that Henry argues that, as a woman, the Virgin ought to be even better provided with medical acumen than a man;[46] indeed, he praises women for their capacity to attend the sick through hands-on caring: 'Et c'est bone custume qe, quant l'en est durement desheitez, qe un femme est ordené a estre delez luy, car plus suef et plus graciousement le manye et toutz choses ly fait plus plesantement qe ne ferroit une homme' [And it is sound practice that, when someone is seriously ill, a woman is appointed to be beside him, for she handles him more tenderly and more gently, and in all things treats him far more agreeably, than would a man].[47]

Henry's use of medical metaphors and understanding of the symbiotic relationship between medicine and religion illuminate the extent to which medical concepts had permeated the discourse of well educated aristocrats by the fourteenth century. In his deployment of carefully crafted medical metaphors throughout his book, Henry, a wealthy nobleman, betrays a basic grasp of medical theory and practice that was based not only on classical medicine but also on contemporary anatomy and surgery.

Before the development of surgery in the thirteenth and fourteenth centuries, however, the theory and practice of medieval medicine were primarily centred on the humoral theory of Hippocratic and Galenic medicine, combined with the Aristotelian idea of moderation. The classical idea maintains that the human being is made up of humours and that disease is caused by the imbalance of these humours. This idea was smoothly translated into the context of Christian history, in which the best weapon against disease was understood to be a healthy system of physical and spiritual care.[48]

44 *Livre de Seyntz Medicines*, p. 207.

45 See an altarpiece of c. 1500 from the Collegiate Church of Laufen near Basel, reproduced in Carole Rawcliffe, 'Hospital Nurses and Their Work', in *Daily Life in the Late Middle Ages*, ed. Richard Britnell (Stroud, 1998), pp. 43–64 (p. 60).

46 See *Livre de Seyntz Medicines*, p. 207.

47 *Livre de Seyntz Medicines*, p. 233.

48 Rawcliffe, *Leprosy in Medieval England*, p. 71. For scholastic discussion, see Joseph

Clearly, this concept of humoral harmony accorded well with the teachings of the Church which explained that the chief cause of sickness was Original Sin – a result of Eve's disobedience in tempting Adam with the apple of forbidden knowledge. Adam and Eve possessed a perfect mixture of humours in Paradise. With the advent of sin, however, that perfect balance was destroyed and diseases entered the world.[49] This, in turn, suggests that Christ is himself in perfect balance, while sinful humanity must constantly endeavour to keep a good humoral balance. However, as St Augustine explained, it was the coming of Christ to recapture that precious harmony of body and soul which proved so effective a medicine against the malignant effects of the Fall.[50] Yet, humoral balance was vulnerable to the deadly sins, resulting in abuse of the six so-called 'non-naturals': loosely grouped under the categories of ambient air, exercise and rest, sleeping and waking, food and drink, evacuation and repletion and the passions or accidents of the soul.[51] As 'each of the deadly sins carried a humoral penalty',[52] humanity had to strive to avoid the sins and keep a good humoral balance through the proper management of the six non-naturals, preserving the health of both the body and soul.

In this cultural milieu, medieval medicine advanced in Italian universities during the twelfth century, owing to the rediscovery of ancient medical texts and translations from Greek and Arabic medical writings into Latin. As a result, works like Avicenna's *Canon of Medicine* and Aristotle's writings on natural science were introduced to university syllabuses. Importantly, many physicians trained in medical schools such as Salerno, Montpellier and Paris went on to seek 'a higher degree in theology – a phenomenon that peaked in the second half of the fourteenth century'.[53] Medical knowledge, therefore, was disseminated outside the universities primarily through learned clerics, who had come to appreciate the important connection between medicine and religion. For example, armed with a solid grasp of medical ideas, theologians often drew on a complex and sophisticated explanation of physiology, based on the Galenic theory of humours, when taking confession. William of Auvergne, who examined the spiritual implications of physiology, believed

Ziegler, 'Medicine and Immortality in Terrestrial Paradise', in *Religion and Medicine in the Middle Ages*, ed. Peter Biller and Joseph Ziegler (York, 2001), pp. 201–42 (pp. 212–15).

49 Ziegler, 'Medicine and Immortality', p. 209.

50 Augustine, *The City of God Against the Pagans*, trans. R. W. Dyson (Cambridge, 1998), bk. 10, ch. 27, p. 432.

51 See further Pedro Gil-Sotres, 'The Regimens of Health', in *Western Medical Thought from Antiquity to the Middle Ages*, ed. Mirko D. Grmek (Cambridge, MA, 1998), pp. 291–318.

52 Christopher Bonfield, 'The *Regimen Sanitatis* and its Dissemination in England, *c.* 1348–1550', unpublished doctoral thesis, University of East Anglia, 2006, p. 90.

53 Dyan Elliott, *Proving Woman: Female Spirituality and Inquisitional Culture in the Later Middle Ages* (Princeton, 2004), p. 204.

that 'a person's humoral makeup – that is to say, complexion – informed his or her spiritual aptitude'.[54]

The authority of learned medicine was such that the issue with disease was understood as an attempt to make and control meaning and to convey knowledge persuasively by means of humoral discourse. As David Harley points out:

> Humoral medicine [became] a network of signs and meanings which structured the experience of sickness as a disorder of the individual's constitution through the effects of contra-natural or non-natural factors. Whatever the causes, most therapy was not directed at the disease but at the restoration of the balance. The species of disease had to be invented, propagated, and defended.[55]

The popularity of learned medicine is witnessed at the highest level of ecclesiastical authority in the early thirteenth century. More than seventy doctors were serving popes and cardinals at times during the century and Innocent III (1160/1–1216) retained a doctor who had a privileged association with the Salerno school of medicine.[56] The pope's interest in medicine is not only attested by this appointment, but also by his use of medical terms in his sermons, such as the one delivered on the important occasion of the opening of the Fourth Lateran Council. Innocent III's pontificate also stimulated the dissemination of medical works within his cultural circles and the papal curia.[57] As Agostino Paravicini-Bagliani argues, the papal court eventually became 'an important center for the production of medical works and their diffusion throughout Europe'.[58] This keen interest in medicine shown by the highest level of the Church may well have precipitated the spread of medical knowledge among the learned clerical practitioners who served the social elite in Italy and beyond.

The laity's concern for the health of the body and the soul increased even more following the outbreak of plague in 1347, a catastrophic event which expanded the marketplace for literature of medical advice. From 1347–50 onwards, translations of guides to health, such as the *Secreta secretorum* (Secret of Secrets) and its close relation, the *Regimen sanitatis Salerni* (Salernian Regimen of Health), and plague tracts were produced for a large audience. These texts were based on the Hippocratic and Aristotelian ideas of *regimen sanitatis* (regimen of health) which advocated a holistic approach

54 Elliott, *Proving Woman*, p. 206.

55 David Harley, 'Rhetoric and the Social Construction of Sickness', *Social History of Medicine* 12 (1999), 407–35 (p. 416).

56 Agostino Paravicini-Bagliani, *The Pope's Body*, trans. David S. Peterson (Chicago, IL and London, 1994), p. 186. Paravicini-Bagliani also argues that medical knowledge was linked to promotion to the cardinalate.

57 Paravicini-Bagliani, *The Pope's Body*, p. 188.

58 Paravicini-Bagliani, *The Pope's Body*, p. 192.

to health.[59] Most plague tracts like these were composed to explain the disease and educate people in prevention and treatment. A popular treatise by Johannes de Burgundia, entitled *Tractatus de morbo epidemiæ* (1365), was translated into English and became a best seller,[60] revealing the high level of concern about health in contemporary society.[61] Indeed, this genre of medical literature, known as the *regimen sanitatis*, developed in the medieval West to provide advice for those anxious about falling ill. The *Secreta secretorum* and the *Regimen sanitatis Salerni*, written in verse and containing material from the *Secreta*, were two of the most popular works of advice circulating in late medieval England.[62] The *Regimen sanitatis Salerni* was reputedly composed for an English king by the physicians of Salerno and its popularity is attested by the fact that there are over 100 extant versions which were disseminated across Europe.[63] The preface to the *Secreta secretorum* indicates that the text originated in a regimen Aristotle wrote for Alexander the Great:[64] it was a mirror for princes, a manual for ruling a healthy state and a healthy royal body, grounded in the concept of the human body as a microcosm of the macrocosmic state,[65] and advising the king on how to act and rule as well as advising him personally on his health throughout the year. With frequent references to such medical authorities as Hippocrates, Galen and Aristotle, it soon gained popularity throughout medieval Europe and was translated into a number of vernaculars.[66] The pseudo-Aristotelian *Secreta secretorum* was

59 The *Secreta secretorum* was translated from the Arabic *Kitāb sirr al-asrār* (*The Book of the Secret of Secrets*) at some point in the first half of the twelfth century. See *Secretum secretorum: Nine English Versions*, ed. M. A. Manzalaoui, vol. 1, EETS o.s. 276 (Oxford, 1977), p. v; Hippocrates, *Hippocrates with an English Translations*, trans. W. H. S. Jones, 4 vols (London, 1948), vol. 4, 'Regimen in Health' and 'Regimina, I-III'. Galen synthesised Hippocratic and Aristotelian ideas in his treatise, *De regimine sanitatis*: see Gil-Sotres, 'The Regimens of Health', pp. 293–4. See also Melitta Weiss-Adamson, '*Regimen sanitatis*', in *Medieval Science, Technology, and Medicine: An Encyclopedia*, ed. Thomas Glick, Steven J. Livesey and Faith Wallis (New York and Abingdon, 2005), pp. 438–9.

60 H. S. Bennett, 'Science and Information in English Writings of the Fifteenth Century', *Modern Language Review* 39 (1944), 1–8 (p. 3).

61 Middle English manuscript anthologies containing medical recipes illuminate that 'medical material circulated very flexibly, often being incorporated in manuscripts containing a variety of material intended for household use': see Elma Brenner, Liz Herbert McAvoy and Patricia Skinner, 'Care and Cure: Diseases, Disabilities and Therapies: Conference Report', *Wellcome History* 51 (2013), 26–7 (p. 26). This is based on a lecture delivered by Julia Boffey which focused on National Library of Wales, MS Brogyntyn II.I.

62 Bonfield, 'The *Regimen Sanitatis* and its Dissemination in England', p. 11.

63 Rawcliffe, *Urban Bodies*, pp. 56–7.

64 *Lydgate and Burgh's 'Secrees of Old Philisoffres': A Version of the Secreta Secretorum*, ed. Robert Steele, EETS e.s. 66 (London, 1894), p. 16.

65 Bonfield, 'The *Regimen Sanitatis* and its Dissemination in England', p. 16.

66 Personalised versions of the *regimen sanitatis* were tailored for the social elite to regulate their life style. Humphrey of Gloucester (d. 1447), who had a collection of medical

adapted and simplified for a popular market by John Lydgate (1370–1449), Thomas Hoccleve (1369–1426) and William Forrest (fl. 1530–81).[67] The text was famously incorporated into Lydgate's 'Dietary'[68] and the related 'A Doctrine for Pestilence', both of which contain a medical section with advice based on the 'six non-naturals'.[69] As Carole Rawcliffe argues of the 'Dietary', 'the poem's repeated emphasis upon sensible eating habits and practical information about the six non-naturals [had] about it a timeless, pragmatic quality',[70] which no doubt contributed to its considerable success.

The purpose of the 'Dietary' was also a charitable one: Lydgate wished to help all readers avoid illness, including those unable to afford the aid of apothecaries: 'This receiht bouht is of non appotecarie, / Off Maister Antony, nor of Maister Hewe; / To all indifferent richest dietarie!'[71] Just as the translators of medieval English medical texts saw their vernacular translations as 'a kind of medical sermon, with a pastoral, indeed charitable, function in mind',[72] so Lydgate must have been conscious of his duty to translate useful information from Latin to English.[73] As medicinal cure was translated into the vernacular, the text itself assumed the role of medicine for the masses.[74] In manuscript contexts, we also witness an increasingly wide distribution of

books in his library, benefited from his close connection with Gilbert Kymer, the Oxford chancellor, priest and physician, who composed a special regimen for his patron.

67 *Lydgate and Burgh's 'Secrees of Old Philisoffres'*; *The Minor Poems of John Lydgate*, ed. Henry Noble MacCracken, 2 parts, EETS o.s. 107, o.s. 192 (London, 1911–34); *Hoccleve's Works, III: The Regement of Princes, A.D. 1411–12 from the Harleian MS. 4866, and fourteen of Hoccleve's minor poems from the Egerton MS. 615*, ed. Frederick J. Furnivall, EETS e.s. 72 (London, 1897), pp. 1–197; for William Forrest's *The Pleasant Poesye of Princelie Practise*, see *Secretum secretorum*, pp. 390–534.

68 Max Förster states that the *Dietary* is a translation of the twelfth-century Latin *Regimen sanitatis Salernitanum* or *Flos medicinae*: 'Kleinere Mittelenglische Texte', *Anglia* 42 (1918), 145–224 (p. 179).

69 As it was much easier to memorise than prose, medical advice in verse may have become more generally disseminated: see Francis R. Packard, 'History of the School of Salernum', in Sir John Harington et al., *The School of Salernum: Regimen sanitatis Salernitanum/ The English Version by Sir John Harington; History of the School of Salernum by Francis R. Packard; and a note on the prehistory of the Regimen sanitatis by Fielding H. Garrison* (New York, 1920; repr. 1970), p. 31.

70 Rawcliffe, *Medicine and Society*, p. 39.

71 *The Minor Poems of John Lydgate*, part 2, p. 707 (lines 166–8).

72 Faye Marie Getz, 'Charity, Translation, and the Language of Medical Learning in Medieval England', *The Bulletin of the History of Medicine* 64 (1990), 1–17 (p. 9).

73 For the popularity of Lydgate's 'Dietary' in the context of late medieval translation and book production, see Naoë Kukita Yoshikawa, 'The Translation of the *Regimen Sanitatis* into a Handbook for the Devout Laity: a New Look at the *Kalender of Shepherds* and its Context', in *Medieval Translator XV: In Principio Fuit Interpres*, ed. Alessandra Petrina (Turnhout, 2013), pp. 303–15.

74 For the translation into English of medical texts, plague tracts and guides to healthy living following the plague, see Rawcliffe, *Urban Bodies*, pp. 48–9, 60–2.

medical texts alongside spiritual texts, a phenomenon which provided the milieu to nurture a merging concept of the health of body and soul.

Meanwhile, medical concepts and language had been further absorbed into religious discourse, as suggested at the start of this Introduction. In addition to the Exeter confessional manual mentioned above, Robert Mannyng of Brunne's *Handlyng Synne* (c. 1303), a popular vernacular guide to spiritual health adapted from the Anglo-Norman *Mannuel de pechiez* (c. 1260), ministers to unlettered souls, drawing on metaphors selected from the regimens and other medical writings.[75] Robert's attempt to translate the text suggests that he presumes some level of medical knowledge of his audience, in spite of their being 'unlettered'. By the beginning of the fourteenth century, preachers also began to employ medical topics in religious discourse. The fourteenth-century Franciscan *Fasciculus morum*, a popular handbook for preachers, is replete with medical metaphors such as 'blood letting of confession' and 'diet of fasting and penance'.[76] Since preaching was one of the major means of mass communication in late medieval society, it helped the language of medicine to become common currency for a lay urban audience as well as for the nobility, again indicating the compatibility of religious and medical language during the period. Thus, by the beginning of the fourteenth century, medicine had become a potent metaphor for both religious and the laity, and, as Joseph Ziegler maintains, 'had acquired a cultural role in addition to its traditional function as a therapeutic art'.[77]

As mentioned above, however, that cultural role and traditional function were deeply gender inflected. Indeed, as many recent studies have shown, the medieval response to the female body was essentially highly ambivalent.[78] On one hand, the healing powers of the Virgin encapsulated those of women as nurses and nourishers, as we have seen. On the other, the Church not only dismissed women as daughters of Eve or, in the famous words of Tertullian (d. c. 235) as 'the devil's gateway', but it also explained their weakness by means of Hippocratic (Galenic) medical theories. Arguing that women's damp and fleshly bodies make them phlegmatic, theologians supported stereotypes of female inferiority and disseminated such misogynistic ideas throughout Christendom. Nevertheless, since women were valued for bearing offspring, their health was a serious concern both for family and society, and therefore

75 *Robert of Brunne's 'Handlyng Synne'*, ed. F. J. Furnivall, 2 parts in 1 vol., EETS o.s. 119, 123 (London, 1901, 1903).

76 For example, it informs the audience of the therapeutic and purgative functions of confession. See *Facsciculus Morum: A Fourteenth-Century Preacher's Handbook*, ed. and trans. Siegfried Wenzel (University Park, PA, 1989), pp. 254–7, 594–7.

77 Joseph Ziegler, 'Medical Similes in Religious Discourse: The Case of Giovanni di San Gimignano OP (ca. 1250–ca. 1333)', *Sciences in Context* 8 (1995), 103–31 (p. 103).

78 See note 28.

the therapeutics related to fertility and procreation remained a vital part of medieval medicine.[79]

So important was this reproductive function that medieval women were often conceived of synecdochically in terms of the uterus. According to the Hippocratic tradition, the uterus was capable of moving throughout the body.[80] As Monica Green explains, 'such movement was thought to be caused by retention of the menses, excessive fatigue, lack of food, lack of (hetero)sexual activity, and dryness or lightness of the womb (particularly in older women)'.[81] The wandering uterus induced a typical female disease known as uterine suffocation, a condition intimately associated with a medical assumption that women needed regular sexual activity to maintain their health.[82] The curse of menstruation was also linked to women's disease. Although menstrual blood was thought to nourish the embryo during pregnancy and to be turned to milk after childbirth, medieval medicine explained that menstruation was designed to get rid of harmful humours in the body and defined menstrual blood as poisonous.

One of the most important medieval texts on women's medicine is the *Trotula*, the compendium which emerged in Salerno in the late twelfth century. This collection of gynaecological and cosmetic texts consists of three parts, the first and the third of which, *On the Conditions of Women* and *On Women's Cosmetics*, were anonymous.[83] A prologue to *On the Conditions of Women* reveals that it is a product of a Christian culture: by recasting the creation story of Genesis into Galenic physiological terms, 'the prologue explains how woman's subjugation to man allows reproduction to take place, which in turn is the chief cause of illness in the female body'.[84] Importantly, the authority for the second text, *On Treatments for Women*, is named in the earliest manuscripts as Trota, a Salernitan woman healer (*medica*), and there is plenty of evidence to suggest that women practised medicine in Salerno in the eleventh and twelfth centuries.[85] Indeed, although the world of bookish, academic medicine was primarily monopolised by university-trained physicians, women were actively participating in care and cure elsewhere, too.[86]

79 For an overview of women and medicine, see Rawcliffe, *Medicine and Society*, chapters 8, 9.

80 Soranus of Ephesus (fl. early second century) insisted that the womb did not wander, so did Galen, yet their views were not able to suppress the popular beliefs: see *The Trotula: An English Translation of the Medieval Compendium of Women's Medicine*, ed. and trans. Monica H. Green (Philadelphia, 2001), 'Introduction', p. 24.

81 *The Trotula*, 'Introduction', p. 22.

82 *The Trotula*, 'Introduction', p. 26.

83 *The Trotula*, 'Preface', p. xii.

84 *The Trotula*, 'Introduction', p. 36.

85 *The Trotula*, 'Preface', p. xii; 'Introduction', p. 48.

86 Nevertheless, medical history was predominantly a history of great men, written by retired doctors who were less interested in women's activities or folk remedies.

They were expected to supervise the health and welfare of their families, at least, and played a notable part in medical treatment, which usually began at home in the kitchen where food was prescribed in accordance with humoral therapy. Moreover, since childbirth and childrearing were centred on women, it is not surprising that midwives played a prominent role in women's medicine. For example, Soranus of Ephesus (d. c. 129), a Greek physician who practised in Rome and whose work on gynaecology proved influential throughout the medieval period, had a high opinion of midwives for their professional, unperturbed attitude, placing great importance upon their education.[87] There is plenty of iconography dating from the late Middle Ages too which bears witness to the way childbirth was supported by a midwife and a group of women.[88] With a solid grasp of the theory and practice of obstetrics and childcare, midwives were committed to the welfare of mother and child. Moreover, their responsibility was sometimes extended to priestly duty: midwives occasionally baptised a child in the event s/he was born dead or dying, and heard the confession of a dying mother.[89] In this context, they were agents of the Church, administering the care of the soul on behalf of a parish priest.

Importantly, towards the end of the Middle Ages, as noted above, women's medicine converged with popular devotion to the Virgin Mary and other female members of the Holy Kindred (notably St Anne).[90] As holy women throughout Europe became devotional patrons and exemplars for medieval women, they were increasingly enlisted for intercession, protection and miraculous cure. And, of course, it was very often pregnant women who desperately sought out holy women to intercede on their behalf. Terrified of the 'curse of Eve', they also frequently made use of a birth-girdle upon which were written charms, prayers, accounts of Christ on the cross, the Life of St Margaret, patron saint of childbirth etc. to help them cope with the dangers of childbirth. These examples point towards women's medicine as an obvious site for the convergence of religion and medicine, providing, too, a paradigm for the main themes addressed in this volume: while popular devotion in terms of women's medical care is reflected in the proliferation of the images of holy women in childbed, these images can also help to unpack the socio-political

87 *Sources for the History of Medicine in Late Medieval England*, ed. and trans. Carole Rawcliffe (Kalamazoo, MI, 1995), p. 106; Rawcliffe, *Medicine and Society*, p. 195.

88 See, for example, Albrecht Dürer's woodcut, 'Birth of the Virgin' for childbirth and female solidarity.

89 John Mirk, *Instructions for Parish Priests*, ed. Edward Peacock, EETS o.s. 31 (London, 1868), pp. 3–4.

90 The late medieval proliferation of devotion to the Virgin and female saints might also underscore the growing power of medieval women in the realities of family life. For a recent study on popular devotion, see Carole Hill, *Women and Religion in Late Medieval Norwich* (Woodbridge, 2010).

meanings of gender divisions embedded in late medieval culture.[91] Therefore, although this volume is not centred on women's medicine specifically, the highly gendered nature of medicine and the discourses it generated offers a nuanced context for many of the concerns intrinsic to this collection of essays.

*

The essays in this volume interrogate the convergence of medical and devotional discourse broadly and in a number of different ways: textually, conceptually, historically, socially and culturally. They are organised in terms of four thematic groups, although the concerns naturally overlap. The first three groups – 'Mary the Physician', 'Female Mysticism and Metaphors of Illness' and 'Fifteenth-Century Poetry and Theological Prose' – concern themselves predominantly with English textual contexts. The essays included here discuss complex, nuanced responses to the bodily and spiritual illnesses, in which the intersection between spiritual and physical discourses were strengthened and crystallised by the use of medical hermeneutics in religious and secular literature, along with their gendered trajectories. The fourth group – 'Disfigurement, Disability' – includes two essays offering detailed case-studies regarding blindness and leprosy, respectively.

The exploration begins with two essays that focus on Mary the Physician. Centred on the importance of the widespread belief in Mary's healing power in late medieval England, Diane Watt's essay contextualises the female role as healer in both hagiographical/mystical and secular traditions. Arguing that the Virgin had a complex association with healing that went beyond her more generally recognised association with childbirth, Watt explores the interaction of spiritual and bodily health in writings by and about late medieval English women. Focusing on *The Life of Christina of Markyate*, *The Book of Margery Kempe* and the letters of the Paston women, the essay demonstrates the firmly-established tradition of women as healers and the connection between their performance of this role and their devotion to and emulation of the Virgin Mary through the later Middle Ages.

Also focussing on Mary the Physician, Roberta Magnani's essay explores the complex dialectic between spiritual and religious discourses in the works of Geoffrey Chaucer. Deploying Michel Foucault's theory of 'bio-power', the essay examines Chaucer's extensive engagement with Marian literary

91 See Elizabeth L'Estrange, *Holy Motherhood: Gender, Dynasty, and Visual Culture in the Later Middle Ages* (Manchester, 2008): L'Estrange has shown that the postpartum scenes depicted in late medieval manuscript miniatures are linked more to larger dynastic concerns than to gendered ideas. In her study on human dissection in late medieval Italy, Katharine Park focuses on an increasing attention to female sexuality and generation, and reveals the centrality of gender in the development of human anatomy: see *Secrets of Women: Gender, Generation, and the Origins of Human Dissection* (New York, 2006). See also Green, 'Integrative Medicine', pp. 1229–30.

tropes and the concept of Mary the Physician as the assistive agent in the dissemination of desirable Christian subjugated positions. Magnani also investigates Chaucer's complex stance on authority in terms of gender hierarchies, particularly through the Doctour of Phisik's Tale. Here, Chaucer's Doctour interrogates the dominance and validity of male clerical authority by discussing a textual space in which Mary the Physician, and femininity more generally, can be imagined as an alternative and superior form of incarnated authority, thereby renewing the notion of Mary as an assistive agent.

Part Two turns its focus to the female mysticism and metaphors of illness alluded to in the essays of Watt and Magnani. Concentrating on female-authored mystical writing, Naoë Kukita Yoshikawa examines the layers of medical allusions in the revelations of Mechtild of Hackeborn, translated from the Latin into Middle English in the early fifteenth century. Mechtild's earthly experience as a chantress stimulates her longing for mystical union with God, a union conceived of in terms of the health of her soul. Embedded in her revelations is the cult of the Sacred Heart that developed at Helfta: Mechtild deploys an array of allegories representing the heart to convey her understanding of mystical union. Yoshikawa argues that this, in particular, invites the modern reader to appreciate an intricate interplay between eucharistic symbolism, popular piety and the emergent discourse of medicine.

Following on from Yoshikawa, Liz Herbert McAvoy's essay looks at the development of anchoritic medical discourse and examines the 'medicinal' role played by penance and contemplation within the anchoritic life, both as a *regimen sanitatis* for the spiritual health of the anchorite and as a 'prescribed' cure for the spiritual ills of the Christian community. Focusing especially on the revelations of Julian of Norwich, McAvoy argues that Julian's development of the Motherhood of God is predicated in part upon the medicinal discourse common to some of her sources or her writing's anchoritic precursors such as *Ancrene Wisse* and – in Germany – Grimlaicus of Metz's *Regula Solitariorum* (Rule for Solitaries). She argues that the sustained image of a blood sacrifice of a maternal God illuminates the shift in hermeneutics from the male anchorite as 'medical practitioner' of the soul in the early medieval anchorhold, to the female-focused spirituality and healing associated with late-medieval piety and its practices.

This part concludes with Juliette Vuille's essay on Julian of Norwich and Margery Kempe, whose writings are explored this time from psychological and psychiatric perspectives. Vuille analyses in detail the importance of the historical and cultural context to understand better the issue of medieval madness. She takes to task those commentators who have recently applied modern psychiatric diagnoses to the 'madness' of medieval, literary accounts of visions, such as those experienced by Julian of Norwich and Margery Kempe in their encounters with the divine. Arguing against such interpretations, Vuille demonstrates how the 'holy insanity' of the two visionaries enabled them to acquire authority via the practice of *discretio spirituum* and thus attain their divinely ordained identities within the medieval spiritual community.

The third part of this volume concerns itself with the cultural force of medical tropology in fifteenth-century religious poetry and prose. Takami Matsuda's essay unpacks the pervasiveness of medical tropes in John Audelay's poems, which are replete with references to spiritual illness and its cure. Arguing that the corpus of Audelay's writing is characterised by the close link between physical and spiritual illness at both literal and metaphorical levels, Matsuda explores how the poet transforms bodily illness into a means of healing spiritual illness, both for himself and for the reader. Underpinned by the concept of Purgatory both as a specific locale and as a metaphor for penance in this world, he argues that penance is transformed into a long-term medical treatment that begins in this life as an earthly purgatory. For Audelay, as Matsuda demonstrates, Purgatory is not only a system and place in which to complete due penance, but also the realm in which the process of spiritual healing may be effected with growing hope.

The predominance of medical tropes in late medieval vernacular literature is further investigated in Louise Bishop's essay, which explores the theme of meditative reading as cure and medicine, with a focus on figurative language and body politics centred on the heart. She examines Reginald Pecock's Middle English prose, such as the *Reule of Cristen Religion*, and argues that 'literal and metaphoric hearts intertwine with medieval ideas about the heart as seat of understanding, the role of the passions concerning health, the effects of reading, and the reach of English politics in the fifteenth century'. By comparing Pecock's vernacular work with the *Doctrine of the Hert*, Bishop explores the conceptions of the heart as a centre of health and a centre of reading, and draws an analogy between the physical and spiritual functions of the heart. Bishop also asserts that Pecock conceived the healthy heart as the locus of healing for the body and soul, and thus revises modern assumptions about hearts and understanding, turning our attention to the fact that heart-centred knowledge and healing can profitably affect our reading of medieval literature.

The next two essays, in the fourth group, both explore a merging discourse of spiritual and physical health in the context of medieval disability and disfigurement. Irina Metzler looks at medieval etiologies of congenital physical and mental impairment. As inseparable from notions of religion, and especially of sin, Metzler argues that congenital disability provides an ideal site for an investigation within philosophical, theological, moral and medical frameworks. By investigating factors that caused congenital disability, Metzler shows that such medieval notions were highly gendered and that people understood such disability as a theological idea of human fallacy in a postlapsarian world.

Focussing on gendered categories, Skinner's essay further explores deformity inflicted on the female body. As the essay unfolds, the tense relationship between religion and medicine is found embedded in hagiographic texts where gender plays a crucial part in the ways hagiographers constructed their stories of the mutilations. Skinner examines three holy women, each of whose lives feature an episode of actual or near-mutilation of the face. Building on Valentin Groebner's analysis of violent punishments inflicted on the female face,[92] Skinner investigates how facial mutilation functioned both as punitive for moral lapses and penitential for the daughters of Eve.

The last two essays present case studies on the perception of two distinct illnesses – leprosy and blindness. Joy Hawkins's essay is centred on the theme of blindness and visual impairments within the context of late medieval England. Exploring the extent to which theologians and medical writers agreed upon the causes of eye disease and the course of action to be undertaken, she argues that medieval attitudes towards the blind were often ambivalent: blindness could be the result of specific sins or misdemeanours, but it was also understood to be a mark of divine grace. As a divine gift, good Christians who accepted their fate with humility hoped to be spared a worse ordeal in Purgatory. The examination of historical documents illuminates that caring for the blind was considered to be a form of spiritual medication which strengthened the health and well-being of those who performed such charitable acts. Grounded in a solid grasp of medical theory and practice, Hawkins reveals a variety of understandings of and responses to blindness.

This volume's final essay, by Elma Brenner, focuses on the historical practice of healing the physical body with regard to the symptoms of leprosy to illuminate the ways in which religious beliefs may have influenced pragmatic/medical measures for dealing with the disease. She explores the intersection between bodily and spiritual care within and outside of *leprosaria*, particularly in the region of Normandy in the high and late Middle Ages. *Leprosaria*, which were often monastic institutions, provided spiritual facilities for their leprous residents but also tended the bodies of the sick, through dietary regulation, bathing, bloodletting and other measures. Brenner's investigation extends from communities to the experience of leprous individuals, which was shaped by their gender and social status. By examining a range of sources, including the statutes of leper houses, medical texts and accounts of leprosy examinations, Brenner elucidates a dedication to the long-term bodily and spiritual care of lepers, which reflects 'stigma and fear, but also compassion and a sense of duty towards the chronically ill'. Ultimately, along with Hawkins's case study, this essay shows that the dominant interrelationship of physical and spiritual healing in medieval society is duly supported by historical evidence.

*

The essays in the present volume therefore argue for an inextricable, intricate relationship between the physical and the spiritual in accounts of health, illness

92 Valentin Groebner, *Defaced: the Visual Culture of Violence in the Later Middle Ages*, trans. Pamela Selwyn (New York, 2004).

and disability, deploying diverse and varied methodologies, and demonstrate how medical and religious discourses, particularly those inflected by contemporary gendered ideologies, were integrated in medieval culture. Through the Reformation and concomitant turbulent changes during the Early Modern period, Descartes and his followers asserted the idea that the body and the soul were separate entities, as a result of which the post-Cartesian society lost the co-relation between theology and medicine.[93] Therefore, the essays included this volume argue that a refocusing on the Middle Ages provides a way of re-thinking and understanding a far more united concept of psychological and corporeal well-being. Furthermore, keenly aware of the fact that the medical and the literary methodologies overlap and complement each other in unique and sometimes contradictory ways, its contributors pursue a wide range of approaches to these themes. Through active interdisciplinary discussion, it examines the role of medicine as a cultural agent within medieval cultural discourses.

Ultimately, the volume's wider aim is to consolidate the developing momentum behind the new, interdisciplinary, theoretically and internationally debated issues surrounding medicine, religion and gender. It is our wish that this interdisciplinary foray into medieval discourses of various kinds will inspire further work in this area and promote new dialogue between scholars about the ways in which medicine, religion and gender interact and how they fit into the broader field of cultural history. Much remains to be ploughed and unearthed in this complex field. To paraphrase the words of Galen in this context, we may be 'sightless moles' whose eyes are yet to open,[94] but it is hoped that this volume leads the way from sightlessness to vision, casting light on the fused discourses of religion, medicine and gender in the Middle Ages.

93 For Descartes and Cartesianism, see Roy Porter, *Blood and Guts: A Short History of Medicine* (London, 2002), pp. 65–8.

94 Laqueur, *Making Sex*, pp. 27–8.

PART I

MARY THE PHYSICIAN

1

MARY THE PHYSICIAN: WOMEN, RELIGION AND MEDICINE IN THE MIDDLE AGES

Diane Watt

The idea of Christ the Physician was widespread in the Middle Ages because cure of the soul was seen as an essential aspect of medical care. Yet for women in particular, the Virgin Mary seems to have had associations with medicine that went beyond her more generally recognised associations with intercessory healing and with childbirth. One of the defining and distinctive qualities of women's visions in the post-Conquest period is the increasing importance of the role played by the Virgin Mary, and some of these visions illustrate vividly Mary's medical role. At the same time, the Virgin Mary was central to the everyday religious life of women in the late medieval household, and prayers to Mary and other forms of Marian devotion were connected not only to motherhood but also to healthcare more broadly. This essay explores the interaction of spiritual and physical health in writing by and about late medieval English women. It argues that the belief in *Mary as Physician*, in Mary as a doctor of medicine, in late medieval England was closely linked to, and indeed validated, the role of the woman as healer.

The importance of Christ the Physician is examined in Naoë Kukita Yoshikawa's study of the connections between health of the soul and health of the body in the writings of the two late medieval European women visionaries, Marie d'Oignies and Margery Kempe. As Yoshikawa explains:

> The basis of this type of convergence between the Christian faith and medieval medicine is the concept of *Christus medicus*, or Christ the physician, which was firmly established during the Middle Ages. This concept dates back to the synoptic gospels where Christ was conceived as the physician of both soul and body. St Augustine (c. 354–430), among others, made frequent use of the idea of *Christus medicus*. He saw the Passion of Christ as the best medicine through which man might recover his spiritual and physical health.[1]

1 Naoë Kukita Yoshikawa, 'Mysticism and Medicine: Holy Communion in the *Vita of Marie d'Oignies* and *The Book of Margery Kempe*', in *Poetica* 72, Special Issue, *Convergence/Divergence: The Politics and Late Medieval English Devotional and Medical*

Yoshikawa's primary focus is on the importance to late medieval female visionary experience of the belief in the 'medicinal qualities of the Eucharist'.[2] Nevertheless, at the same time, Yoshikawa also addresses the centrality to women's mystical writings of visions of and meditations on the Purification of the Virgin. Here I take Yoshikawa's argument further and offer evidence for a belief in Mary as Physician, or *Maria medica,* in late medieval England.[3] After providing a brief introductory overview of the role of women as providers of healthcare in the Middle Ages, this essay will explore devout women's attitudes to, and understandings and management of, physical and mental illness, focusing on examples taken from *The Life of Christina of Markyate* and *The Book of Margery Kempe*, and paying particular attention to the importance of the Virgin Mary. The essay will then go on to contrast these texts with evidence taken from secular women's writing, namely the fifteenth-century letters of the Paston women, to demonstrate the continuation of the tradition of women as healers and the connection between their performance of this role and their devotion to the Virgin Mary through the later Middle Ages.

MEDIEVAL WOMEN AS PROVIDERS OF HEALTH CARE

Women's involvement in medical practice in the Middle Ages has been the focus of some scholarly attention in recent decades. Groundbreaking studies in this field include Monica Green's essays 'Women's Medical Practice and Health Care in Medieval Europe' (published in 1989) and 'Documenting Medieval Women's Medical Practice' (1994), Carole Rawcliffe's *Medicine and Society in Later Medieval England* (published in 1995), and Green's monograph, *Making Women's Medicine Masculine* (2008).[4] Green's 'Bibliography on Medieval Women, Gender, and Medicine (1980–2009)' provides a comprehensive survey of work in the field.[5] While a formal education in medicine was the preserve

Discourses, ed. Denis Renevey and Naoë Kukita Yoshikawa (Tokyo, 2009), 109–22 (p. 113).

2 Yoshikawa, 'Mysticism and Medicine', p. 113.

3 This argument also links to Yoshikawa's article exploring the idea of the Virgin Mary as nurse in Henry of Lancaster's *Le Livre de Seyntz Medicines*: 'Holy Medicine and Diseases of the Soul: Henry of Lancaster and *Le Livre de Seyntz Medicines*', *Medical History* 53, 3 (2009), 397–414. For Mary's role as physician, see also Roberta Magnani, 'Chaucer's Physicians: Raising Questions of Authority' and Takami Matsuda, 'Purgatory and Spiritual Healing in John Audelay's Poems' in this volume.

4 Monica H. Green, 'Women's Medical Practice and Health Care in Medieval Europe', *Signs* 14, 2 (1988-89), 434–73; Monica H. Green, 'Documenting Medieval Women's Medical Practice', in *Practical Medicine from Salerno to the Black Death*, ed. Luis Garcia-Ballester, Roger French, Jon Arrizabalaga, and Andrew Cunningham (Cambridge, 1994), pp. 322–52; Carole Rawcliffe, *Medicine and Society in Later Medieval England* (Stroud, 1995); Monica H. Green, *Making Women's Medicine Masculine: The Rise of Male Authority in Pre-Modern Gynaecology* (Oxford, 2008).

5 Monica H. Green, 'Bibliography on Medieval Women, Gender, and Medicine (1980–

of men in the Middle Ages, and women were not licensed, not all medical practitioners were academically trained and Green warns rightly against only recognising the activities of 'explicitly labelled practitioners'.[6] In England, an example of a woman saint being described as 'benedicta medica' [the blessed doctor] can be found in Goscelin of St Bertin's late eleventh-century account of the visionary healing from scrofula of Ælfgifu, abbess of Wilton, by the royal saint Edith of Wilton (d. c. 986).[7] However this is a posthumous miracle, and Goscelin does not attribute the title or similar healing activities to Edith in his earlier narrative of her life. Nevertheless, even if women medical practitioners were seldom formally recognised in such terms, women did contribute to scholarly discourse on medicine. While the attribution of women's health care texts to the putative female physician Trotula of Salerno is problematic, the abbess and visionary Hildegard of Bingen is famous for two medical works: an encyclopaedia of the natural world, *Physica*, which includes an extensive herbarium, or description of the medicinal properties of plants; and her compilation of medical advice, *Causae et Curae*.

The twelfth century however seems to have been exceptional in this respect, and according to Green in *Making Women's Medicine Masculine*, women's engagement with medical *textual* culture declined in the later Middle Ages, and their access to handbooks on healthcare was severely limited. While some exceptional women, including the mid fourteenth-century Cecilia of Oxford, employed by Philippa of Hainault, wife of Edward III, even practised as surgeons,[8] most engaged in a range of medical practices that were not identified in professional terms, including midwifery, wet nursing and nursing. The fifteenth-century *Book of Margery Kempe* includes a now well known account of Kempe's experiences as an unwilling nurse in a domestic setting:

> It happyd on a tyme þat þe husbonde of þe sayd creatur [Kempe], an man in gret age passyng thre scor ȝer, as he wolde a comyn down of hys chambyr bar-foot & bar-legge, he slederyd er ellys faylyd of [lost] hys fotyng & fel down to þe grownd fro þe gresys [stairs], & hys heuyd [head] vndyr hym greuowsly brokyn & bresyd. … Þan sche toke hom hir husbond to hir & kept hym ȝerys aftyr as long as he leuyd & had ful mech labowr wyth hym, for in hys last days he turnyd childisch a-ȝen & lakkyd reson þat he cowd not don hys owyn esement to gon to a sege [he could not go to a seat to relieve himself], er ellys he wolde not, but

2009)', at http://www.sciencia.cat/biblioteca/documents/Green_CumulativeBib_Feb2010.pdf.

6 Green, 'Documenting Medieval Women's Medical Practice', p. 329.

7 A. Wilmart, 'La légende de Ste Édith en prose et vers par le moine Goscelin', *Analecta Bollandiana* 56 (1938), 265–307 (p. 294).

8 Thomas Benedek, 'The Roles and Images of Medieval Women in the Healing Arts', in *The Roles and Images of Women in the Middle Ages and Renaissance*, ed. Douglas Radcliffe-Umstead (Pittsburgh, PA, 1975), pp. 145–59 (p. 152).

as a childe voydyd his natural digestyon [relieved himself] in hys lynyn clothys þer he sat be þe fyre er at þe tabil, wheþyr it wer, he wolde sparyn no place. And þerfor was hir labowr meche þe mor in waschyng & wryngyng & hir costage in fyryng [expense in keeping a fire] & lettyd [distracted] hir ful meche fro hir contemplacyon þat many tymys sche xuld an yrkyd [would have disliked] hir labowr saf sche bethowt hir how sche in hir ȝong age had ful many delectabyl thowtys, fleschly lustys, & inordinat louys to hys persone.[9]

Margery Kempe provides a particularly interesting, and potentially anomalous or atypical, example of the sort of expectations that circulated around female involvement in health care in late medieval England, because although Kempe was a married laywoman, she had a conversion experience as an adult, and thereafter lived a deeply religious life, which was expressed in her distinctive dress, her diet, her frequent pilgrimages, her prayers and her visions and affective piety. In this respect, and similar to vowesses, beguines and lay anchoresses, Kempe blurs the boundary between the laywoman and the woman religious. Her *Book* records in considerable detail the hostility that her unconventional religious life generated, and her treatment of her husband is no exception. When the increasing frail John Kempe fell down stairs, his wife was blamed for neglecting him and thus for failing in her duties: 'And þan þe pepil seyd, ȝyf he deyd [died], hys wyfe was worthy to ben hangyn for hys deth, for-as-meche as sche myth a kept hym & dede not.'[10] Kempe represents caring for her senile husband – in typical effective detail – not as a vocation, but as an act of penance, but the reality must have been that nursing was a key element of medieval housewifery, and that fulfilling this role was expected of women.

Women within the household also engaged in practices sometimes termed unlearned or popular, such as herbalism. Indeed, as we will see later in this article in the examples found in the Paston letters, the kitchen garden or herber was a major source of supplies for medieval medical treatments. In late medieval England, hospitals were usually housed in or linked to religious houses,[11] and looking after those who were ill or dying was seen as a particular vocation for nuns as well as for laywomen who served as hospital nurses. In the late thirteenth-century *Golden Legend*, St Elizabeth of Hungary is represented as exemplary in this respect. We are told that, following the death of her husband, she founded a hospital and took it upon herself to tend to the patients. William Caxton's 1483 English translation of this text is particularly illuminating:

And then this blessed Elizabeth received the habit of religion and put herself diligently to the works of mercy, for she received for her dower two hundred

9 *The Book of Margery Kempe*, ed. Sanford Brown Meech and Hope Emily Allen, vol. 1, EETS o.s. 212 (Oxford, 1940), ch. 76, pp. 179–81.

10 *The Book of Margery Kempe*, ch. 76, p. 179.

11 Rawcliffe, *Medicine and Society*, p. 207.

> marks, whereof she gave a part to poor people, and of that other part she made a hospital, and therefore she was called a wasteress and a fool, which all she suffered joyously. And when she had made this hospital she became herself as an humble chamberer in the service of the poor people, and she bare her so humbly in that service, that by night she bare the sick men between her arms for to let them do their necessities, and brought them again, and made clean their clothes and sheets that were foul. She brought the mesels [lepers] abed, and washed their sores and did all that longed to a hospitaller.[12]

Like every hagiography, the life of Elizabeth of Hungary is highly conventional, and the extreme virtue of the subject is inevitably described in stereotypical terms, yet this passage has a verisimilitude that gives the account some plausibility. There is no suggestion here that Elizabeth miraculously healed all who came to her – the miracle, in so far as there is one, lies in the fact that the saint, who was born a princess, in her humility willingly embraces menial tasks, and endures the scorn of her critics. Caxton's choice of language is revealing: Elizabeth is a 'chamberer'—that is, a 'servant' – but she is also a 'hospitaller', in other words a religious dedicated to the care of the sick. However, the word 'hospiteler' or 'hospitaller' usually referred specifically to the Knights Hospitaller, the male religious and chivalric order that has its origins in caring for sick pilgrims in the Holy Lands.[13] In translating this text for an English audience in the fifteenth century, Caxton seems to have been uncomfortable with the saint undermining her own aristocratic status, and in referring to her as a 'hospitaller' Caxton elevates her role significantly above that of a servant or nurse, and in so doing genders her role masculine.

Because care for the body and care for the soul were seen to be inextricably linked, the practices of medicine and religion were entwined. From the early medieval period onwards, physical illness was often associated with sinfulness, as seen in the following passage, describing the death of the saintly Anglo-Saxon abbess Æthelthryth of Ely in the seventh century, from Bede's *Ecclesiastical History* (completed 731):

> Sed certiori notitia medicus Cynifrid, qui et morienti illi et eleuatae de tumulo adfuid, qui referre erat solitus quod illa infirmata habuerit tumorem maximum sub maxilla. 'Iusseruntque me' inquit 'incidere tumorem illum, ut effiueret noxius umor qui inerat. Quod dum facerem, uidebatur illa per biduum aliquanto leuius habere, ita ut multi putarent quia sanari posset a languore. Tertia autem die prioribus adgrauata doloribus et rapta confestim de mundo, dolorem omnem ac mortem perpetua salute ac uita mutauit. …' Ferunt autem quia, cum praefato tumore ac dolore maxillae siue colli premeretur, multum delectata sit hoc genere infirmitatis, ac solita dicere: 'Scio certissime quia merito

12 Jacobus de Voragine, *The Golden Legend or Lives of the Saints,* trans. William Caxton, ed. F. S. Ellis, published online in Internet History Sourcebooks at http://www.fordham.edu/halsall/basis/goldenlegend/GoldenLegend-Volume6.asp#Elizabeth.

13 MED, s.v. 'hospiteler'.

> in collo pondus languoris porto, in quo iuuenculam me memini superuacua moniliorum pondera portare; et credo quod ideo me superna pietas dolore colli uoluit grauari, ut sic absoluar reatu superuacuae leuitatis, dum mihi nunc pro auro et margaretis de collo rubor tumoris ardorque promineat.'
>
> [But more certain proof is given by a doctor named Cynefrith, who was present at her [Æthelthryth's] death-bed and at her elevation from the tomb. He used to relate how, during her illness, she had a very large tumour beneath her jaw. 'I was ordered', he said, 'to cut this tumour so as to drain out the poisonous matter within it. After I had done this she seemed to be easier for about two days and many thought that she would recover from her sickness. But on the third day she was attacked by her former pains and was soon taken from the world, exchanging pain and death for everlasting health and life. ...' It is also related that when she was afflicted with this tumour and by the pain in her neck and jaw, she gladly welcomed the said pain and used to say, 'I know well enough that I deserve to bear the weight of this affliction in my neck, for I remember that when I was a young girl I used to wear an unnecessary weight of necklaces; I believe that God in His goodness would have me endure this pain in my neck in order that I may thus be absolved from the guilt of my needless vanity. So, instead of gold and pearls, a fiery red tumour now stands out upon my neck.'][14]

Whereas for Margery Kempe in the fifteenth century the task of nursing is the act of penance, for Æthelthryth in the seventh century, the tumour itself is a physical sign of former sin, and the patient endurance of this plague is an act of atonement. However Bede's account is more multilayered than this analysis suggests. As Bede's life of Æthelthryth recounts, the abbess had been twice married before becoming a nun. While Bede insists that Æthelthryth's marriages were unconsummated, his narrative betrays anxiety about her status as a virgin, which is only resolved when her body is exhumed in order to be moved to another burial site, and found to be uncorrupted – with the wound on her neck where the tumour was removed miraculously healed, and only a faint scar remaining. For the physician Cynefrith, and for Bede himself, the evidence of the uncorrupted corpse was proof that Æthelthryth remained pure in her lifetime, but the scar, as a reminder of the suffering caused by her tumour, indicates that by the time of her death Æthelthryth had fully atoned for her former imperfections, which include her marriages as well as her vanity.

While physical illnesses were often, although not necessarily, linked to sinfulness, mental illness in particular was associated with possession by devils. Treatment of both therefore might be directed at the soul as well as the body or the mind and, alongside prayer, charms, incantations and invocations were used for healing. Prayers to Christ and the saints, including the Virgin Mary, were seen to be particularly effective, and might be combined with

14 *Bede's Ecclesiastical History of the English People*, ed. and trans. Bertram Colgrave and R. A. B. Mynors (Oxford, 1969), pp. 394–7.

other devotional acts such as pilgrimage. The health benefits of visiting Our Lady at Walsingham were spelled out in a poem describing the origins of the shrine, known as the 'Pynson Ballad' because it was first published in a short pamphlet by the printer Richard Pynson in the late fifteenth century:

> Many seke ben here cured by Our Ladyes myghte
> Dede agayne revyved, of this is no dought,
> Lame made hole and blynde restored to syghte,
> Maryners vexed with tempest safe to porte brought
> Defe, wounded and lunatyke that hyder have sought
> And also lepers here recovered have be
> By Oure Ladyes grace of their infyrmyte
>
> Folke that of fendys have had acombraunce
> And of wycked spyrytes also moche vexacyon
> Have here be delyvered from every such chaunce,
> And soules greatly vexed with gostely temptacion,
> Lo, here the chyef solace agaynst all tribulacyon
> To all that be seke, bodely or goostly,
> Callynge to Oure Lady devoutly.[15]

By the Reformation the Shrine of Our Lady at Walsingham in Norfolk, which was founded in the eleventh century, was one of the most important pilgrimage destinations not only in England, but in Western Christendom. The fame and significance of the shrine served to reinforce the reputation of the Virgin Mary, if not as physician, then certainly as intercessory healer.

MARIA MEDICA: MARY AS HEALER IN *THE LIFE OF CHRISTINA OF MARKYATE*

The specific association of the Virgin Mary with healing is a feature of revelatory texts in particular. One of the defining and distinctive qualities of women's visions in the post-Conquest period is the increasing importance of the role played by the Virgin Mary. A key devotional text that includes extensive discussion of a woman's experience of illness, combined with a strong Marian focus, is the anonymous twelfth-century *Life of Christina of Markyate*. Born in the late eleventh century (just over forty years after the shrine at Walsingham was founded), Christina of Markyate was from a noble Anglo-Saxon family. In her infancy, Christina made the resolution to devote herself to God, but conflict with her family arose when they forced her into marriage. In the end, Christina fled from her new husband and went into hiding, where, with the help of a network of supporters, she was able to live as

15 The ballad is reproduced in its entirety online in the Walsingham Archives at http://www.walsinghamanglicanarchives.org.uk/pynsonballad.htm. The sole surviving copy of the pamphlet is Cambridge, Magdalene College, Pepys Library 1254.

a recluse before eventually, following the dissolution of her marriage, taking her vows and establishing her own small religious community. There are clear parallels here with the example of the formerly married Æthelthryth, and the wider tradition of female Anglo-Saxon saints who left their husbands for God, and it is partially within this tradition that Christina situates herself.

Embedded within Christina's *Life* are accounts of the terrible illnesses she endured for many years, following her enclosure in a cramped corner of the cell of her spiritual guide Roger, a revered hermit monk of St Albans. After Roger's death, Christina took over his hermitage in Markyate, and gathered around her a group of devout women. The *Life* records two Marian visions which occurred at Markyate in which Christina herself was divinely healed – one from physical sickness, the other from an intense spiritual as well as physical burden that apparently resulted from her anxiety about whether she had succeeded in preserving her virginity. The ambivalence with which illness and physical and mental suffering were regarded in the Middle Ages is illustrated in these two examples. In the first it seems that Christina's illness functions as a form of aestheticism, albeit one from which she is cured; but in the second it is associated with what are seen, by Christina at least, as possible transgressions in her earlier life, and more specifically her marriage. In this case, the cure suggests that she has atoned for her faults or that the faults did not exist in the first case.

The first of Christina's Marian healing visions centres on a near-death experience, when she became paralysed down one side of her body. According to the *Life*, male physicians were called in to treat Christina, but their treatments, which included blood-letting as well as medicinal compounds, made her illness worse rather than better. The narrator records that 'nam humana industria quicquid artis habebat in curam illarum nequicquam temptaverat' ['For everything known to human science had been tried in vain'].[16] Christina's eventual recovery followed a dream experienced by one of her female companions of the 'magne auctoritatis matronam' ['woman of great authority']:

> Et cum cedisset ante lectum egrote: proferre pixidem in qua lectuarium attulerat insolite fragrancie. Quod cum delicatissime prepararet. ut cibaret illam: omnes simul eam corripere. dicendo cum lacrimis. Noli domina noli lectuarium et laborem tuum perdere. quia vidimus illam quam curare satagis per simile lectuarium quo utebatur heri vix mortem evasisse. Illa vero pro nichilo ducere ignorancium verba. et propter quod venerat sicut ceperat lectuario porrecto sanare languidam.
>
> [When (the woman of great authority) had sat down on the patient's bed, she took out a small box in which she had brought an electuary of unusual fragrance. While she was daintily preparing to give it to her, all of them with

[16] *The Life of Christina of Markyate: A Twelfth Century Recluse*, ed. and trans. C. H. Talbot (Toronto, 1998), pp. 122–3.

> tears in their eyes warned her, saying: 'Do not waste both your lozenge and your labour, lady, because we saw the woman you are trying to cure barely escape death after taking a similar electuary yesterday.' But she took no notice of what they were saying, and, carrying out the errand on which she had come, gave the lozenge to the sick woman and cured her.][17]

The writer goes on to identify the woman of great authority as the Virgin Mary. This vision then, experienced by Christina's companion, served to confirm the miraculous nature of Christina's recovery, and specifically Mary's role not simply as intercessory healer but in this case as the physician who successfully cured Christina.

The second healing vision was witnessed by Christina herself. It can be dated to shortly before Christina made her profession as a nun in St Albans abbey before Alexander, bishop of Lincoln, in 1131 or thereabouts. Significantly, the vision took place on the seventh day of the Feast of the Assumption of the Blessed Virgin Mary. As she prepared to take her vows, Christina, who, as mentioned above, had had to be released from an enforced betrothal, and who had herself also struggled with reciprocated sexual desire for an unnamed cleric, experienced great anxiety concerning her status as a virgin and sought reassurance from the Virgin Mary. Having waited patiently for several days for a response to her prayers, she was rewarded with a vision in a confirmation of her piety and sanctity that resonates strongly with the Annunciation and the Assumption of the Virgin. Christina awoke and found her female companions still sleeping, having apparently failed to rise for nocturnes. Suddenly angels surrounded Christina, addressing her with the words 'ave … virgo Christi' ['Hail, virgin of Christ'],[18] and placed a crown on her head.

> Tunc enim angelis sese recipientibus in celum: illa secum remansit. indubitanter agnoscens per celestem coronam quod Christus eam mente et corpore virginem usque servaverat. Preterea se repperit ita sanam ut infirmitatum quibus ante laboravit. nec minimam quidem deinceps sentiret molestiam.
>
> [Then, as the angels withdrew to heaven, she remained alone, knowing for certain from the heavenly crown that Christ had preserved her chaste in mind and body. Furthermore, she felt so strong in health that never afterwards did she feel the slightest twinge from those maladies which had afflicted her earlier on.][19]

While the crowning of Christina places her within the tradition of legendary virgin martyrs such as Margaret of Antioch, and the miraculous healing affirms her blessed state, the divine verification of her chastity reinforces not only her devotion to but also her identification with Mary as Physician as well as Mary as Mother of God.

17 *The Life of Christina of Markyate*, pp. 124–5.
18 *The Life of Christina of Markyate*, pp. 128–9.
19 *The Life of Christina of Markyate*, pp. 128–9.

Tellingly, these Marian visions are prefaced in the *Life* by an account of Christina herself playing a role in the cure of a young woman who was suffering from 'gutta caduca' ('falling sickness')[20] or epilepsy. The young woman had been blessed with a revelation of Margaret of Antioch, who instructed her to visit Christina and to drink from water blessed by Christina, promising that this would result in her recovery. The epileptic woman duly approached Christina and told her about her illness and vision, and also described her *culpa* or 'fault', thus forging a link between her condition and her own sinfulness.[21] Tom Licence has argued that in the case of miracles and revelations associated with recluses such as Christina, 'visions reveal the favourable conditions of souls dwelling in the anchorites' prayers' but they do not assert directly 'that the prayers secured those conditions'.[22] While Licence is talking specifically about revelations of salvation, a similar point can be made about healing miracles. When approached by the epileptic woman, Christina's initial reaction was to refuse her request and to suggest to her that her vision was false. However, eventually she agreed to bless the water for the woman, but insisted that she would do this in the chapel at the same time as the priest was celebrating mass and the congregation were at prayer. Christina further distanced herself from the miracle by insisting that during the mass a man appeared to her, whom she identified as the Apostle, presumably St John the Evangelist.[23] The efficacy of Christina's intercession might thus be diluted – the mass, the prayers of the others, the appearance of the Evangelist, all contributed to the miracle – but the anonymous author of her *Life* nevertheless goes on to describe her as 'Christina ipsa que celitus procurabat salutem aliis' ['Christina, who obtained cures for others from heaven'].[24] Although a number of saints, including Valentine and Vitus, as well as St John the Baptist, and less commonly St John the Evangelist, are associated with the cure of epilepsy, the Virgin Mary was also often evoked in this context. The most notable, and infamous, example from England is the public healing of the early sixteenth-century visionary, the Holy Maid of Kent, Elizabeth Barton, whose early prophetic visions were accompanied by seizures which were attributed to epilepsy by some (hostile) eyewitnesses as well as later commentators.[25] Before a large audience, Barton prostrated herself before an image of Our Lady in the small chapel of Court-at-Street in Kent, following a revelation that this would result in her cure. While it is Margaret of Antioch and St John rather than the Virgin Mary who are

20 *The Life of Christina of Markyate*, pp. 118–19.

21 *The Life of Christina of Markyate*, pp. 120–1.

22 Tom Licence, *Hermits and Recluses in English Society, 950–1200* (Oxford, 2011), p. 169.

23 *The Life of Christina of Markyate*, p. 120 n.1.

24 *The Life of Christina of Markyate*, pp. 120–1.

25 See Diane Watt, *Secretaries of God: Women Prophets in Late Medieval and Early Modern England* (Cambridge, 1997), pp. 57–65.

directly involved in the miraculous cure of the epileptic woman in Christina of Markyate's *Life*, in juxtaposing the account with the Marian visions that resulted in the healing of Christina herself, in one of which Mary unambiguously assumes the authority of the physician or doctor of medicine, Christina's own role as intercessory healer is closely linked to her emulation of the Virgin Mary.

THE VISIONARY AS PHYSICIAN IN *THE BOOK OF MARGERY KEMPE*

The argument that a belief in Mary as Physician was widespread in the later Middle Ages is not immediately supported by the example of *The Book of Margery Kempe*, written almost 300 years after *The Life of Christina of Markyate*. As is well known, Margery Kempe's semi-autobiographical *Book* opens with an account of the mental illness Kempe experienced in her early twenties following the birth of her first child. Kempe had had a difficult pregnancy and a painful labour. Fearing that she was going to die, and worrying about a secret sin that she had never revealed, she sent for her priest in order to make her confession. Unfortunately the priest's response was such that she was unable to complete her confession, and, suffering complete suicidal despair, she went out of her mind. It is striking that the narrative of Margery Kempe's recovery from this period of insanity, which from a modern perspective would seem to be a form of postpartum depression, makes *no* reference to the Virgin Mary. Rather it is a very beautiful Jesus Christ who appears to Margery Kempe at her lowest point and offers her compassion and consolation. And indeed it is Jesus Christ with whom Margery Kempe is identified in her suffering. We are told:

> Sche bot [bit] hir owen hand so vyolently þat it [the bite mark] ws seen al hir lyfe aftyr. And also sche roof [ripped] hir skyn on hir body a-ȝen hir hert wyth hir nayles spetowsly [pitilessly], for sche had noon oþer instrumentys [implements].[26]

Even though Kempe describes herself as being tormented by devils and evil spirits, it is clear that the wounds she inflicts upon herself in her hand and near her heart represent a form of stigmata, and as such are an indication of her sanctified status.

Yet even though the Virgin Mary is not mentioned in the account of Kempe's own miraculous healing, the idea of Mary as Physician, or at any rate as intercessory healer, may well underlie it. Yoshikawa, in her analysis of this episode, points to a possible gap in the narrative, and suggests that Margery Kempe's 'complete recovery, though not mentioned in her book, must have

26 *The Book of Margery Kempe*, ch. 1, p. 8.

been realised when she went through the rite of purification at her parish church'.[27] As Yoshikawa explains,

> For ordinary women the rite of purification concludes a period of physical recovery of the newly delivered mother who was considered unwell. This notion of the newly parturient mother's sickness was related to the ceasing of menstruation, something which was considered to affect her humoral balance. Closely associated with women's health, the Purification is thus a symbolic threshold which readmits women to receive the sacramental Host, for medieval canon law prohibited women after childbirth from receiving the sacraments because they were considered symbolically and ritually impure. In addition to the physical trauma of childbirth, women had to endure the spiritual trauma induced by the virtual exclusion from the Christian ritual.[28]

The link between the healing of Margery Kempe and the Virgin Mary is implicit but nonetheless compelling. If the Virgin Mary is not mentioned here, her intercessory presence can nevertheless be felt. The Purification of the Virgin, which is celebrated at Candlemas, valorises late medieval woman's experience of childbirth, and, as Yoshikawa points out, is itself celebrated in Kempe's subsequent visions. Furthermore, in an episode much later in the *Book*, which closes the opening sequence, Kempe herself takes on the role of healer in relation to another women experiencing postpartum depression. At the request of the woman's husband, Kempe attended to her:

> And þe sayd creatur [Kempe] went to hir iche day onys er twyis at þe lest wey [at least]. … And þe sayd creatur preyid for þis woman euery day þat God xulde, ȝyf it were hys wille, restoryn hir to hir wittys a-geyn. And owr Lord answeryd in hir sowle & seyd, 'Sche xulde faryn ryth wel.' Þan was sche mor bolde to preyin for hir recuryng [recovery] þan sche was be-forn, & iche day, wepyng & sorwyng, preyid for hir recur [recovery] tyl God ȝaf hir hir witte & hir mende a-ȝen. And þan ws sche browt to chirche & purifijd as oþer women be, blyssed mote God ben.[29]

The anonymous scribe of *The Book of Margery Kempe* records that those who saw this act of healing celebrated it as 'a ryth gret myrakyl' and he identifies himself as an eye-witness: never before had he seen a woman so out of her mind as this woman, and afterwards he saw her 'sad & sobyr a-now' [well-behaved and sober enough].[30] Yet, even though no saints appear in visions either to the woman or to Margery Kempe, and even though Kempe prays for the woman without the support of others, Kempe, like Christina of Markyate, is careful to attribute the miracle not to her own efforts, but to God. Margery

27 Yoshikawa, 'Mysticism and Medicine', p. 115.
28 Yoshikawa, 'Mysticism and Medicine', p. 112.
29 *The Book of Margery Kempe*, ch. 75, p. 178.
30 *The Book of Margery Kempe*, ch. 75, p. 178–9.

Kempe may be intercessor and mediator, but the gradual recovery of the woman is the result of divine intervention alone. Furthermore, and crucially, in this passage the importance of the purification ceremony or churching as signifying the return to spiritual as well as physical health is made explicit. Thus, even though the Virgin Mary is not *explicitly* evoked in this passage, her importance is again implied by the reference to the purification ceremony. The striking parallels with the earlier episode describing Margery Kempe's own postpartum crisis suggest that Margery Kempe's intercession on the woman's behalf is akin to that of the Virgin in her own healing, and that in intervening in the life of this very distressed and ill woman, Margery Kempe was emulating the Virgin's care for the sick.

WOMEN AND MEDICINE IN THE MEDIEVAL HOUSEHOLD

Did the idea of Mary as Physician extend into a secular context? The third set of examples I would like to consider here are taken from the Paston letters, which were written in Norfolk in the fifteenth century. Increasingly, throughout the Middle Ages and Renaissance, the practice of medicine moved from the female realm into the male: a transition which was of course particularly marked in the case of midwifery, but true of other areas. A petition to parliament by a group of surgeons in 1421 attempted to introduce greater regulation and included the recommendation 'That no woman use the practyce of fisyk [medicine]' on pain of imprisonment and the imposition of a heavy fine.[31] Elaine Whitaker has argued that 'the Paston women intuitively perceived their displacement as authorities on health maintenance.'[32] It is certainly the case that Margaret Paston regarded doctors with some suspicion, telling her husband in 1464 to 'be ware what medesynys ye take of any fysissyanys of London', adding that she will never trust them in the light of her family's past experience.[33] However, I argue that their letters indicate that women within the late medieval household continued to play important roles when it came to healing as well as caring for the sick. The Paston women's responsibilities in health care extended from nursing to treating ailments and to prescribing and dispensing medicines.

Here is an example taken from a letter from Margaret Paston to the family chaplain, James Gloys:

[31] 'A Petition to the Parliament of 1421 for Protective Legislation', in *Rotuli Parliamentorum*, ed. J. Strachey et al. (London, 1767–77), vol. 4, p. 158. Quoted in Carole Rawcliffe, *Sources for the History of Medicine in Late Medieval England* (Kalamazoo, MI, 1995), pp. 62–4 (p. 63).

[32] Elaine E. Whitaker, 'Reading the Pastons Medically', *English Language Notes* 31 (1993), 19–27 (p. 19).

[33] *The Paston Letters and Papers of the Fifteenth Century*, ed. Norman Davis, 2 parts, EETS s.s. 20, 21(Oxford, 1971, 1976), part 1, p. 291.

> I am soré [sorry] þat my cosyn Bernay is seke, and I pray you yeff [give] my white wine, or ony of my wateris [essences], or ony othere thyng that I haue þat is in youre awarde [keeping] may doo hym ony comforth, lette hym haue it. … And I remembere þat water of mynte or water of millefole [mint or milfoil essence] were good for my cosyn Bernay to drynke for to make hym to browke [tolerate food]; and yeue thei send to Dame Elesebeth Callethroppe, þer ye shall not fayill of the tone or of bothe. Sche haith othere wateris to make folkis to browke [She has other herbal essences to make people tolerate food].[34]

Although no receipt or recipe books belonging to Margaret Paston have survived, in which she would have kept a record of her medicines, their uses, and how to prepare them, it is evident from letters such as these that Margaret Paston, in common with other medieval housewives, kept her own supply of medical remedies. Indeed in one letter, Margaret Paston asks her son to purchase theriac for her in London; theriac is a medicinal compound that was used as an antidote to poison and as a general panacea.[35] These medicines were not only for household use: clearly Margaret Paston was also consulted by or on behalf of more distant kin, such as Berney in the letter quoted above, neighbours, and friends. And of course, women in different households exchanged recipes and medicine: here Margaret is confident that Elizabeth Calthorpe will be willing to supply any essences lacking in her own collection.

Another example is found in a letter by John Paston III, writing to his wife Margery. Given the brevity of the letter, and the insight into medieval medical practices in the household that it provides, it is worth quoting the letter in its entirety:

> Mastress Margery, I recomand me to yow, and I prey yow in all hast possybyll to send me by the next swer [sworn] messenger that ye can gete a large playster of your *flose vngwentorum* [a large compress of your best ointment] for the Kynges Attorney Jamys Hobart; for all hys dysease is but an ache in hys knee. He is the man that brought yow and me togedyrs, and I had lever then xl li. ye koud wyth your playster depart hym and hys peyne [I would rather you were able to rid him of his pain with your compress than have £40]. But when ye send me the playster ye must send me wryghtyng hough it shold be leyd to and takyn fro [applied to and removed from] hys knee, and hough longe it shold abyd on hys kne vnremevyd, and hough longe the playster wyll laste good, and whethyr he must lape [wrap] eny more clothys a-bowte the playster to kepe it warme or nought.
>
> And God be wyth yow.
>
> Your JOHN PASTON[36]

[34] *The Paston Letters*, part 1, pp. 370–1.

[35] *The Paston Letters*, part 1, p. 243.

[36] *The Paston Letters*, part 1, p. 628.

What is striking about this letter is the connection that John III makes between the request for medical supplies – the compress and the ointment, which would have been lime-based, and instructions about how to use them (the exhaustive list of questions indicates that medicine is something of a mystery to him), and the important role that the patient played in the marital union of John and Margery. John recognises perhaps that Margery will be unwilling to part with her medical recipe and therefore seeks to reassure her that they are both personally indebted to the patient.

Previous scholarship has paid some attention to those letters of the Paston women that relate to child-bearing. Wendy Harding has argued that pregnancy was an 'unwritten women's discourse', something that was part of a female oral sphere but which could only be hinted at, rather than addressed directly, in the women's correspondence with men.[37] Around 1441, Margaret Paston wrote to her husband:

> Elysabet Peverel hath laye seke xv or xvj wekys of þe seyetyka [sciatica], but sche sent my modyr word be Kate þat sche xuld come hedyr wanne God sent tyme, þoov sche xuld be crod in a barwe [even if she must be wheeled in a barrow].[38]

Harding's commentary is apposite: 'By virtue of her new state, Margaret has joined a circle of women – her mother, Kate (a family servant), and the midwife – who communicate by word of mouth and who are linked through their concern with the maternal body.... Only a trace of this unwritten discourse remains in Margaret's letter.'[39] Nevertheless, what Harding does not acknowledge are the elements of playful teasing of Margaret's husband, as recipient of this letter.

Similar teasing is also found in another, slightly later, letter from Margaret to her husband which alludes, again indirectly, to the experience of childbirth; a letter in which, significantly, there are also references to the Virgin Mary. In this letter, however, Margaret's primary concern is for the health of her husband, as he is recovering in London, from a period of illness:

> Ryth worchipful hosbon, I recomande me to yow, desyryng hertely to here of your wilfare, thanckyng God of your a-mendyng of þe grete dysese þat ye have hade; and I thancke yow for þe letter þat ye sent me, for be my trowthe my moder and I wer nowth in hertys es fro the tyme þat we woste [knew] of your sekenesse tyl we woste [knew] verely of your a-mendyng. My moder hat be-hestyd a-nodyr ymmage of wax of þe weytte of yow to Oyur Lady of Walsyngham [My mother promised another image of wax, of your weight, to Our Lady of Walsingham], and sche sent iiij nobelys to þe iiij orderys of frerys

[37] Wendy Harding, 'Medieval Women's Unwritten Discourse on Motherhood: A Reading of Two Fifteenth-Century Texts', *Women's Studies* 21 (1992), 197–209.

[38] *The Paston Letters*, part 1, p. 217.

[39] Harding, 'Medieval Women's Unwritten Discourse', p. 200.

> at Norweche to pray for yow; and I have be-hestyd to gon on pylgreymmays to Walsyngham and to Sent Levenardys for yow. Be my trowth, I had neuer so hevy a sesyn [so sorrowful a time] as I had fro þe tyme þat I woste of your sekenesse tyl I woste of your a-mendyng, and ȝyth myn hert is in go grete esse, ne nowth xal be tyl I wott þat ȝe ben very hol [completely better].[40]

Here once again, the Virgin Mary is associated with intercessory healing, in this care through the double reference to the Shrine of Our Lady at Walsingham. It would appear that Margaret Paston had great faith in the efficacy of the Shrine at Walsingham: near the end of her life, when her own health was failing, she made another pilgrimage to that destination.[41]

In his recent study, *Margaret Paston's Piety*, Joel Rosenthal is somewhat sceptical about the sincerity of the concern felt for John Paston's health by either his wife Margaret or his mother Agnes. He says of the letter quoted above, 'neither wife nor mother seems to have contemplated a trip to London to offer personal succor, let alone nursing care'.[42] Rosenthal, however, misses the point of the reference to the priory of St Leonard in Norwich. St Leonard's was also a popular pilgrimage site, and it had a famous image of the Virgin, but the reason Margaret may have chosen to visit the priory of St Leonard specifically may have been that St Leonard is the patron saint of pregnant women. Later in the letter it becomes clear that the reason that Margaret Paston was not in a position to travel to London to attend to or to nurse her husband was because she was expecting their second child:

> I xal sende my moder a tokyn þat sche toke [gave] me, for I sopose þe tyme is cum þat I xulde sendeth here yf I kepe þe be-hest [promise] þat I have made—I sopose I have tolde yow wat it was. I pray yow herterly þat ye wol wochesaf to sende me a letter as hastely as ȝe may, yf wrytyn be non dysesse [harm] to yow, and þat ye wollen wochesdaf to sende me worde quowe your sot dott [promise to send me news of your health]. Yf I mythe have hade my wylle I xulde a seyne yow er dys tyme. I wolde ȝe wern at hom, yf it were your ese and your sor myth ben as wyl lokyth to here as it tys þer ȝe ben now, lever dan a new gounne, þow it were of scarlette. [I would rather you were at home, if your comfort and illness could be as well looked after as it is where you are now, than have a new gown, even though it were of scarlet.] I pray yow, yf your sor be hol and so þat ȝe may indure to ryde, wan my fader com to London þat ȝe wol askyn leve and com hom wan þe hors xul be sentte hom a-ȝeyn; for I hope ȝe xulde be kepte [looked after] as tenderly herre as ȝe ben at London.[43]

From this it is clear that, even when pregnant, Margaret embraces her role as nurse to her sick husband. It is interesting to speculate about the nature of the

40 *The Paston Letters*, part 1, p. 218.

41 *The Paston Letters*, part 1, p. 640.

42 Joel T. Rosenthal, *Margaret Paston's Piety* (New York, 2010), p. 62.

43 *The Paston Letters*, part 1, p. 218.

'token' that Margaret Paston sent to her mother, to indicate her pregnancy. Sue Niebryzdowski has recently written about the importance of the Virgin Mary in discourses about pregnancy in the Middle Ages. As Niebryzdowski points out, 'Although Mary's somatic experience of childbirth was unique (she remained, after all, virgin post-partum), women were able to appropriate those aspects of Mary's pregnancy and childbirth with which they might empathise.'[44] Strips of parchment on which the Virgin's name was inscribed, or scrolls with the text of the Magnificat written on them, worn during childbirth, were thought to help in the experience of labour.[45] Margaret Paston may well have sent her mother some sort of Marian artefact, such as a necklace or ring, which would signify her hope for the safe delivery of her first child. For Margaret Paston and her family, the Virgin Mary offered protection and assistance to pregnant women, but might also cure the sick, and ease the suffering of the elderly. The Virgin Mary's role here seems to be that of intercessory healer rather than physician: she was a member of the community of women responsible for healthcare in medieval England. For Margaret, her husband and her sons, the medical support offered by herself, and by other female members of her family and social network, like that offered by the Virgin Mary, was to be trusted above that of the physicians of London.

CONCLUSION

The evidence of the Paston letters supports the argument that the idea of the Virgin *Maria medica* or Mary as Physician alongside her more widely recognised role as intercessory healer and her associations with childbirth validated women's roles as healers in both religious and secular contexts. In England, the idea of the Virgin as healer was strengthened by the importance of her shrine in Walsingham. As the examples taken from *The Book of Margery Kempe* and the letters of Margaret Paston illustrate, the Virgin Mary had particularly strong associations with what we now think of as women's health. Nevertheless, as *The Life of Christina of Markyate* reveals, *Maria medica* – the woman of great authority – was not limited to assisting with intercessory healing, pregnancy, childbirth, and postpartum conditions, but included the practice of medicine. Furthermore, it is clear from the two visionary texts considered here that, in acting as healers themselves, mystics such as Christina of Markyate and Margery Kempe were in some sense imitating the Virgin Mary. If the term 'medica' or its equivalents was not applied even

44 Sue Niebryzdowski, 'Marian Literature', in *The History of British Women's Writing, 700–1500*, ed. Liz Herbert McAvoy and Diane Watt (Basingstoke, 2012), pp. 112–20 (p. 116).

45 *The Knowing of Woman's Kind in Childing: A Middle English Version of Material Derived from the Trotula and Other Sources*, ed. Alexandra Barratt (Turnhout, 2001), lines 369–74.

to saintly women much beyond the twelfth century, the strong connection between women and medicine as well as midwifery is illustrated well into the fifteenth century in the letters of Margaret Paston, a woman who had great confidence in her own medical authority, even as she disdained the knowledge and abilities of the (male) experts in the city.

2

CHAUCER'S PHYSICIANS: RAISING QUESTIONS OF AUTHORITY

Roberta Magnani

As Naoë Kukita Yoshikawa indicates in the introduction, this volume is situated in the dialectic space created by the intersection of a number of coterminous discourses: medicine, religion and gender. The concepts of *Christus medicus* and Mary the Physician testify to the interconnectedness of spirituality and medical practice, while posing questions about authority and power hierarchies that are overtly gendered, as the Virgin assumes an equal healing or salvific potency in relation to the Trinity. In the works of Geoffrey Chaucer, the interconnection of these three coextensive discourses and the ensuing preoccupation with authority and truth become apparent in the centrality of Marian figurations. This essay, which is structured in three parts, aims at exploring and exploding received ideas of authority, whether spiritual, medical, textual or gendered. After engaging with Chaucer's orthodox depiction of Mary as nurse, that is, as assistive and exemplary agent whose ideological function is to disseminate a *regimen* of desirable subject positions, I will attend to Chaucer's heterodox representations of the Virgin. In line with variant strands of Mariology, which Diane Watt examines in detail in her essay above, the poet's texts open up to a dramatisation of the Virgin's power that transcends her feminine assistive role and aligns her to the visions of Mary the Physician narrated in Christina of Markyate's *Life*. Chaucer's unravelling of the absolute authority of patriarchal structures that underpin the Trinity and orthodox doctrines of salvation culminates in the portrait and Tale of his secular Physician. Consistent with his training in speculative and discursive disciplines such as theology, the Doctour of Phisik weaves a fractured narrative in which concepts of truth and authority are rigorously interrogated. In his search for a stable physical and spiritual *regimen sanitatis*, the Physician identifies the Virgin's feminine potency as principle of truth.

Roberta Magnani

THE VIRGIN MARY: THE ASSISTIVE AGENT OF 'BIO-POWER'

Since the fifteenth century Chaucer's literary reputation has been profoundly imbricated in his devotion to the Virgin Mary. As part of his personal tribute to 'fadir' and 'maistir Chaucer' in *The Regiment of Princes*, Thomas Hoccleve associates the poet's moral and literary excellence to his Marian output:

> As thow wel knowist, o blessid Virgyne,
> With lovyng herte and hy devocioun,
> In thyn honour he wroot ful many a lyne.
> O now thyn help and thy promocioun!
> To God thy sone make a mocioun,
> How he thy servant was, mayden Marie,
> And lat his love floure and fructifie.[1]

An examination of the extant manuscripts of Hoccleve's works indicates the relevance and the extent of the dissemination of Chaucer's Marian devotion, as these lines are positioned on the same folio in which the portrait of Chaucer is situated. This well known likeness of the poet, part of the Harley-Ellesmere tradition of portraiture, dominates the margins of both London, British Library, MS Royal 17.D.iv (fol. 93v) and, more famously, British Library, MS Harley 4866 (fol. 88r). It captures Chaucer in a solemn authorising gesture which directs the audience's attention to Hoccleve's text. While asserting the patriarchal authority of Father Chaucer, Hoccleve describes Mary's role in purely assistive terms: the Mother of Christ is a mediating agent between God and mankind ('help'; 'promocioun'; 'mocioun'), as well as an object of profound devotion; however, within Hoccleve's literary and spiritual patrilinearity (Chaucer/Hoccleve; God/Christ), the Virgin is firmly positioned as subordinate to the superior authority of the Trinity.

The Virgin's assistive function is echoed and expanded in the first stanza of the *ABC*, a Marian lyric which Chaucer adapts from *Le Pèlerinage de la vie humaine*, a French text composed by Guillaume Deguileville:

> Almighty and al merciable queene,
> To whom that al this world fleeth for secour,
> To have relees of sinne, of sorwe, and teene,
> ...
> Help and releeve, thou mighti debonayre,
> Have mercy on my perilous languor.[2]

1 Thomas Hoccleve, *The Regiment of Princes*, ed. Charles R. Blyth (Rochester, NY, 1999), lines 4985–91.

2 Geoffrey Chaucer, *An ABC*, in *The Riverside Chaucer*, ed. Larry D. Benson, 3rd edn (Oxford and New York, 1987), lines 1–3, 6–7. All further references to Chaucer's works will be taken from this edition and will be given in parentheses in the text.

The dominant rhetoric of care and comfort ('help'; 'releeve'; 'secour') in the suppliant speaker's address to the 'queene' is predicated on a dialectic relation between spiritual and medical discourses, as he/she searches for a cure for both 'langour', or physical disease, and the spiritual malady of 'sinne'. More overtly, in the tenth stanza of Chaucer's *abecedarium*, the trope of Mary the Physician and the interconnection between medical practice and spiritual care/cure become apparent:

> Now, queen of comfort, sith thou art that same
> To whom I seeche for my medicyne,
> Lat not my foo no more my wounde entame;
> My hele into thin hand al I resygne. (77–80)

Mary is here addressed as the healer of wounds and the provider of remedies aimed at the body and the soul. As Carole Rawcliffe argues in her study of medieval medicine, the epistemological equivalence of sin and disease underpins the concept of *Christus medicus* whose suffering on the Cross is seen as curative and redemptive by theologians like St Augustine.[3]

Henry, duke of Lancaster's *Livre de Seyntz Medicines* (1354) is an extended reflection on the idea of Christ the Physician. Yoshikawa has studied Henry's engagement with the trope of the *Christus medicus* in the *Livre* and the related image of the Virgin Mary as attentive nurse:

> Employing wounds as a dominant metaphor, Henry envisions himself as mortally wounded by sin and pleads for urgent medical help. The subsequent meditations show how his wounds are healed by Christ the physician and the Virgin, who acts as a nurse in the service of her Son.[4]

In line with contemporary homiletic and theological modes of expression, Henry deploys a rhetoric of physical illness which functions as an extended metaphor for sin and describes the path to salvation as a sustained treatment of ailments. In this context an attention to prophylaxis becomes central; following dominant medical theories based on humoral balance, the devout Christian has to seek strategies to govern his/her body to prevent perilous excesses of choler, phlegm, black bile and blood, which can be read as physiological manifestations of diseases of the soul. As Yoshikawa explains, after articulating his confession through medical metaphors ('that I might with my tongue heal the foul wound of my mouth'), Henry devises a therapeutic and penitential *regimen* aimed at curing his moral malady.[5] His prophylaxis

3 Carole Rawcliffe, *Medicine and Society in Later Medieval England* (Stroud, 1997), pp. 17–19.

4 Naoë Kukita Yoshikawa, 'Holy Medicine and Diseases of the Soul: Henry of Lancaster and *Le Livre de seyntz medicines*', *Medical History* 53, 3 (2009), 397–414 (p. 398).

5 Quoted in Yoshikawa, 'Holy Medicine and Diseases of the Soul', p. 402.

culminates in the Virgin's dressing of the duke's wounds, a medical-spiritual metaphor that resonates powerfully with the *ABC*'s speaker's plea not just for comfort, but also for purgation and moral cleanliness ('entame'):

> The bandaging of the sores and wrapping them in fair white cloths signifies, most sweet Lord, that the precious medicines – as are the blessed milk, the holy tears, and the precious blood – should be well and firmly bandaged by the resolute intention for a good and pure life; and good intention shows itself in deed, in word and in thought.[6]

Henry's therapeutic remedy consists of a diet of desirable behaviours and Christian virtues, such as purity and wholesomeness, which the Virgin administers through her cleansing tears and life-giving milk.

As Chaucer's Prioress points out in the Prologue to her Tale, which she constructs as a Marian *supplicatio* and *elogium*, the Virgin is central to any prophylactic *regimen*, as she is 'soules boote' (VII. 466). Indeed, her assistive function transcends the curative properties of her tears and milk, as well as her 'natural' feminine role as carer and nurse, as she is the vehicle through which dominant ideological subject positions are reproduced and disseminated. In particular, Christian orthodoxy is fostered through a *regimen sanitatis* whose aim is to avow humoral excesses and the coextensive sinful intemperance of the soul; the often-incompliant body and soul necessitate, therefore, a series of dietary dictates and strategies of containment whose boundaries are policed by agents of 'bio-power' such as Mary. In his *History of Sexuality* Michel Foucault describes 'bio-power' as an ideological tool of domestication of the body to force its subjection to hegemonic values and, consequently, facilitate political control, or, as Foucault would put it, 'governmentality':

> The old power of death that symbolised sovereign power was now [in the classical age] carefully supplanted by the administration of bodies and the calculated management of life. ... there was an explosion of numerous and diverse techniques for achieving the subjugation of bodies and the control of populations, marking the beginning of an era of "bio-power".[7]

Within this Foucauldian conceptual framework, the Virgin is evoked as an agent of surveillance and the harbinger of orthodoxy. In the *ABC*, in particular, the contrite speaker recognises and welcomes Mary's spiritual and physical acts of surveillance, as he/she pleads '[r]edresse me, mooder, and me chastise' (129). According to the *Middle English Dictionary*, the verb 'redressen' conflates medical and spiritual discourses: Mary is asked to remedy the speaker's suffering while correcting, directing and restraining

6 Quoted in Yoshikawa, 'Holy Medicine and Diseases of the Soul', p. 412.

7 Michel Foucault, *The Will to Knowledge: History of Sexuality*, vol. 1, trans. Robert Hurley (Harmondsworth, 1998), pp. 139–41.

moral excesses.[8] Much as Henry of Lancaster's *regimen* requires the care of Mary-the-nurse, the *ABC*'s petitioner prays for the enlightening policing of the Mother of Christ.

The function of the Virgin as agent of surveillance and guiding principle for the penitent is augmented by the use of a traditional convention of the Marian literary *elogium*. In line with the findings exposed in Piero Boitani's detailed survey of Marian tropes in medieval literature, Mary is associated with the semantic field of light and fire, encapsulated in the Dantean image of the 'maris stella', or the beatific vision that accompanies Dante in the final stages of his spiritual journey towards the Jerusalem Celestial in *Paradiso*.[9] In *The Man of Law's Tale* Custance's *supplicatio* to the Virgin is resolutely inscribed in this tradition through the triple repetition of the *stella* trope: 'the mayde bright, Marie', 'lady bright', 'brighte sterre of day' (II. 841, 850, 852). At the desperate time when Custance faces exile alongside her innocent child, Mary represents hope, mercy, comfort and stability. The only response to Custance's spatial displacement, the Virgin provides material and spiritual guidance. As the herald of light, Mary is, therefore, constructed as a hermeneutic principle. In the *ABC* not only is she addressed through the vocative 'O verrey light of eyen that ben blynde' (105) and identified as the purveyor of orthodox theology or spiritual truth, but she is also interpellated as a figure of textuality:

> Kalenderes enlumyned ben thei
> That in this world ben lighted with thi name,
> And whoso goth to yow the righte way,
> Him thar not drede in soule to be lame. (73–6)

Here the poem establishes an analogy between Mary and liturgical texts; as evidenced in the Church calendars, increasingly popular books aiding the reader to commemorate saints and celebrate important dates in the liturgical year, the Virgin becomes a textual sign, that is, an element of the decorative programme in the material space of the manuscript leaf.[10] As a codex's illumi-

8 *Middle English Dictionary*, http://quod.lib.umich.edu/cgi/m/mec/med-idx?type=id&id=MED36356 [accessed 12 January 2014]. The MED provides, among others, the following glosses for the verb 'redressen' whose possible significations combine spiritual and physical cure: '1 (b) to relieve (distress); find a remedy for (grief, wretchedness); (c) to improve (a condition); restore (the body, a building). 2 To correct (sb., one's will), reform (sb.); save (man's soul); lead (sb.) back to the right path; also, *fig.* redeem (sb.). 3 (a) To make (sth.) straight; (b) to put or keep (sth.) in order; arrange (sth.), achieve; restrain (excess)'.

9 Piero Boitani, 'His desir wol fle withouten wynges: Mary and Love in Fourteenth-Century Poetry', in *Chaucer's Frame Tales*, ed. Joerg O. Fichte (Cambridge, 1987), pp. 83–128 (pp. 87, 98).

10 A discussion of Church calendars in relation to Chaucer's work can be found in Laurel Broughton, 'Chaucer and the Saints', in *Chaucer and Religion*, ed. Helen Phillips (Cambridge, 2010), pp. 111–31 (p. 111).

nations guide the reader through its content, Mary functions as hermeneutic principle policing 'the righte way' for the penitent in search of a therapeutic spiritual and material *regimen.*

In her theoretical reflection on the virginal woman, Luce Irigaray describes the virgin's subject position in terms that are remarkably germane to the medieval construction of Mary as function of hermeneutics presented in Chaucer's adaptation of Deguileville's Marian text:

> She is nothing but the possibility, the place, the sign of relations among men. In and of herself, she does not exist: she is a simple envelope veiling what is really at stake in social exchange. In this sense, her natural body disappears into its representative function. ... woman, for her part, as medium of exchange, is no longer anything but *semblance.*[11]

According to Irigaray, the virgin is a textual sign and a 'representative function' in the economy of exchange, but also, I would add, in the structures of 'bio-power', as desirable subject positions are written on her as 'simple envelope', as vacant surface to be inscribed with ideological content. As Sherry Reames points out, *The Prioress's Prologue* offers a 'standard' portrayal of the Virgin in which her moral excellence is celebrated as exemplary: [12]

> Lady, thy bountee, thy magnificence,
> Thy vertu and thy grete humylitee
> ...
> Thou goost biforn of thy benyngnytee,
> And getest us the lyght, of thy preyere,
> To gyden us unto thy Sone so deere. (VII. 474–5, 478–80)

This enumeration of Christian virtues writes orthodoxy on the figure of Mary who becomes a tissue of tropes and an ideological construct. She is, in other words, exemplary and magnificent, but also a '*semblance*', that is a sign which offers the devout a diet of graciousness and submissiveness to the ultimate authority of God. The Virgin is here the cure and the *regimen*: a textual 'envelope' that provides a hermeneutic path towards the salvific vision of the Son.

A similar figuration of virginal exemplarity and Irigarayan *semblance* is apparent in the character of Virginia, the female protagonist of the Physician's tale, who is described as textual sign or incarnated exemplar:

> For in hir lyvyng maydens myghten rede,
> As in a book, every good word or dede
> That longeth to a mayden vertuous,

11 Luce Irigaray, *This Sex which is not One*, trans. Catherine Porter with Carolyn Burke (Ithaca, NY, 1985), p. 186.

12 Sherry Reames, 'Mary, Sanctity and Prayers to Saints: Chaucer and Late-Medieval Piety', in *Chaucer and Religion*, ed. Phillips, pp. 81–96 (p. 87).

She was so prudent and so bountevous.
Bothe of hir beautee and hir bountee wyde,
That thurgh that land they preised hire echone
That loved vertu, save Envye allone,
That sory is of oother mennes wele
And glad is of his sorwe and his unheele.
(The Doctour maketh this descripcioun). (VI. 107–17)

The establishment of a prophylactic regimen is therefore a textual exercise to be written and read in a book. The Virgin Mary and Virginia, her literary counterpart, are textual strategies of 'bio-power' or, in other words, of dissemination of orthodox constructs of feminine Christianity: meek, prudent, restrained, virginal. As incarnated grammars of ideal femininity, their orthodoxy is sanctioned through a dual strategy of authorisation, since both the text and the paratext confirm the received authority of this construct: the 'Doctour'. A number of manuscripts, in fact, append 'Augustinus' to the line that invokes the 'Doctour' as the *auctor* from whom the Physician's words derive.[13] The explanatory notes to *The Physican's Tale* in *The Riverside Chaucer* link St Augustine's authority to the final part of the description of Virginia's exemplary excellence in which the text introduces a quasi-proverbial reference to envy.[14] I would, however, argue that it is not at all implausible that the gloss encompasses the passage as a whole and attributes the entire praise of the young virgin's honour to St Augustine. The Church Father's pronouncements on the superior status of virginity are, of course, a well known tenet of his theological thinking:

> But we, according to the faith and sound doctrine of holy Scriptures, both say that marriage is no sin, and yet set its good not only below virginal, but also below widowed continence; and say that the present necessity of married persons is an hindrance to their desert, not indeed unto life eternal, but unto an excellent glory and honor, which is reserved for perpetual continence: and that at this time marriage is not expedient save for such as contain not; and that on the tribulation of the flesh, which comes from the affection of the flesh, without which marriages of incontinent persons cannot be, the Apostle neither wished to be silent, as forewarning what was true, nor to unfold more fully, as sparing man's weakness.[15]

13 The Latin gloss 'Augustinus' can be found in a number of authoritative manuscripts such as San Marino, CA, Huntington Library, MS Ellesmere 26 C 9, Aberystwyth, National Library of Wales, MS Hengwrt 154 (Peniarth 392D), Cambridge University Library MS Dd.iv.24 and London, British Library, MS Egerton 2864. For more details on manuscript glosses, see *The Text of The Canterbury Tales Studied on the Basis of All Known Manuscripts*, vol. 3, ed. John M. Manly and Edith Rickert (Chicago, IL, 1940), p. 515.

14 Larry D. Benson, 'Explanatory Notes: *The Physician's Tale*', in *The Riverside Chaucer*, pp. 901–4 (p. 903). Benson explains the Latin gloss as a reference to the definition of envy that St Augustine provides in *Enarrationes in Psalmos*.

15 St Augustine, *De virginitate*, ch. 21, in *Nicene and Post-Nicene Fathers*, vol. 3, ed. Philip Schaff (New York, 2007), p. 424.

In this passage from *De Virginitate* St Augustine mounts a defence of chastity through a rhetoric of containment and continence; the temperance of the virginal body and soul resonates with the medico-spiritual discourse found in a *regimen sanitatis* such as Henry of Lancaster's *Livre*. The Virgin and Virginia are therefore textual sites, 'simple envelopes' on which an orthodox *regimen* of containment of excesses is written and disseminated.

CHAUCER'S VOICING OF THE 'WOMAN OF GREAT AUTHORITY'

Chaucer's dramatisation of the docile body of Mary is, as Reames argues, evidence of the orthodox Mariology articulated in his works. She asserts that the poet conforms to dominant Christian doctrine, since he avoids 'the theological error of setting her in competition with the Trinity, as if she were a goddess, a supernatural being with power all of her own'.[16] Notwithstanding Reames's convincing argument, textual evidence suggests that, instead of enclosing Mary within the ideological walls of an inescapable doctrine, Chaucer's texts open up a debate on Mariology with a specific concern for her status, power and agency in relation to Christ and the Trinity in general. Alongside Marian doctrinal orthodoxy, founded on the concept of the merciful 'vicaire' of God, the poet's work appears to accommodate variant doctrinal stances which are largely dependent on the emerging cultic standing of Mary in the later Middle Ages, especially within the practices of affective piety. This development is testified, for instance, in the establishment of the cultural and theological trope of Mary the Physician. As Diane Watt explains in her essay for this collection, the emergence of this trope is consistent with women's heavy involvement in healing practices, so much so that Carole Rawcliffe, among others, points out that 'in an age before the establishment of a professional monopoly wise women, empirics and herbalists actually constituted the great majority of practitioners at work'.[17] Monica Green's survey of medieval female practitioners reaches a similar conclusion on the ubiquity of women in the care of patients:

> Although they were not represented on all levels of medicine equally, women were found scattered throughout a broad medical community consisting of physicians, surgeons, barber-surgeons, apothecaries, and various uncategorizable empirical healers.[18]

Although her work focuses on the Early Modern period, Margaret Pelling's findings on the role played by women in 'medical families' give insights into a

16 Reames, 'Mary, Sanctity and Prayers to Saints', p. 86.

17 Rawcliffe, *Medicine and Society*, p. xv.

18 Monica H. Green, 'Women's Medical Practice and Health Care in Medieval Europe', *Signs* 14, 2 (1989), 438–73 (p. 439).

socio-cultural context that undoubtedly started to develop in the Middle Ages and is therefore relevant to the times in which Chaucer was writing his Marian texts. Pelling gathers compelling evidence that supports a re-assessment of the influence that women exerted on male members of their families during the domestic formative years that preceded their formal training as physicians.[19]

Despite their ubiquity, the cultural and professional standing of women as providers of care and cure was decidedly inferior to many of their male counterparts and was met with much resistance from the medical academic establishment and society in general. For instance, in his categorisation of medical practitioners, Huling E. Ussery places women among the 'lesser practitioners' and, more specifically, among the 'unlicensed and unaffiliated practitioners' such as leeches, midwives, 'wise women', herbalists and quacks.[20] Notwithstanding her attempt to re-assign agency to Early Modern women in medical practice, Pelling concedes that, precisely because of the profound interconnection between domesticity and medical care, women's engagement with medical practice remains largely confined to the domestic space. Far from being a result of women's lack of skill in matters of care and cure, their professional subordination to male physicians is largely due to ideological and institutional resistance to women's access to the profession.[21] The gendered rationale behind such resistance becomes apparent in the petition presented before Parliament in England in 1421 demanding that 'no Woman use the practyse of Fisik'.[22] Validated by theological and scientific discourse, hostility to recognising the centrality of women's contribution to medical practice is illustrated by Bruno of Calabria's contemptuous pronouncement that 'vile and presumptuous women usurp the office to themselves and abuse it, since they have neither learning nor skill'.[23] Clerical and professional homosociality traps women in an ambiguous professional position in which their agency is undermined. As the posthumous representations and mis-representations of Trotula of Salerno testify, women at the heart of the cure and care of the sick were ostracised and their authority usurped by male practitioners. As Green demonstrates, from the Middle Ages onwards women were gradually excluded from medical practice and, in the areas of care traditionally associated with female practitioners, such as midwifery and gynaecology, they were 'gradually restricted to a role as subordinate and controlled assistants in matters where,

19 Margaret Pelling, 'The Women of the Family? Speculations around Early Modern British Physicians', *The Society for the Social History of Medicine* 7, 3 (1995), 383–401, especially p. 397.

20 Huling E. Ussery, *Chaucer's Physician: Medicine and Literature in Fourteenth-Century England*, Tulane Studies in English 19 (New Orleans, LA, 1971), p. 6.

21 Pelling, 'The Women of the Family?', p. 386.

22 Quoted in Green, 'Women's Medical Practice and Health Care', p. 449.

23 Rawcliffe, *Medicine and Society*, p. 186. This quotation is taken from Bruno of Calabria's *Magna Chirurgia* (c. 1250).

because of socially constructed notions of propriety, men could not practice alone'.[24]

This is, therefore, a gender-specific issue of authority and power which resonates with the doctrinal debate on orthodox Mariology to which I alluded earlier. Despite institutional hostility to women and their subordinate professional status, Watt's essay shows that the trope of Mary the Physician advanced the cause of female medical practitioners by giving female acts of care a devotional prominence. In fact, the Virgin's assistive function dramatised in Custance's prayer to Mary in *The Man of Law's Tale* or in the *ABC* positions Chaucer's texts within doctrinal orthodoxy, but does not account for the heterogeneity of the late medieval debate on Mary's authority. Hilda Graef's extensive mapping of Marian theology demonstrates that, if eminent Christian thinkers such as Aquinas rejected the very possibility of endowing Mary and the Trinity with equal agency, St Bonaventure and other medieval *auctores* argued for the Virgin partaking in God's redemptive plan.[25]

A much earlier precedent to Chaucer's engagement with this variant Marian doctrine is the experience of Christina of Markyate, a twelfth-century English visionary and hermit. In the account of her life we find further evidence of the cultural currency of Mary's authority. In her essay for this collection, Watt discusses an event narrated in the *Life of Christina of Markyate* which unequivocally frames the interconnection between spiritual and medical practices within a discourse of power. Afflicted by illness, Christina was tended to by a number of male physicians who, however, failed to cure her. Healing could only be effected by a female practitioner who appeared as a vision to one of Christina's companions while she was dreaming. The text describes the physician as an agent of authority and power whose medical skills clearly exceed those of her male counterparts. The 'magne auctoritatis matronam' [woman of great authority] is firmly identified as the Virgin Mary, as Watt explains. While the vision preserves Mary's traditional feminine attentiveness in the act of providing care ('Quod cum delicatissime prepararet. ut cibaret illam' ['While she was daintily preparing to give it to her']), her power is articulated through her silent *gravitas* and self-assured disregard for warnings about an inevitable failure of the cure.[26]

24 Green, 'Women's Medical Practice and Health Care', pp. 460, 472. For a comprehensive overview of scholarship on Trotula of Salerno, see a section of Monica Green's Academia.edu page, 'Trota and the "Trotula"': https://independent.academia.edu/MonicaGreen1/Trota-and-the-%27Trotula%27#add.

25 Hilda Graef, *Mary: A History of Doctrine and Devotion* (New York, 1963; repr. Notre Dame, IN, 2009). A discussion of St Bonaventure's and Thomas of Aquinas's Marian doctrines can be found on pp. 219–27. See also Hilda Graef, 'Devotion to Our Lady', *Twentieth-Century Encyclopedia of Catholicism*, vol. 45 (New York, 1963), p. 44.

26 *The Life of Christina of Markyate: A Twelfth-Century Recluse*, ed. and trans. C. H. Talbot (Toronto, 1998), pp. 124–5.

It is in this context of multifarious Marian devotion that Chaucer's heterodox Mariology can be situated. In her analysis of the *ABC*, Reames normalises Chaucer's 'extravagant' attempts to endow Mary with redemptive authority by restoring his orthodox credentials: 'he resists the most serious excesses of Marian piety ... the temptation to set Mary against God, to glorify her at His expense'.[27] I would, instead, contend that, rather than dramatising mere 'extravagant' exceptions, Chaucer's literary Mariology engages with the heterogeneous debate on Mary's authority and presents the reader with a vision of the Virgin that is strikingly consistent with Christina's 'woman of great authority'. The *ABC* opens with an invocation to the Virgin that unequivocally endows her with a degree of authority normally only associated with God: 'Almighty and al merciable queene' (1).[28] Also, Chaucer's verse accommodates slippages in meaning that open up the text to counter-hegemonic descriptions of Mary's power and agency:

> Soth is that God ne granteth no pitee
> Withoute thee; for God of his goodnesse
> Foryiveth noon, but it like unto thee.
> He hath thee maked vicaire and maistresse
> Of al this world, and eek governouresse
> Of hevene, and he represseth his justise
> After thi wil; and therfore in witnesse
> He hath thee corowned in so rial wise. (137–44)

Grammatically and ideologically, the Virgin's agency is obliterated by identifying God/'he' as the subject of sentences describing Mary's function rather than Mary/'thee' who is, instead, the object of such clauses ('He hath thee maked'; 'He hath thee corowned'). At the same time, however, the text speaks her authority, since she dominates a secular and spiritual hierarchy of which she is both 'maistresse' and 'governouresse'. Most importantly, her will appears to inform God's justice, as the verb 'represseth' suggests a variant power relation in which the Creator chooses to position Himself as a subject to Mary's authority. In other words, the *ABC* dramatises a doctrinal stance on the Virgin that can be aligned to the emerging Marian piety in the tradition of Christina of Markyate's vision. In *The Prioress's Prologue* this strand of Mariology becomes apparent: 'For she hirself is honour and the roote / Of

27 Reames, 'Mary, Sanctity and Prayers to Saints', p. 92.

28 Although, as I have pointed out, Reames dismisses this innovation as 'an isolated and puzzling anomaly' ('Mary, Sanctity and Prayers to Saints', p. 91), she acknowledges that, at least in part, Helen Phillips re-considers the potential significance of these lines. Phillips argues that the first stanza of the *ABC* illustrates the hiatus between popular manifestations of Marian devotion and clerical orthodoxy: see 'Chaucer and Deguileville: The *ABC* in Context', *Medium Aevum* 62 (1993), 1–19. In this essay I hope to demonstrate that by the late medieval period, as evidenced in Chaucer's works, the concept of Mary as powerful agent began to establish itself beyond popular piety.

bountee, *next hir Sone*, and soules boote' (VII. 465–6 my emphasis). The 'soules boote' and Mother of Christ is here portrayed not in the assistive role of Mary the nurse, as Henry of Lancaster posits, but as Mary the Physician who partakes in God's salvific plan in an equal position of power.

Mary's authority, nonetheless, distinguishes her from the vengeful and aloof God represented in the *ABC*. The speaker addresses Mary because God appears unreachable for the mortal sinner trapped in a secular world; the Virgin, on the contrary, is the 'vicaire' or incarnated divinity. The extract from the *ABC* which I quoted above articulates Mary's dual potency through the use of anaphora, as she is at once '[o]f al this world' and '[o]f hevene'. The incarnational power of Mary is also apparent in *Pearl*, a key example of literary Marian figuration in the Middle Ages. In her analysis of the poem, Teresa Reed identifies the Virgin as a devotional *locus* in which the spiritual and the carnal can be negotiated as one: '[i]n the same way that Mary articulated the Word – that is, gave it intelligibility by giving it the jointed form of the human body – this poem attempts to make the transcendent intelligible through the physicality of form and sound'.[29] In *The Prioress's Prologue* such physicality is endowed with an unmistakably carnal connotation:

> O mooder Mayde, O mayde Mooder free!
> Of bussh unbrent, brennynge in Moyses sighte,
> That ravyshedest doun fro the Deitee,
> Thurgh thyn humblesse, the Goost that in th'alighte. (VII. 467–70)

Chaucer's text liberates Mary from the Irigarayan 'envelope', a docile text perpetually written and re-written, and stripped of agency. Here she transcends her configuration as mere *semblance* to become a chiasmus, that is, a space open to multiple, often paradoxical subject positions; she is at once mother/maiden and maiden/mother, the burning bush of hope and the un-burnt (untouched) virgin, and humble yet capable of ravishing the Ghost. In sum, in *The Prioress's Prologue* Mary is the meek virgin inducing spiritual ecstasy, but also the woman of great authority exerting sensual power.

LOCATING AUTHORITY: CHAUCER'S PHYSICIAN ON MARY AS PRINCIPLE OF TRUTH

It is, however, Chaucer's Physician who presents the most elaborate allegory of Mary's potency. It is particularly fitting that a Tale preoccupied with authority, whether medical, textual, parental or spiritual, should attend to such a current concern with Marian piety and, more specifically, with the

[29] Teresa Reed, *Shadows of Mary: Reading the Virgin Mary in Medieval Texts* (Cardiff, 2003), p. 123.

Virgin's agency in God's salvific plan. One of Chaucer's numerous original narrative accretions to the tragic story of Virginia is the Physician's digression on Nature as principle of authority.[30] Specifically, I would argue that one of the strategies of articulation of Mary's potency in operation in Chaucer's Tale is the alignment of the Virgin with the classical goddess Natura. As Miri Rubin reminds us in her account of Mariology in the period 1200–1400, natural imagery is central to the representation of the Virgin primarily because of the association between perfection and natural beauty established in *The Song of Songs* and the commentaries it generated.[31] Nonetheless, evidence of a direct identification of Mary with Nature is hard to come by. To the best of my knowledge, neither Rubin nor George D. Economou, in his extensive study of the goddess Natura in medieval literature, provides examples of such direct alignment. Notwithstanding such paucity of overt examples, the characterisation of Natura, from its Greek origins to its Latin incarnations and subsequent Christian re-appropriations, resonates in profound ways with medieval literary and devotional representations of the Mother of Christ. In Economou's words, thanks to the work of twelfth-century Chartrian philosophers such as Alan de Lille, Natura was Christianised and fixed as 'an aggregate of ideas':

> It could stand for the Platonic intermediary between the intelligible and material worlds; or for the divinely ordained power that presides over the continuity and preservation of whatever lives in the sublunary world; or for a creative principle directly subordinated to the mind and will of God.[32]

In her oblique identification with a Christianised (assistive and maternal) Nature, Mary remains an allegory, that is a rhetorical construct or envelope to be over-written with meaning. Following the Platonic and Neoplatonic tradition, much like Mary, Nature is 'vicaire' or an intermediary at the service of the superior power of God, the ultimate patriarch. By silently and obliquely aligning Natura with Mary, I contend that Chaucer's narrative recuperates the agential potency of which the classical goddess was progressively divested in her Christian re-imaginings. According to Economou,

> Statius' Natura is an important phase in the tradition from which developed the medieval goddess. A deity … in whose name the righteous may act, she represents the order of the entire universe, a fact that sharply distinguishes

30 A detailed and useful breakdown of Chaucer's narrative accretions can be found in Ussery, *Chaucer's Physician*, p. 129. Ussery acknowledges Chaucer's debt to the *Roman de la Rose* in the Physician's comments on Nature, but specifies that they are a synthesis and adaptation of the French material. The description of Virginia is, however, 'generally agreed to be original with Chaucer' (p. 129).

31 Miri Rubin, *Mother of God: A History of the Virgin Mary* (London: 2009), pp. 260–1.

32 George D. Economou, *The Goddess Natura in Medieval Literature* (Cambridge, MA, 1972), p. 3.

her from the Christian vicaria Dei whose cosmic powers are more limited and subordinated to God.[33]

An erudite scholar of philosophy, Chaucer's Physician articulates and reinstates the Virgin's creational authority through her formidable classical counterpart.

Specifically, in line with the incarnational Mariology found in the *ABC* and *The Prioress's Prologue*, Nature's power appears to be coextensive with literary figurations of the Virgin:

For He that is the formere principal
Hath maked me his vicaire general,
To forme and peynten erthely creaturis
Right as me list, and ech thyng in my cure is
Under the moone, that may wene and waxe. (VI. 19–23)

In the Physician's Tale, as 'vicaire general' and agent of care and cure, whose practices are informed by lunar movements, Nature's characterisation chimes resonantly with the theological and medical authority which Mary typically exerts in Chaucer's Marian texts. By equating Mary with Nature, the Physician cements her positioning as incarnated divinity, that is, not as unreachable spiritual principle, but as 'natural' and material presence for the devout. Nonetheless, as I hope to demonstrate in the final section of this essay, through the association with Nature, the authority of God's 'vicaire' and Mary the Physician is augmented, as creational potency is added to her salvific agency:

For Nature hath with sovereyn diligence
Yformed hire in so greet excellence (VI. 9–10)

Despite having a most excellent father ('[f]ulfild of honour and worthynesse'; VI. 3) and a mother, mentioned briefly in her reproductive role, Virginia is ultimately the fruit of Nature's creative agency. To a rhetoric of power ('sovereyn'), the Physician adds the attributes of distinction and prowess. In other words, in *The Physician's Tale*, although Nature/Mary acknowledges being made by God, she positions herself as an equal in relation to the male divinity: 'My lord and I been ful of oon accord' (VI. 25).

Moreover, her authority is overtly gendered and specifically feminine. As Laurel Braswell argues, although 'the position and orientation of the moon [is] a basis for medical practice, principally with reference to Galenic humoral theory', in medieval medical culture the moon is seen as a signifier of femininity.[34] Also, Nature defines her authority as antagonistic to male agents of artistic creation. In particular, she embarks upon an invective against a

33 Economou, *The Goddess Natura*, p. 46.

34 Laurel Braswell, 'The Moon and Medicine in Chaucer's Time', *Studies in the Age of Chaucer* 8 (1986), 145–56 (p. 145). For a discussion of the interconnection between

number of classical sculptors whose aesthetic endeavours she deems vastly inferior to hers:

> Lo! I, Nature,
> Thus kan I forme and peynte a creature,
> What that me list; who kan me countrefete?
> Pigmalion noght, though he ay forge and bete,
> Or grave, or peynte; for I dar wel seyn
> Apelles, Zanzis, sholde werche in veyn
> Outher to grave, or peynte, or forge, or bete. (VI. 11-17)

The numerous manuscript glosses appended to this passage have the dual function of signposting the erudite references to classical artists and, almost certainly unwittingly, of bringing into focus the gender politics informing their works. The Latin annotation accompanying Pygmalion's name points the reader in the direction of Ovid's *Metamorphoses* and the one elucidating the reference to Apelles and Zeuxis quotes Cicero's *De Inventione*.[35] It is barely necessary to remind ourselves of Ovid's rendition of Pygmalion's love of Galatea, a sculpture he forges and then turns into a woman. Perhaps a little less known to the non-classicist reader is Cicero's account of Zeuxis's creative techniques deployed specifically when sculpting a female subject:

> While, therefore, he was admiring the figures of the boys and their personal perfection very greatly; "The sisters," say they, "of these boys are virgins in our city, so that how great their beauty is you may infer from these boys." "Give me, then," said he, "I beg you, the most beautiful of these virgins, while I paint the picture which I promised you, so that the reality may be transferred from the breathing model to the mute likeness."[36]

Whether merely visible vicariously through male beauty or inanimate objects of the male gaze, in the works of the artists vilified by Nature women are again positioned as Irigarayan 'envelopes' and pure *semblance*. Similarly, in Chaucer's text, the conspicuous repetition of verbs belonging to the semantic field of artistic pursuit ('to grave, or peynte, or forge, or bete') draws attention to their artificiality as forgeries in the inferior hands of male artists and their derivative creations. Nature's superior creative authority is instead predicated upon the establishment of a matrilineal descent which usurps male artists of

astrology and medicine, and the alignment of femininity with the moon, see Rawcliffe, *Medicine and Society*, p. 83.

35 The Latin glosses appended to this passage read: 'Quere in Methamorphosios' or 'Pigmalion Appollus and Zephirus' (in Oxford, Bodleian Library, MS Arch. Selden B.14); and 'Apelles fecit mirabiule opus in tumulo darij vide in alexandro libro I° de Zanz in libro Tulij'. These glosses can be found in the same manuscripts listed in note 13.

36 *Cicero: De Inventione*, trans. C. D. Yonge, 2.1–3. http://classicpersuasion.org/pw/cicero/dnv2-1.htm [accessed 19 December 2013].

their mastery over female subjects. In the Physician's Tale, femininity, Virginia in particular, is figured not through the objectifying male gaze, but through Nature's divinely sanctioned creative agency. In fact, the Physician specifies that Virginia is a creature whose moral excellence and extraordinary beauty derive from Nature. Virginius 'hadde' her, as he has parental control over his daughter, but Nature 'peynted' her; in other words, as her name suggests, Virginia is aligned to the Virgin Mary and to Nature, her allegory, whose maternal/creational authority co-opts patriarchy.

In this matrilineal line of descent Virginia partakes in Nature's superior authority and in the Virgin's incarnated piety. J. D. W. Crowther puts forward a convincing argument in which he delineates the similarities between Virginia's narrative and the lives of women martyr saints. In his article he remarks on her lack of agency, since death is imposed upon her by her father's authority rather than being a deliberate choice to preserve the saint's purity.[37] Although his case is compelling, in the space of Chaucer's Physician's Tale Virginia is afforded an authoritative voice which, albeit limited, is presented as a principle of truth. Unlike the male aesthetic artificiality denounced by Nature, according to the Physician, Virginia's speech is pure and unembellished, and its overt femininity is ostensibly juxtaposed to the forgery of male-generated art:

> Hir facound eek ful wommanly and pleyn,
> No countrefeted termes hadde she
> To seme wys. (VI. 50–2)

Although the Physician's words appear to confine Virginia within the trope of the acquiescent female subject, Chaucer's language indicates a much greater level of agency. Her parlance is no ordinary speech, but it is 'facound' and therefore marked by eloquence and rhetorical elegance. Such sophistication is firmly opposed to the 'countrefeted' endeavours of male artists and it is clearly gendered as 'wommanly'. As female agent of *logos*, her words are 'pleyn'; of course, this adjective can point to a common and artless speech, but, as the *MED* indicates, it can also signify an unambiguous, truthful and unaffected use of language.[38] Much like the Virgin Mary is incarnated truth,

[37] J. D. W. Crowther, 'Chaucer's *Physician's Tale* and its "Saint"', *English Studies in Canada* 8, 2 (1982), 125–37 (pp. 126–30).

[38] *Middle English Dictionary*, http://quod.lib.umich.edu/cgi/m/mec/med-idx?type=id&id=MED33561 [accessed 12 January 2014]. The MED provides, among others, the following glosses for the adjective 'plain': '4a. (a) Clear, explicit; unambiguous, unmistakable; also, evident, overt; (b) of a planet's orbit: fixed; (c) of a gem: clear, transparent, or translucent; (d) free from deception or distortion; actual, real, true; ~ account; ~ cas (mening, soth, treuth); (e) of persons, the heart, the will: candid, honest, sincere, truthful; reliable, dependable; open, frank, forthright; of the countenance: having a sincere expression or an honest appearance; hole and ~; ~ conscience, a clear conscience; ~ withouten gile (ipocrisie); (f) simple, pure, absolute; paradise ful ~, ?utter paradise; (g) as noun: at ~,

hermeneutic and spiritual intermediary between the transcendental and the carnal, Virginia and Nature represent the potency of the material presence of the feminine: candid voice, pure body and divine authority.

In John A. Pitcher's words, *The Physician's Tale* is 'a tour de force of rhetorical indirection and fractured speech' and it 'crucially politicises the function of discourse in the reproduction of medieval gender hierarchies'.[39] Discourse, rhetoric, literariness, authority and gender politics are indeed the central concerns that the Physician articulates in his Tale. In *The General Prologue* he is portrayed as a man of exceptional erudition:

> In al this world ne was ther noon hym lik,
> To speke of phisik and of surgerye,
> For he was grounded in astronomye.
> ...
> Wel knew he the olde Esculapius,
> And Deyscorides, and eek Rufus,
> Olde Ypocras, Haly, and Galyen,
> Serapion, Razis, and Avycen,
> Averrois, Damascien, and Constantyn,
> Bernard, and Gatesden, and Gilbertyn. (I. 412–14; 429–34)

The cumulative effect of enumeration ensures that the Physician is immediately recognised as an outstanding medical practitioner. According to Russell Hope Robbins, the list of *auctores* known to the Physician encompasses, but also exceeds, the number of authorities found in his survey of medieval medical manuscripts, as Aesculapius, Dioscorides, Hali and Rufus are included in books available to doctors less frequently than others.[40] Chaucer's Physician is, therefore, a man of rare erudition and his comprehensive training aligns him more closely to the prestigious Faculties of Medicine established on the Continent than to the more haphazard provision offered by Oxford and Cambridge. While Continental medical authorities advocated the study of surgery, physic and astronomy, in England medical training was mainly speculative and discursive, as medical doctorates were designed for the formation of clerics and theologians.[41] However, despite suggesting that his practical training matched his theoretical knowledge, the language of *The General Prologue* signifies the dominance of discursivity and speculation in

in (short and) ~, plainly; the ~, the plain case; the short and ~, the long and the short of it, briefly, concisely.'

39 John A. Pitcher, *Chaucer's Feminine Subjects: Figures of Desire in The Canterbury Tales* (New York, 2012), p. 7.

40 Russell Hope Robbins, 'The Physician's Authorities', in *Studies in Language and Literature in Honour of Margaret Schlauch*, ed. Mieczyslaw Brahmer, S. Helsztynski and J. Krzyzanowski (New York, 1971), pp. 335–41 (pp. 340–1).

41 For a detailed study of medieval medical training both on the Continent and in Britain, see Rawcliffe, *Medicine and Society*, especially pp. 83–118.

the Physician's medical practice, as his prowess lies in his ability 'to speke' of his discipline rather than to practise it.[42]

It is, I would argue, the disembodied authority of 'phisik' that draws him to dramatise the corporal and incarnated potency of femininity in a Tale that explores the relation between patriarchal power and female agency. Despite being dismissed as a lesser Tale often on the basis of its unsuitability to its teller, *The Physician's Tale* offers a powerful illustration of the professional, intellectual and ethical anxieties of the medical profession in the Middle Ages.[43] Harold F. Brooks defines the Physician as a 'completely unlocalised figure' because of the international quality of his professional profile, but also, I would add, because of his fluid subject position.[44] In the first instance, Chaucer's Physician is presented as disengaged with theological and spiritual matters. In *The General Prologue* it becomes apparent that '[h]is studie was but litel on the Bible' (I. 438). Unlike most doctors of medicine at the time of Chaucer, who undertook medical training to have access to a prestigious clerical career, the Physician's interests are secular and intellectual. Linguistically, the 'verray, parfit praktisour' (I. 422) of physic is aligned to the 'verray, parfit gentil knyght' (I. 72); yet, all this alignment does is to reinforce the juxtaposition between the ascetic knight and the secular doctor. Similarly, the richness of his clothing is a manifestation of professional success and his preoccupation with emerging proto-capitalist values such as monetary gain and social promotion:

> In sangwyn and in pers he clad was al,
> Lyned with taffata and with sendal.
> And yet he was but esy of dispence;
> He kepte that he wan in pestilence.
> For gold in phisik is a cordial,
> Therefore he lovede gold in special. (I. 439-44)

As Carole Rawcliffe explains, wearing expensive clothing was an important self-promoting strategy for the medieval physician; however, the elaborate robes sported by Chaucer's Doctour also manifest his cultural otherness.[45] In Laura Hodges's words, the sophistication of exotic materials 'symbolically

42 The centrality of discourse to *The Physician's Tale* is investigated in Daniel Kempton, '*The Physician's Tale*: The Doctor of Physic's Diplomatic "Cure"', *Chaucer Review* 19, 1 (1984), 24–38.

43 The narrative structure of the Tale, which is often perceived as disjointed and haphazard because of its emphasis on digressions, for instance, is discussed in Anne Middleton, '*The Physician's Tale* and Love's Martyrs: "Ensamples Mo Than Ten" as a Method to the *Canterbury Tales*', *Chaucer Review* 8 (1973), 9–31. An early example of such critique is John M. Manly, 'Chaucer and the Rhetoricians', *Proceedings of the British Academy* 12 (1926), 95–113.

44 Harold F. Brooks, *Chaucer's Pilgrims: The Artistic Order of the Portraits in the Prologue* (London, 1962), p. 31.

45 Rawcliffe, *Medicine and Society*, p. 108.

evoke a recognition of both the physical and economic reality of medical practice as well as the eastern origin of and influence on medieval medicine'.[46] The associations of 'pers' with Persia and eastern culture emphasise the alterity and fluidity of his subject position while cementing the construction of Chaucer's Physician as a figure of extraordinary intellect.

In his liminal position between clerical vocation and secular profession, western and eastern medical cultures, care of the body and intellectual prowess, the Physician seeks an unmovable principle of authority, or a *regimen* that provides a grammar of balance and unity between conflicting cultural imperatives. In one of his narrative accretions, he digresses and addresses governesses and parents in charge of the care and cure of innocent children:

> And ye maistresses, in youre olde lyf,
> That lordes doghtres han in governaunce,
> … therfore, for Cristes sake,
> To teche hem vertu looke that ye ne slake.
> … Ye fadres and ye moodres eek also,
> Though ye han children, be it oon or mo,
> Youre is the charge of al hir surveiaunce,
> Whil that they been under youre governaunce.
> Beth war, if by ensample of youre lyvynge,
> Or by youre necligence in chastisynge,
> That they ne perisse. (VI. 72–3, 81–2, 93–9)

As I argued in the first part of this essay, the rhetoric of 'bio-power' ('surveiaunce'; 'governaunce'; 'chastisynge') which dominates this passage resonates with the prophylactic *regimen* of Henry of Lancaster's *Livre* and much Marian material found in Chaucer's texts. The expurgation of excesses and the surveillance of guardians are meant to provide a hermeneutic of moral and physical order, that is, an authoritative 'diet' through which the preservation of innocence can be achieved. In *The General Prologue* the Physician is defined as a temperate man who prescribes and abides by strict strategies of governance of the body through a 'diete mesurable' (I. 435). Nonetheless, the hermeneutic authority of his *regimen* proves fallible, as Virginia succumbs to the deviant impulses of Apius. Parental authority, to which she meekly surrenders her agency ('Dooth with youre child youre wyl'; VI. 250), paradoxically obliterates her innocence instead of protecting it.

In the process of dramatising a stable principle of spiritual authority, the Physician's Tale, instead, fragments itself into a narrative that unveils its own constructedness instead of its hermeneutic consistency. Far from being the 'pleyn' discourse attributed to Virginia, the Doctour's text is overtly artificial. The most notable and subversive example of his deconstruction of authority

46 Laura Hodges, *Chaucer and Clothing: Clerical and Academic Costume in the General Prologue to The Canterbury Tales* (Cambridge, 2005), p. 201; see also pp. 215–16.

is the narrative framing within which Nature's speech is situated. In spite of her superior salvific and creative potency, and her being harbinger of truth, Nature's invective against the forgery of human artistic endeavour is structurally and conceptually enclosed with a paradigm of fictionality and discursivity: '[a]s though she wolde seyn' and '[t]hus semeth me that Nature wolde seye' (VI. 11, 29). Nature's pronouncement on her ultimate authority is articulated as a narrative imagined by the Physician.

As the Tale concludes with not one but three interpretative voices (the Physician's, the Host's and the Pardoner's), the Physician's exploration of authority and pursuit of order open up the text to multiple slippages that disperse a stable vision of truth, whether spiritual or intellectual. In line with Chaucer's engagement with heterodox forms of Mariology, Mary the Physician, invoked through the allegory of an omnipotent Nature, is, however, at least momentarily, the site where truth and authority can be found.

PART II

FEMALE MYSTICISM AND METAPHORS OF ILLNESS

3

HEAVENLY VISION AND PSYCHOSOMATIC HEALING: MEDICAL DISCOURSE IN MECHTILD OF HACKEBORN'S *THE BOOKE OF GOSTLYE GRACE*

Naoë Kukita Yoshikawa

The Booke of Gostlye Grace is the Middle English translation of *Liber specialis gratiae*, the revelations of Mechtild of Hackeborn, a German mystic and chantress of the Benedictine/Cistercian convent of Helfta at the end of the thirteenth century.[1] The *Liber* is thought to have been compiled by Gertrude the Great and Helfta nuns during the last decade of the thirteenth century, but it was soon shortened and abridged by an anonymous redactor.[2] The *Liber* was widely circulated in various versions throughout Europe, and then translated into a variety of vernaculars. *The Booke* is the only extant text from Helfta to have been translated into Middle English. The translation dates to the early fifteenth century: this was the same period that Bridget of Sweden's *Liber Celestis* and Catherine of Siena's *Dialogo* were being translated into English in a Carthusian or Birgittine milieu.

The Middle English translation is based on an abridged version of the Latin text which concentrates on visions connected with the Church's liturgy and those associated with Mechtild's personal piety. Nevertheless, it retains the

1 *The Booke of Gostlye Grace of Mechtild of Hackeborn* (hereafter *The Booke*), ed. Theresa A. Halligan (Toronto, 1979). All references to *The Booke of Gostlye Grace* will be from this edition, followed by part, chapter and page number. The Middle English translation survives in two fifteenth-century manuscripts, London, British Library, MS Egerton 2006 (upon which Halligan's edition is based) and Oxford, Bodleian Library, MS Bodley 220, which are similar except that the former contains rubrics preceding chapters. The earliest Latin manuscript of the *Liber specialis gratiae* (hereafter the *Liber*) containing all seven books is Wolfenbüttel (Guelferbytanus), Herzog August Bibliothek, codex 1003, copied in 1370 by Albert, vicar of St Paul in Erfurt. Although it has some editorial problems, the only Latin edition available today is *Revelationes Gertrudianae ac Mechtildianae* (hereafter *Revelationes*), ed. Dom Ludwig Paquelin, 2 vols (Paris, 1875–77), vol. 2, pp. 1–422.

2 See Margarete Hubrath, 'The *Liber specialis gratiae* as a Collective Work of Several Nuns', *Jahrbuch der Oswald von Wolkenstein Gesellschaft* 11 (1999), 233–44.

framework of the original version and the translator has followed the contents of the revelations 'als thay stande in the booke' (I, [translator's prologue], 65). Part I contains Mechtild's vision arranged around the seasons and holy days of the liturgical year; Part II lists the special graces bestowed on her; Part III gives guidance for 'the helthe of manys sawle'; Part IV offers instruction to religious men and women; and Part V concerns prayers for the deceased.[3]

Behind the Middle English translation of the *Liber* lies the politico-religious tension of the late fourteenth and early fifteenth centuries, reflected in Arundel's *Constitutiones* of 1409/1410. As Vincent Gillespie argues,

> [o]ne of the unintended consequences of Arundel's decrees may have been a new impetus to the translation into English of older texts with an impeccably orthodox pedigree or an unimpeachable authorial reputation, and Syon was probably a leading centre in the production of such texts.[4]

The Booke of Gostly Grace is therefore one of those books that may well be connected to Syon, known for its interest in contemplative experience and '[reflecting] the orthodox reform agenda of the English church and the house that became its metonymy'.[5] *The Booke* was disseminated as one of the approved texts of vernacular, mystical materials in fifteenth-century England and its reader included the female nobility, such as Cecily Neville, duchess of York.

Mechtild's spirituality and the context of Helfta and its social and religious milieu have been explored by Caroline Walker Bynum and Mary Jeremy Finnegan, while the popularity and circulation of Mechtild's revelations in fifteenth-century England have been examined by Rosalynn Voaden and C. Annette Grisé.[6] The Middle English text itself has generally escaped widespread scholarly attention, however, with the exception of Theresa Halligan's introduction to her edition of *The Booke* and a few other studies.[7]

3 *The Booke of Gostlye Grace*, ed. Halligan, 'Introduction', p. 38. Nevertheless, as Voaden argues, categorising the *Liber* (and *The Booke*) in this way might 'obscure the sheer aesthetic power of the revelations (p. 436)': Rosalynn Voaden, 'Mechtild of Hackeborn', in *Medieval Holy Women in the Christian Tradition, c. 1100–c. 1500*, ed. Alastair Minnis and Rosalynn Voaden (Turnhout, 2010), pp. 431–51.

4 Vincent Gillespie, '1412-1534: Culture and History', in *The Cambridge Companion to Medieval English Mysticism*, ed. Samuel Fanous and Vincent Gillespie (Cambridge, 2011), pp. 163–93 (p. 174).

5 Gillespie, 'Culture and History', p. 173.

6 Caroline Walker Bynum, *Jesus as Mother: Studies in the Spirituality of the High Middle Ages* (Berkeley, CA, 1982), pp. 209–27; Mary Jeremy Finnegan, *The Women of Helfta: Scholars and Mystics* (Athens, GA, 1991); Rosalynn Voaden, 'The Company She Keeps: Mechtild of Hackeborn in Late-Medieval Devotional Compilations', in *Prophets Abroad: The Reception of Continental Holy Women in Late-Medieval England*, ed. Rosalynn Voaden (Cambridge, 1996), pp. 51–69; C. Annette Grisé, 'Continental Holy Women and the Textual Relics of Prayers in Late-Medieval England', in *The Medieval Translator*, vol. 10, ed. Jacqueline Jenkins and Olivier Bertrand (Turnhout, 2007), pp. 165–78.

7 *The Booke of Gostlye Grace*, ed. Halligan, 'Introduction'; Barbara Kline, 'The Discourse

This essay will focus on Mechtild's highly somatic revelations and explore the convergence of medical and devotional discourses in terms of the theory and practice of the medieval *regimen sanitatis*. Mechtild's revelations display a convergence of the senses, where her entire body is restored to health through sensory experience. As we shall see, Mechtild's revelatory experience illuminates the way in which she appropriates her medical knowledge to convey her mystical encounter with the divine.

A recognised authority at a time of spiritual upheaval and renewal, Mechtild's revelations unfold orthodox and Christocentric theology: they are especially characterised by a focus on the material reality of the Sacred Heart, a cult that developed at Helfta and was disseminated throughout Europe. Mechtild's descriptions of mystical union frequently convey a strong sense of oneness with God, envisioned as taking place in Christ's heart. The trope of the physical and metaphorical hearts serves to generate devotional aspiration.[8] A sophisticated array of allegories representing the heart demonstrates Mechtild's conceptualisation of spiritual interiority and invites us to appreciate an intricate interplay between eucharistic symbolism, popular piety and the emergent discourse of medicine, a discourse that contributes to the progress of Mechtild's understanding of mystical union in terms of spiritual health.

I would argue that the uniqueness of Mechtild's revelations lies especially in the convergence of medical and devotional discourses which permeate the *Booke* and that religious, medical tropes were well received by the audiences of both Latin and vernacular texts in late medieval England, where concerns with the health of body and soul were increasing.[9] In her vision of Black Monday (Easter Monday), for example, Mechtild uses the widespread concept of *Christus medicus*, or Christ the physician. Her frequent use of medical imagery might be partly explained by her own experience of disease and pain.[10] Christ tells her that he will act as a physician to cure her sickness and promises inseparable union between them: 'Botte ʒif þowe be syeke, y am the wyseeste leeche whiche schalle heyle the fro alle syekenes ande betwyx the ande me schalle no dyuysioun be, botte ane euerlastynge couple ande an

of Heaven in Mechtild of Hackeborn's *Booke of Gostlye Grace*', in *Imagining Heaven in the Middle Ages: A Book of Essays*, ed. Jan Swango Emerson and Hugh Feiss (New York, 2000), pp. 83–99; Voaden, 'Mechtild of Hackeborn'. For an earlier interest in Mechtild's revelations, see Karma Lochrie, *Margery Kempe and Translations of Flesh* (Philadelphia, 1991), pp. 76–88.

8 A variety of themes and images in the *Booke* are of interest from a devotional perspective. Some figurative tropes, such as the kitchen imagery in part one, find affinity with those in approved devotional treatises: see, for example, *The Doctrine of the Hert: A Critical Edition with Introduction and Commentary*, ed. Christiania Whitehead, Denis Renevey and Anne Mouron (Exeter, 2010).

9 For the increasing interest in bodily and spiritual health, see my introduction to this volume.

10 See, for example, *The Booke*, II, 13, 344; II, 32, 387.

vnyoun inseperable' (I, 43, 197). In her vision, Mechtild sees Christ being taken up on the cross, clothed with 'a reede coote fulle of holys', and she hears Christ saying to her: 'Þus was my bodye in the passioun tyme oueralle peersede ande alle to-rente with sorowfulle paynes insoomoche þat þare was no place of helth in me fro the soole of my foote to the heyght of my heede' (II, 12, 343). Since the suffering body of the crucified Christ is frequently a site of self-identification for mystics, Mechtild must have identified the bodily afflictions of her own body with Christ's suffering during his Passion in which there was 'no place of helth'(II, 12, 344). She understands this revelation as a token that she would shortly suffer from a disease herself.

Mechtild is not unique in deploying medical imagery and discourse. The language of medicine is common currency in late medieval mystical writing. Just as Christ identifies himself as 'magnus medicus' in Hildegard of Bingen's *Scivias*, the analogy of Christ the Physician becomes a staple in discussing medicine for the soul, and related medical discourse frequently appears in late medieval devotional literature.[11] In England, the author of *Ancrene Wisse* conceives of sickness as a kind of divine gift and enumerates the gracious effects of sickness: it '(i)wescheð þe sunnen þe beoð ear iwrahte, (ii) wardeð to3ein þeo þe weren towardes, (iii) pruueð pacience, (iii[i]) halt in eadmodnesse, (v) muchleð þe mede, [(vi)] eueneð to martir þene þolemode' ['(i) washes away the sins that have already been committed, (ii) protects against those that were about to be, (iii) tests patience, (iv) maintains humility, (v) increases the reward, (vi) makes whoever bears it patiently equal to a martyr'].[12] Predicated upon the inseparability of body and soul, this kind of discourse was prevalent in late medieval religious texts.

Mechtild's use of medical metaphors suggests, however, that she had a basic grasp of the theory and practice of medieval medicine. When she envisions Christ seated on the throne with one foot resting on a sapphire, 'she remembers that as the sapphire has the virtue of driving out malign humours, so the soul is purified through the wounds of Christ':[13] 'Ryght als a saphyere be his vertewe voydes wykkede humours, ryght so my woundys puttys awaye the venyme of þe sawle ande purifieth itt fro alle fylth. Ande als a garnette gladdys a mans herte, ryght so my wondeys makes a soule ioye in me eftere þat he es amendede of hys synne.' (II, 1, 325).[14] It must be emphasised that Mechtild

11 Hildegard of Bingen, *Scivias*, I, 3: see *Scivias*, trans. Columba Hart and Jane Bishop (New York, 1990), p. 104. For Henry of Lancaster's use of 'Christ the Physician', see Naoë Kukita Yoshikawa, 'Holy Medicine and Disease of the Soul: Henry of Lancaster and *Le Livre de Seyntz Medicines*', *Medical History* 53, 3 (2009), 397–414 (p. 399).

12 *Ancrene Wisse: A Corrected Edition of the Text in Cambridge, Corpus Christi College, MS 402 with variatnts from other manuscripts*, ed. Bella Millett, 2 vols, EETS o.s. 325, 326 (Oxford, 2005–06), vol. 1, Part 4. 7, p. 69; *Ancrene Wisse: Guide for Anchoresses*, trans. Bella Millett (Exeter, 2009), p. 69.

13 Finnegan, *Women of Helfta*, pp. 49–50.

14 Christ reveals that all precious stones heal bodily sickness just as his wounds are

not only demonstrates her knowledge of lapidary and humoral theory but as she compares Christ's wounds with the medicinal quality of gems, she also emphasises the therapeutic power of Christ's body, thereby incorporating medical ideas into mystical discourse.

Indeed, the late medieval devotion to Christ's humanity shown by his sufferings during the Passion stimulated the related devotion to his blood, heart and wounds, all of which symbolised the Eucharist.[15] Moreover, devotion to the eucharistic body of Christ was increasingly emphasised in the wake of the Fourth Lateran Council. The driving purpose of the Council was to stress the centrality of the mass, and the sacrament was considered to be the protection against and remedy for both spiritual and bodily ills. The mass became 'in every sense a *medicina sacramentalis*, suffused with occult power',[16] and exposure to the Host, even without reception, was perceived to have a beneficial effect on bodily infirmities.[17] As Christ confides in Mechtild, his blood was deemed to be the 'medycine of sawles heyle' (I, 35, 178) while his fresh red wounds are 'verrey medycine of heyle to mannys sawle' (I, 38, 183).

Alongside eucharistic medicine, throughout the Middle Ages medical theory was founded upon the ancient idea of the proper management of the 'six non-naturals'.[18] Based on Hippocratic and Galenic theory, medieval medicine recommended that the best weapon against disease was a healthy system of physical and spiritual care, the ethos of which was based upon Christian morality. Indeed, classical medicine and the teaching of the Church were smoothly integrated through the translation of the classical theory of humours into the context of Christian history. Since St Augustine (c. 340–430), the Church had maintained that in Paradise Adam and Eve possessed a perfect mixture of humours. With the advent of sin, however, the balance was destroyed and diseases entered into the world.[19] This, in turn, meant that the chief cause of sickness was Original Sin – a result of Eve's

profitable for man's soul: see the *Booke*, III, 21, 529. For the medicinal use of sapphire in late medieval England, see *English Mediaeval Lapidaries*, ed. Joan Evans and Mary S. Serjeantson, EETS o.s. 190 (London, 1933), pp. 100–3.

15 For a study of the Eucharist in medieval culture, see Caroline Walker Bynum, *Wonderful Blood: Theology and Practice in Late Medieval Northern Germany and Beyond* (Philadelphia, 2007).

16 Carole Rawcliffe, *Leprosy in Medieval England* (Woodbridge, 2006), p. 339.

17 John Mirk, for example, claimed that anyone who saw the Host at the moment of elevation would be safe for the rest of the day from death and blindness: John Mirk, *Instructions for Parish Priests*, ed. E. Peacock, EETS o.s. 31 (London, 1868), p. 10; Peregrine Horden, 'A Non-Natural Environment: Medicine without Doctors and the Medieval European Hospital', in *The Medieval Hospital and Medical Practice*, ed. Barbara S. Bowers (Aldershot, 2007), pp. 133–45 (p. 141).

18 See the Introduction to this volume, p. 13.

19 Joseph Ziegler, 'Medicine and Immortality in Terrestrial Paradise', in *Religion and Medicine*, ed. Joseph Ziegler and Peter Biller (York, 2001), pp. 201–42 (p. 209).

disobedience in tempting Adam with the apple of forbidden knowledge. The coming of Christ allowed humankind to recapture the harmony of body and soul by reversing the malignant effects of the Fall.[20] Grounded in the *regimen sanitatis*, the Galenic system maintained that the body's humoral balance could be affected by the 'non-naturals' – variable aspects of the environment and of human behaviour, which, based on Galenic rules of hygiene, were loosely grouped under the categories of ambient air, exercise and rest, sleeping and waking, food and drink, evacuation and repletion, and the passions of the soul, or accidents of the soul.[21] One could also understand these non-naturals according to a spiritual model, by means of which the body's humoral balance was vulnerable to the deadly sins, acting both externally and internally. Therefore, one ought to endeavour to avoid sin and keep a good humoral balance through the proper management of the six non-naturals, thus preserving the health of both body and soul.

The interconnection between physical and spiritual health was reinforced around the time of the Gregorian Reform and the Fourth Lateran Council (1215). Canon 21 (Omnis utriusque sexus) demanded annual confession and communion, enabling the Christian penitent to achieve reconciliation with God and restore humoral imbalances by eliminating anxiety and the fear of damnation.[22] Thus, an underlying concern of pastoral instruction was the teaching of appropriate behaviour and attitudes to enable Christians to maintain a clean, good soul.[23]

The theory and practice of the *regimen sanitatis* spread across Christendom largely through the *Isagoge* [Introduction to medicine], a succinct explanation of key determinants of health, written by Hunayn in Arabic and translated into Latin by Constantinus Africanus at Monte Cassino between c. 1075 and 1085.[24] Among the six non-naturals, Hunayn stresses the need for emotional balance to preserve bodily and spiritual health. Commenting on the affections

20 See Augustine, *The City of God Against the Pagans*, trans. R. W. Dyson (Cambridge, 1998), bk. 10, ch. 27, p. 432.

21 See further Pedro Gil Sotres, 'The Regimens of Health', in *Western Medical Thought from Antiquity to the Middle Ages*, ed. Mirko D. Grmek (Cambridge, MA, 1998), pp. 291–318.

22 Lay confession long preceded the Council, but a new emphasis was placed on the sacraments of confession and the Eucharist after 1215: see Sarah Hamilton, *The Practice of Penance, 900–1050* (Woodbridge, 2001), pp. 5, 7, 10.

23 See *Fasciculus morum: A Fourteenth-Century Preacher's Handbook*, ed. and trans. Siegfried Wenzel (University Park, PA, 1989), pp. 254–7, 594–7.

24 *Isagoge* laid a foundation of how to diagnose a patient and organise therapy, but emphasis on the six non-naturals as key determinants of health and illness had a particular influence on western medical thinking. *Isagoge* was later included in a popular compendium of medical texts, the *Articella* or *Little Art of Medicine*. See Vivian Nutton, 'Medicine in Medieval Western Europe, 1000–1500', in *The Western Medical Tradition, 800 BC to AD 1800*, ed. Lawrence I. Conrad, Michael Neve, Vivian Nutton, Roy Porter and Andrew Wear (Cambridge, 1995), pp. 139–205 (pp. 141–2).

of the mind, he writes that such affections as those 'which bring the natural heat from the interior of the body to the outer parts or the surface of the skin'[25] produce a corresponding effect within the body. This happens suddenly, as with anger, or gently and slowly, as with delight and joy, while some affections, such as grief, 'disturb the natural energy both internal and external'.[26] Unless properly managed, such emotions as anger, fear, joy and sorrow could cause damage to the soul. Thus, as Peregrine Horden argues, 'emotions fall within the sphere of medicine' and '[t]he salutary importance of moderating emotions such as joy and sadness was made familiar to the whole medieval audience of medical learning through its inclusion in many medical treatises, theoretical and practical, even surgical ones'.[27] Advice literature (or advice manuals), such as *Secreta secretorum* and *Regimen sanitatis Salerni*, also emphasised the moderation of the accidents of the soul.

The theory and practice of the medieval *regimen sanitatis* is the key to understanding Mechtild's highly sensory, somatic revelations. Alongside her emphasis on eucharistic medicine, Mechtild's revelations are replete with such delights as heavenly music, smells or images – all of which become the means by which her entire body is restored to health. Mystical texts often display a convergence of the senses: mystics convey their experience as accompanied by sweet smells[28] and pleasant sounds, and, famously, Richard Rolle describes divine love as a burning fire and God's voice as secret sweet music.[29] But Mechtild further links the visionary language of sensation with healing by using sensory metaphors to narrate the experience. Postulated upon the belief that the accidents of the soul were crucial factors influencing the state of both body and mind, Mechtild complements her revelations with medical theory about the passions of the soul, and particularly stresses that music is a powerful therapeutic tool to moderate these passions. As a chantress of her community, who directed the music of the mass and led the singing, Mechtild must have benefited from the daily celebration of the mass and the prayers of the canonical Hours, in which the liturgical music and smell of incense

25 *A Source Book in Medieval Science*, ed. Edward Grant (Cambridge, MA, 1974), p. 708.

26 *A Source Book in Medieval Science*, p. 709.

27 Horden, 'A Non-Natural Environment', p. 135.

28 Catherine of Siena, in the *Dialogue*, speaks of tasting the fragrance of the sacrament: cited in Caroline Walker Bynum, *Holy Feast and Holy Fast: The Religious Significance of Food to Medieval Women* (Berkeley, CA, 1987), p. 174. Conversely, Julian of Norwich describes her temptation by the devil as a feverish state in which Julian, in her sickbed, smells his stench. See *A Vision Showed to a Devout Woman* (known as her short text), in *The Writings of Julian of Norwich: A Vision Showed to a Devout Woman and A Revelation of Love*, Medieval Women: Texts and Contexts 5, ed. Nicholas Watson and Jacqueline Jenkins (Turnhout, 2006), section 23, lines 18–22.

29 *The Incendium Amoris of Richard Rolle of Hampole*, ed. Margaret Deanesly (Manchester, 1915), cap. 15, pp. 187–91.

would have energised the spirits[30] and moderated the accidents of the soul. The healing power of liturgical music is also recounted in the Sister Books, produced by Dominican nuns in Germany between about 1310 and 1350.[31] These books record the spiritual life of women's cloistered communities and bear witness to the way the sisters were deeply consoled by the grace of heavenly music in their illnesses.[32]

As a chantress, Mechtild's earthly experience further stimulated her longing for mystical union with God.[33] As Barbara Kline argues, 'Mechtild's exposure of her face to God is followed by all the company of saints and angels singing, in one voice, a melody that cannot be described by human tongue.'[34] She envisions herself and Christ as ascending to the top of the hill, where she is welcomed by a host of angels with bells of gold 'whiche gaffe a fulle merye swete sowne' (I, 26, 145). Yet, as noted above, it is not only her role as chantress but also her experience of illness that permeates her visions. Her mystical experience is integrated into a discourse of psychosomatic religious healing, in which union with God is conceived of in terms of the health of her soul, where emotion, or accidents of the soul, is crucial. In what follows, I will contextualise Mechtild's revelations within the *regimen sanitatis* and show how she embraces psychosomatic healing in her pursuit of mystical union with God.

Among a variety of means to preserve mental equilibrium, the therapeutic power of music is prominent in Mechtild's revelations. Peter Murray Jones argues that music was thought to be particularly beneficial in treating 'fevers, lovesickness, and mental disorders: among these, melancholy and mania, frenzy and lethargy'.[35] Indeed, the concept of music as medicine, so popular in the late Middle Ages, was rooted in classical theories of medicine. Boethius, who was just as much a musicologist as a philosopher, understood that music is firmly rooted in mathematics and that the body and soul are integrated into musical harmony: in *De institutione musica* [On the institution of music], he

30 It was believed that there were three different spirits in the body: natural, vital, and animal. They were affected by outside influences, and in turn affected every aspect of human behaviour. See further below.

31 Gertrud Jaron Lewis, 'Music and Dancing in the Fourteenth-Century Sister-Books', in *Vox Mystica: Essays for Valerie M. Lagorio*, ed. Anne Clark Bartlett et al. (Cambridge, 1995), pp. 159–69 (p. 163).

32 Jeanne Ancelet-Hustache (ed.), 'Les "vitae sororum" d'Unterlinden: Édition critique du manuscrit 508 de la Bibliothèque de Colmar', *Archives d'histoire doctrinale et littéraire du moyen âge* 5 (1930), 317–517 (pp. 382–3, 458).

33 See especially *The Booke*, I, ch. 26. For the influence that her role as chantress had upon her literary expression, see Kline, 'The Discourse of Heaven', p. 83.

34 Kline, 'The Discourse of Heaven', p. 89.

35 Peter Murray Jones, 'Music Therapy in the Later Middle Ages: The Case of Hugo van der Goes', in *Music as Medicine: The History of Music Therapy since Antiquity*, ed. Peregrine Horden (Aldershot, 2000), pp. 120–44 (p. 135).

states that the Pythagoreans knew that 'the whole structure of [one's] soul and body has been joined by means of musical coalescence. For just as one's physical state affects feeling, so also the pulses of the heart are increased by disturbed states of mind.'[36] Boethius also made a three-fold distinction between *musica mundana* (cosmic music), produced by the motion of celestial bodies, *musica humana* (human music), which unites the rational and irrational parts of the soul and incorporates both to the body and *musica instrumentalis* (instrumental music), which is made by various instruments.[37] The classical tradition held that the emotional power of music could exercise moral and spiritual power over human beings and that music could heal, soothe and even invigorate the body and soul. On the other hand, the power of music could be used for ill: such music could please the devil. In her letter to the prelates at Mainz upon the interdict of the Office, Hildegard tells how Satan was driven to despair by the voice of Adam singing in Paradise and never ceased thereafter to attempt to destroy the sweet beauty of divine praise and spiritual hymns:

> But when the devil, man's great deceiver, learned that man had begun to sing through God's inspiration and, therefore, was being transformed to bring back the sweetness of the songs of heaven, mankind's homeland, he was so terrified at seeing his clever machinations go to ruin that he was greatly tormented. Therefore, he devotes himself continually to thinking up and working out all kinds of wicked contrivances. Thus he never ceases from confounding confession and the sweet beauty of both divine praise and spiritual hymns, eradicating them through wicked suggestions, impure thoughts, or various distractions from the heart of man and even from the mouth of the Church itself, wherever he can, through dissension, scandal, or unjust oppression.[38]

Hildegard reveals the idea of music as a means of recapturing the original joy and beauty of paradise, as well as of music as a way of understanding history.

Moreover, as Barbara Newman points out, Christian theorists added the notion of *musica celestis* to the classical concept of *musica mundana* and *musica humana* and *musica instrumentalis*. *Musica celestis* [celestial music], or the singing of the angels in heaven was a monastic commonplace. Bound up with the moral and spiritual life, music was 'both duty and joy, the continual and sometimes arduous discipline of a monastic community', and it was 'the

36 *Fundamentals of Music: Anicius Manlius Severinus Boethius*, trans. (with introduction and notes) Calvin M. Bower and ed. Claude V. Palisca (New Haven, CT and London, 1989), bk. 1, 1, p. 7.

37 *Fundamentals of Music*, bk. 1, 2, pp. 9–10.

38 Letter 23, in *The Letters of Hildegard of Bingen*, vol. 1, trans. Joseph L. Baird and Radd K. Ehrman (New York and Oxford, 1994), p. 78.

sign of its angelic and supra-mundane life'.[39] More to the point, in compensating for the voice that Adam lost, music and worship could heal the diseased soul and restore celestial harmony.

De institutione musica was a standard text in the undergraduate syllabus.[40] Physicians who studied this work as part of their university training would have understood that 'music and melody gave an insight into human physiology and the close connection between the humours, harmony and health'.[41] The idea of music as medicine seems to have been disseminated through the authority of Boethius: a fifteenth-century vernacular text argues that '[mannes bodily spirites] may with melodious proporciouns of sownes in mvsical instrumentis esily ch*a*unge the desires of mannes soule from the hevynes of ire to joye and myrth, as Boice declarith in the bigynnyng of his Musik'.[42]

Theoretically, Galenic physiology explained that the passions of the soul could easily disturb the vital, animal and natural spirits which, housed in the heart, the brain and the liver respectively, were responsible for life itself. More specifically, it was thought that the animal spirit was responsible for the neurological functions, whereas the vital spirit was for the passions of the soul.[43] Music could invigorate the spirits. In the words of the thirteenth-century encyclopaedist Bartholomaeus Anglicus: 'a swete voys ... schewiþ out þe passiouns of þe soule, and witnes þe strengþe and vertue of spiritualle membres ... and chaungiþ þe affeccioun of þe hierers [humours]'.[44] Indeed, the fourteenth-century vernacular translation of the *Secreta secretorum* explains that music could even reunite the body and soul if they had been temporarily disjoined, as 'the Sowle of a man hath delyte in instrumentys of myrth ... al the body therof streynth takyth'.[45]

The vital spirit, housed in the heart, was deemed to be 'distributed

39 Saint Hildegard of Bingen, *Symphonia: A Critical Edition of the* Symphonia armonie celestium revelationum *[Symphony of the Harmony of Celestial Revelations]*, trans. Barbara Newman (Ithaca, NY and London, 1988), 'Introduction', pp. 20–1.

40 Music was included in the quadrivium, along with arithmetic, geometry and astronomy, in northern European universities.

41 Christopher Bonfield, 'The *Regimen Sanitatis* and its Dissemination in England, *c.* 1348–1550', Ph.D. thesis, University of East Anglia, 2006, pp. 214–15.

42 Linne R. Mooney, 'A Middle English Text on the Seven Liberal Arts', *Speculum* 68 (1993), 1027–52 (p. 1045).

43 Richard Palmer, 'In Bad Odour: Smell and its Significance in Medicine from Antiquity to the Seventeenth Century', in *Medicine and the Five Senses*, ed. W. F. Bynum and Roy Porter (Cambridge, 1993), pp. 61–8 (p. 64).

44 Bartholomaeus Anglicus, *On the Properties of Things: John Trevisa's Translation of Bartholomaeus Anglicus 'De proprietatibus rerum'*, 3 vols, ed. M. C. Seymour et al. (Oxford, 1975-88), vol. 1, bk. 5, p. 213. Just before these words, Bartholomaeus cited Aristotle on a variety of voices.

45 *Three Prose Versions of the Secreta secretorum*, vol. 1, ed. Robert Steele, EETS e.s. 74 (London, 1898), p. 141.

through the arteries to vivify the whole body'.[46] The heartbeat and the pulsation of the arteries helped blood enriched with vital spirit disperse throughout the body.[47] Being '[i]ntermediate between body and soul, the spirits had a certain mobile independence'.[48] The vital spirit might retreat to the heart 'in the experience of fear, or rush from the heart outwards – the sensation of anger'.[49] On the other hand, it could be stimulated to come back into the arterial system by pleasant sound, thereby moderating the passions and revitalising the soul. The *regimen sanitatis* explains that the vital spirit could be 'lured from its hiding place in the heart by the sound of laughter',[50] since 'dyuers Instrumentes of myrthe … oppyn [the] herte and conforte [it]'.[51]

Significantly, the classical explanation of the therapeutic value of music was translated into Mechtild's mystical vision, from which a more potent form of therapy for the health of body and soul emerged. Since Augustine, mystics had understood that music provides direct mystical access to God.[52] It has the capacity to move souls to mystical heights when the devout sing, hear or play an instrument. The power of music to raise the spirits and mitigate emotions would have led mystics to incorporate psychosomatic healing intuitively into their longing for union with God, in which Christ's body becomes the means to spiritual health and salvation.[53]

Indeed, healing is sometimes achieved most comprehensively through the mediation of a musical instrument in the visionary's experience. In Mechtild's vision, Christ's body is envisioned as the instrument with which she can participate in heavenly music and attain union with God. Early in her book, the voice of Christ is compared to a sweet instrument which embraces her with love:

> Than atte laste sche felle downe to the feete of Ihesu ande anone þat swete instrumente, the voyce of Cryste, gaffe a sowne ande saide: 'Ryse vpp my frende, schewe me þi face.' & alle the companye of sayntys ande of aungels whyche was abowne in the hyeste toppe of the hille sange so merylye with oure lorde God ande in God with a fulle swete sange of love as hitt hadde bene oo voyce. Ande

46 Palmer, 'Bad Odour', p. 64.

47 Nancy G. Siraisi, 'The Music of the Pulse in the Writings of Italian Academic Physician (Fourteenth and Fifteenth Centuries)', *Speculum* 50 (1975), 689–710 (p. 696).

48 Palmer, 'Bad Odour', p. 64.

49 Palmer, 'Bad Odour', p. 64.

50 Bonfield, 'The *Regimen Sanitatis*', p. 210.

51 *Three Prose Versions*, pp. 140–1.

52 Robert Boenig, 'St Augustine's *jubilus* and Richard Rolle's *canor*', in *Vox Mystica*, ed. Bartlett et al., pp. 75–86 (p. 77).

53 For an astute discussion of the musical body of Christ during his Passion, see Bruce W. Holsinger, *Music, Body, and Desire in Medieval Culture: Hildegard of Bingen to Chaucer* (Stanford, CA, 2001), ch. 5.

> suche a melodye þare was þat no mannys tonge suffycis to schewe hitt. (I, 26, 143–4)

At the elevation of the Host during the mass, Mechtild envisions a harp coming out from Christ's heart.[54] In identifying the harp with Christ himself and the harp strings with chosen souls, she calls Christ the chanter of all chanters who strikes the harp:

> sche saught anone an harpe come owte fro the deuyne herte whiche hadde many strengys. Þe herpe was oure lorde Ihesu; the herpe strengis ware alle chosene saules whiche bene alle one in God be luffe. Þan the hye chantour of alle chantours, oure lorde Ihesu, smote the herpe, ande alle þe aungells with a delectable sowne intunyde þis songe in duche tonge and sayde; *Regem regum etc.* (II, 3, 334)

In addition to the harp, a trumpet appears in her vision.[55] As an attribute of the angels playing music at Christ's Second Coming, the trumpet becomes a powerful metaphor of salvation as it emerges from the heart of God and stretches to her heart:

> [S]che sawe a trumpe commynge forth fra the herte of God to here herte, ande þan agayne itt was tornede fro this maydene to the herte off God be þe whiche trumpe was betokenede the preysynge ande the herynge of God. Þat trumpe was arayede with knoppes or knottes off golde, ande be þe knottes was betokenede þe blyssede soules whiche nowe preyse ande glorifies oure lorde in hevyne euere withoutyne ende. (II, 1, 328)

Noticeably, the trumpet is decorated with golden ribbons, the blessed souls in heaven; the vision could therefore have helped Mechtild develop a greater sense of assurance in her hope for salvation.

Furthermore, probably stimulated by the liturgy of Trinity Sunday, Mechtild sees a vision in which a psaltery with ten strings comes out from the heart of God to her heart: nine strings betoken the orders of angels, while the tenth string betokens God. As she touches the first string, she gives worship to God and participates in the heavenly choir:

> Also in this same vysione itt semede to here syght þat luffe stode atte þe ryght syde of God ande fro the herte of God schewede owte ane instrumente [of melodye ande of a mery sowne whiche instrument] rechede forth to the herte of þis maydene. Þis instrumente was ane psawtere to syght whiche hadde x strenges,

54 For revelations concerning bride mysticism in terms of the tradition of medieval plucked-string instruments, see Therese Schroeder-Sheker, 'The Alchemical Harp of Mechthild of Hackeborn', *Vox Benedictina* 6, 1 (1989), 40–55. I would like to thank Professor Barbara Newman for drawing my attention to this article.

55 Gertrude the Great has a similar vision in which a musical pipe emerges from Christ's heart. For the somatics of liturgy at Helfta, see Holsinger, *Music, Body, and Desire*, pp. 240–53.

> ande of þat es wretyne in þe psalme of the psawtere: … My God, I schalle synge to the in a psawtrye with x strengeys. Be þe ix strengeys were betokenede þe ix orders of aungellys … Be the tenth strenge was betokenede owre lorde hymselfe. … Þis maydene þan felle downe before oure lorde and softelye towchede the fyrste strenge beneth ande gaffe praysynge ande worschepe to God ande sayde: *Te Deum patrem ingenitum*. (II, 35, 392–3)[56]

The psaltery was considered to be the instrument which David had played with his own hands to rid Saul of the evil spirit. This cure was often regarded as 'an allegory of the role of Christ and the church in curing sin',[57] and it invited moral, tropological interpretations, becoming 'a cosmological metaphor for the moral universe'.[58] In the Old Testament, as in Mechtild's vision, the psaltery is strung with ten strings (Psalms 32.2). Augustine interpreted the strings as the 'Ten Commandments, which may be divided into three for the Trinity and seven for humanity in that [man is] composed of the four elements together with heart, soul, and mind'.[59] Augustine further explained that the strings of the psaltery were 'stretched over the sound board like the sinews of Christ's body on the Cross',[60] identifying Christ's suffering body with this musical instrument. Mechtild's vision of the psaltery thus illuminates its intensely eucharistic implications. Noticeably, her vision is similar to a miniature from the *Speculum humanae salvationis*, a devotional treatise in rhymed prose composed in 1324 by the Dominicans of Strasbourg, in which 'the slack strings of the *psalterium* invite the viewer to complete the typology and put it in motion by imagining the passion itself as a musical performance'.[61] Here the musical body in pain is envisioned as a redemptive sign.

In another vision of Mechtild's, trumpets come forth from the hearts of each angel to the heart of Christ, and create a melody full of mirth:

> [S]che desyredde þat alle the mynistracion whiche schulde be done to here, þay schulde gyffe itt to þe praysynge ande to the worscheppe of here oonly luffere.

56 These verses are from the antiphon of two vespers of Trinity Sunday: see *The Booke of Gostlye Grace*, ed. Halligan, p. 100 n. 393/3–9.

57 Murray Jones, 'Music Therapy in the Later Middle Ages', p. 123.

58 Boenig, 'St Augustine's *jubilus*', p. 79.

59 Boenig, 'St Augustine's *jubilus*', p. 79. For Augustine' interpretation of the strings as analogous to the Decalogue, see *De doctrina christiana* II, xvi, 26, in *Music in Early Christian Literature*, ed. James McKinnon (Cambridge, 1987), p. 165. See also Wilhelm Geerlings, 'The Decalogue in Augustine's Theology', in *The Decalogue in Jewish and Christian Tradition*, ed. Henning Graf Reventlow and Yair Hoffman (New York, 2011), pp. 106–17 (p. 117).

60 Boenig, 'St Augustine's *jubilus*', p. 79.

61 Holsinger, *Music, Body, and Desire*, p. 213 and Figure 11, 'Jubal and Tubalcain/ Raising of the Cross', from *Speculum humanae salvationis*, ch. 23 (Darmstadt, Landesbibliothek, MS 2505, fol. 42v). For patristic and medieval traditions regarding the musicality of the human body, see ch. 1.

> Anone than sche sawe trumpes coome furth fro the hertes of eche aungelle to the herte of God, ande þoo trumpes sownede so merelye a sange þat none erthelye man myght telle þe merth of þat melodye. (II, 20, 360)

Rejoicing in heavenly music, Mechtild is then drawn into the heart of Christ, where she breathes the sweetness of divine grace. She is eventually welcomed into the 'paradyse of euerelastynge delycis', where she dines with Christ:

> After þis þe herte offe Cryste oppenede hymselfe ande he drewe into hym the sawle off this maydene, ande closedde here in hymselfe, ande sayde: 'The ouere partye of myne herte schalle be to the þe softnesse ande þe swetnesse of my devyne spyrite, whiche swettenesse … þow schalte breth vppewarde with þy desyre. þowe schalt also thareto lefte vppe thyne eyen, ande þou schalte open thy mowth ande drawe to the swettenesse of devyne grace. … In the sowth partye [of the heart] þowe schalte see the paradyse of euerelastynge delycis ande thare þowe schalte be with me atte borde. (II, 20, 360–1)

This vision illuminates the extent to which Mechtild conceives of heaven as a place full of health. The medieval *regimen sanitatis* recommended that breathing sweet air and having a proper diet (whether individually or communally) would help one to manage the six non-naturals. It was also believed that food smells were not merely appetising, but also nourishing, since Hippocrates and Galen gave smells a particular role in nutrition, because they were absorbed directly without the need for digestion.[62]

Like music, smell was thought to exert a powerful effect on the natural, vital and animal spirits. Pleasant smells became another therapeutic means of vivifying the spirits and controlling the passions of the soul. Defined by Bartholomaeus Anglicus 'as a smoky vapour arising from the substance of a thing',[63] smell was regarded as a real substance, or corporeal entity, 'somewhere between air and water'.[64] When good smells penetrated into the brain, they would work as healing smells that nourished and restored the spirits and humoral balance effectively.[65] Therefore, aromatic medicines had wide applications. As Avicenna advised, 'where several remedies brought about the same effect, the best one to use was the sweetest and most pleasant smelling'.[66] 'Smells could be used to influence the spirits, and even to move them about the body' when the vital spirit retreated to the heart through fear and anxiety.[67]

The salutary aspect of heaven is further elaborated in Mechtild's vision of a wedding banquet. When her faith was steadfastly confirmed through the

62 Palmer, 'Bad Odour', p. 63.
63 Palmer, 'Bad Odour', p. 63.
64 Rawcliffe, *Leprosy*, p. 227.
65 Rawcliffe, *Leprosy*, p. 227.
66 Palmer, 'Bad Odour', p. 64.
67 Palmer, 'Bad Odour', p. 64.

revelations, she learned that the wedding banquet was soon to be held: 'Ande anone whene sche was thus confortede sche herde the orders of aungels in hevene synge with a grete gladnesse. . . . The maydens herte es conferemede. Ande than sche wente forth to that holye feeste off the excellente Cristes bodye ande precious blode.' (II, 16, 350). This banquet is full of the images of Christ's flesh and blood which recall his suffering in the Passion and the celebration of the mass – a daily re-enactment of the Passion. In another vision, Christ identifies his body as both savoury food and musical instruments for the wedding feast, and reveals that his body is the means for the 'helthe' of body and soul:

> Ande whan the tyme of weddynge was come þat I schulde by the, þan be the luffe of myne owne herte I was solde, ande I gaffe myselfe into brede, flesche, ande drynke for the pryse of þat weddynge feeste. Also in þat feste I was both þe harpe ande organes to gladde þaame alle þat were atte þat feeste, ande þat was þe the comfortable wordys of my mowth. Ande in the lykenesse of players y mekede me before þee feete offe my dyscipyls. (III, 1, 410)

As Caroline Bynum cogently argues, late medieval female mystics frequently envisioned the Christic body as food.[68] Lying behind this metaphor is the theology that identifies the flesh and blood of Christ with the sacramental host and wine. In his gloss on Isaiah 63:3, St Augustine explained that Christ was the grape of the Promised Land who was put into the winepress,[69] and the symbolism spread throughout Europe in sermons and prayers. Medieval theologians observed that '[m]ankind was fed with the blood of Christ, [and] even made drunk from this most precious liquor'.[70] Based on this tradition, Mechtild further deploys Christ's body as holistic medicine for her soul, conforming to medieval dietetics, in which the boundary between food and medicine was permeable.[71] Christ's blood in her vision is a delicious and therapeutic drink 'alle fulle of helth' (II, 18, 352), for the blood flowing from Christ's heart not only quenches her thirst but moderates her emotions by transforming her fear and anxiety into a sense of assuredness:[72]

> Sche anone bowede ande inclynede here to the wounde of þe herte of Cryste, whiche was alle fulle of swetnes, ande suppede þareoffe delicious drynkes ande

68 Bynum, *Holy Feast and Holy Fast*, especially ch. 4.

69 St Augustine, *Enarratio in Psalmum* LV, PL 36, col. 649. See Marilyn Aronberg Lavin, 'The Mystic Winepress in the Mérode Altarpiece', in *Studies in Late Medieval and Renaissance Painting in Honour of Millard Meiss*, ed. Irving Lavin and John Plummer, 2 vols (New York, 1977), vol. 1, pp. 297–301 (p. 299).

70 Nicholas Vincent, *Holy Blood: King Henry III and the Westminster Blood Relic* (Cambridge, 2001), p. 34.

71 The medieval physician was frequently also a cook.

72 For therapeutic uses of wine, see Angela Montford, *Health, Sickness, Medicine and the Friars in the Thirteenth and Fourteenth Centuries* (Aldershot and Burlington, VT, 2004), pp. 181–2.

> swete ande alle fulle of helth, and thare alle here bytternesse was tornede into swetnesse, ande here drede was chaungede into sykernesse [assuredness]. (II, 18, 352)

Furthermore, a familiar metaphor of the crucifix as the chamber of the cross carries a therapeutic overtone when Christ sings for Mechtild in the chamber of love:

> [B]ethenke þe in whate manere ande howe I wente into the chambre of þe crosse Ande [as] spowsis gyffen here cloythes to mynstrallys, ryght so I gaffe mye cloythynge to knyghtes, ande mye bodye to thame þat schuldene crucifie me. Ande than I straykede owte myne aarmes and myne handdys to be naylede with herde nayles, and than I sange songys of a wonderfulle softenesse in þe chambyr of luffe, and þat was on þe crosse. After þis I openede my herte to the for ʒowe schulde come yn, ande þat was whan I toke a slepe of luffe with þe deyenge on the crosse. (III, 1, 411–12)

By associating the crucifixion with a chamber filled with music, Mechtild translates the cross into a bridal chamber where her body and soul are healed and brought to mystical union through heavenly music. This translation reveals that health of body and soul is attained only through redemption, in which Christ consummates his love for humankind.

Mechtild's mystical union takes place in the nuptial chamber of Christ's heart, which he opens so that her soul can enter.[73] Jeffrey Hamburger, who finds close affinities between Mechtild's vision and the drawings produced for the nuns of St Walburg, Eichstätt, in fourteenth-century Germany, also argues that 'the heart is the leitmotif of Mechtild's religious imagination'.[74] Moreover, an image of the heart as house, room and dining room is a topos firmly established in the medieval religious culture.[75] As the organ for subjective experience, the heart provides a place of interiority where Mechtild can withdraw in intimate dialogue with Christ and experience 'euerelastynge sykernesse agayns alle [her] aduersaries' (II, 20, 363) – a

73 Jeffrey F. Hamburger, *Nuns as Artists: The Visual Culture of a Medieval Convent* (Berkeley, CA, 1997). Hamburger finds 'an oblique reference to the wound opened by Longinus's lance (p. 135)' in this vision. For the image of Christ's heart opening and enclosing the soul, see *The Booke*, II, 20, 360.

74 Hamburger, *Nuns as Artists*, p. 134.

75 In an image of 'the heart of a house', made for a nun of St Walburg in about 1500, the heart assumes the form of small house and the nun as the bride rests secure in the embrace of the Trinity: See Hamburger, *Nuns as Artists*, pp. 137–41, figure 85 and plate 12. For the preparation of the heart as a house ready to receive God, see *The Doctrine of the Hert*, bk. 1. For the concept of the 'chamber of the heart' and the rise of affective devotion, see Catherine Innes-Parker, '*The Doctrine of the Hert* and its Manuscript Context', in *A Companion to the Doctrine of the Hert: The Middle English Translation and its Latin and European Contexts*, ed. Denis Renevey and Christiania Whitehead (Exeter, 2010), pp. 159–81 (pp. 161 n. 6, 168).

healthy mental state in which there is no anxiety but everlasting peace and assuredness.

The idea of Christ's heart as medicine is further illuminated by an episode about a fellow nun who confides in Mechtild that she has lost her fervent love for God. Mechtild advises the nun to lift up her heart to God, saying in Latin '"Trahe me post te [in odorem vnguentorum tuorum (Cant. 1.3)]" ("Drawe me after the into the smelle of thyne oyntementz")' (IV, 25, 463). She tells the nun to ponder the word, 'trahe', imagining how Christ said 'ȝiffe I be raysede fro the erth, I schalle drawht alle thynges to me' (John 12:32), and to pray to Christ to draw her heart into him and let her encounter the smells of three ointments, 'whiche flowede owte so laargelye fro that noble sellere [spice chest] of his holye herte insomoche þat þay fulfillede hevene and erth' (IV, 25, 464).

The aromatic ointments in the spice chest of Christ's heart have therapeutic qualities by virtue of the healing scents of medicinal substances. The three ointments are germane to the blood flowing from Christ's heart. The first ointment is rosewater which signifies two sorts of liquid – a dew or juice that was expressed from rose petals, and a distillate.[76] A common medicine both in the monastic infirmary and ordinary household,[77] rosewater was metaphorically conceived as a liquid distilled from the rose petals of Christ's bleeding wounds in his heart.[78] The love of God makes the rose boil in 'þe chymneye of charite (III, 25, 464)', producing an ointment that can wash the face of the nun's soul, wiping away the stains of sins to heal spiritual sickness.

The eucharistic overtone is intensified by the second ointment – the red wine which is pressed, on the cross, out of the wound of Christ's heart. The nun is advised to pray that the face of her soul be coloured with his red blood so that her soul might be made worthy to come to a celestial feast, which Mechtild envisions elsewhere in her revelations as taking place in Christ's heart.[79] The third ointment is the sweetness of the divine heart. Called 'the

76 Terence Scully, *The Art of Cookery in the Middle Ages* (Woodbridge, 1995), p. 164. According to Scully, a distillate was produced more economically and it was used 'as a medicine, as a culinary ingredient, and as a perfume' (p. 165). For the same method of distillation for domestic use, see *Le Menagier de Paris*, ed. Georgine E. Brereton and Janet M. Ferrier (Oxford, 1981), pp. 272–3.

77 Theodoric of Bologna, for example, recommended rosewater cooled over snow to treat burns, because it prevents blistering and keeps the area cool and moist: Theodoric, *The Surgery of Theodoric, ca. A.D. 1267*, trans. Eldridge Campbell and James Colton, 2 vols (New York, 1955), vol. 2, p. 135.

78 The Virgin, who was thought to act as a nurse in the service of her Son, *Christus medicus*, was frequently associated with roses. The link between the Virgin and rosewater enhanced the efficacy of this precious liquid in the minds of the devout. A stained glass window at Browne's Hospital in Stamford, Lincolnshire, for example, depicts her holding red roses and white lilies: see Penny Hebgin-Barnes, *The Medieval Stained Glass of the County of Lincolnshire* (Oxford, 1996), p. 290.

79 See, for example, *The Booke*, II, 16, 347–50.

oyntemente of bawme', it 'passes in swetnes þe sauour of alle othere oyntementys' (IV, 24, 465) and is profitable to spiritual sickness.

At the end of the healing process, Mechtild instructs the nun to pray that this mystical ointment be poured into her suffering soul: 'Tharefore praye þat this oyntemente myght be powrede into the herte of þyne sowle, þat itt mowe taaste & feele howe softe owre lorde es' (III, 25, 465). When she tastes the sweetness, the nun's soul will be well fed and fulfilled with the fatness contained in this ointment until she is incorporated into God, the experience of which 'gaffe [her] suche feedynge be luffe' (IV, 24, 465).[80] Here a sense of oneness with God is imagined in terms of medical treatment by the eucharistic ointments that flow from the medicine chest of Christ's heart. The ointments thus invigorate her entire body, promoting a sense of beatitude and equilibrium in the healthy state of body and soul.

Mechtild's highly somatic revelations are grounded in the basic knowledge of the theory and practice of the medieval *regimen sanitatis*, with an emphasis on the Galenic rules of the six non-naturals. Her revelations display a convergence of the senses, where her entire body is restored to health through sensory experience, replete with such delights as heavenly music, smell or images. Nevertheless, deeply embedded in her psychosomatic experience is devotion to Christ's body, which, envisioned as musical instruments and savoury food, incites her soul to fervent devotion and functions as a means of spiritual therapy. Contextualised within the medieval *regimen sanitatis*, Mechtild's revelations emerge as a psychosomatic healing process from suffering to eternal bliss in her pursuit of mystical union with God. Mechtild's revelatory experience thus bears witness to the way in which the classical medical explanation of the therapeutic value of the six non-naturals was absorbed into the Christian faith, and it illuminates how the late medieval mystic envisioned the salvation of her soul as a process of spiritual therapy. An examination of the medical allusions embedded in Mechtild's revelations reveals the symbiotic relationship between religion and medicine in the late Middle Ages as medical discourse became integrated within mystical spirituality.

80 This ointment is envisioned as something abstract rather than a real substance.

4

BATHING IN BLOOD: THE MEDICINAL CURES OF ANCHORITIC DEVOTION

Liz Herbert McAvoy

In the Short Text account of her revelations, Julian of Norwich admits to having struggled with the concept of human sin, deeply troubled over an ontology of fallenness that prevents her from uniting with God: 'If sin hadde nought bene', she states, 'we shulde alle hafe bene clene and like to oure lorde as he made us.'[1] Elsewhere, she records the 'softe drede' that the fear of sin elicits in her and in its ability to wound and separate a human from the goodness of God. Using the visceral vocabulary of the bodily wounding she has witnessed in her earlier vision of Christ's Passion, Julian attempts to articulate the damage and abjection inflicted by sin upon the human soul:

> Sin is the sharpesete scourge that any chosen saule maye be bette with, whilke scourge it alle forbettes man and woman, and alle forbrekes tham, and noughts thamselfe in thare awne sight, sa fareforth that him thinke that he is noght worthy bot as it ware to sinke into helle.[2]

Such deep anxieties about sin are everywhere manifested in the Short Text, although Julian clearly attempts to dispel them by stating her trust in Christ's promise to her that 'alle shalle be wele'[3] and in her belief that the healing of spiritual wounds can be effected by contrition, confession and penance.[4] Here, of course, as on numerous occasions in her writing, Julian shields

1 Julian's texts detailing her visionary experiences of 1373 are known as the Short Text (*A Vision Shown to a Devout Woman*) and Long Text (*A Revelation of Love*) respectively. The latter is an extended and greatly developed version of the first, with some new additions and interpolations. All references to Julian's text will be taken from *The Writings of Julian of Norwich: A Vision Shown to a Devout Woman and A Revelation of Love*, Medieval Women: Texts and Contexts 5, ed. Nicholas Watson and Jacqueline Jenkins (Turnhout, 2006). All references will be to section/chapter and line number, here *Vision*, 13. 34–5.

2 *Vision*, 17. 22–5.

3 *Vision*, 13. 61.

4 *Vision*, 17. 15.

herself behind the orthodox teachings of the Church – in this case the edict of the Fourth Lateran Council in 1215 which required all Christians to undertake regular confession and penance at least once a year in order to cleanse the soul.[5] In Julian's Long Text, however, the product of some twenty or thirty years of musing on her visionary experiences,[6] Julian adds to this list of orthodox remedies a 'bodely sicknesse of Goddes sending',[7] no doubt fully mindful of her own illness which she had so desired as a young woman, and which was granted her in 1373 when she was just over thirty years of age.[8] This illness, which brings about excruciating pain followed by an almost total paralysis, is one rooted in an abject female body: dependent on others, even to move her into an upright position, Julian gradually loses physical sensation, including her eyesight and the ability to breathe.[9] As she approaches death, she imagines hordes of fiends awaiting her in the darkness and is comforted only by 'the image of the crosse' held before her face, an image that appears to be exuding a 'comon light' that Julian fails to understand at that juncture ('I wiste not how').[10] Julian's illness, dependency and lack of understanding, therefore, all combine to accentuate her feminine vulnerability and abjection, as has been argued at length by a number of commentators.[11] It is this experience of abjection, moreover, that appears to have precipitated the visionary encounter which forms the basis of Julian's ultimate realisation in the Long Text that God is, indeed, our divine Mother,[12] whose relation with humankind is predicated upon an empathy and unconditional love that can ultimately counter sin ('Here may we see that we have verily of kind to hate sinne').[13] From experience, then, and protracted meditation upon it, Julian is

5 On this see, for example, R. N. Swanson, *Religion and Devotion in Europe, c. 1215–c. 1515* (Cambridge, 1995), pp. 25–30.

6 The dating of Julian's texts was revised in 1993 by Nicholas Watson, who argued for a much later date for the Short Text (which had previously been deemed an immediate response by Julian to her 1373 visions), considering it to be a product of the mid 1380s, with the Long Text a product of the 1390s up to Julian's death sometime after 1416. See Nicholas Watson, 'The Composition of Julian of Norwich's Revelation of Love', *Speculum* 68 (1993), 637–83.

7 *Revelation*, 39. 12.

8 'And when I was thirty yere old and a halfe, God sent me a bodily sicknes' (*Revelation*, 3. 1).

9 *Revelation*, 3. 14–30.

10 *Revelation*, 3. 25–6.

11 See, for example, Nicholas Watson, '"Yf women be double naturally": Remaking "Woman" in Julian of Norwich's *Revelation of Love*', *Exemplaria* 8, 1 (1996), 1–34. See also Liz Herbert McAvoy, *Authority and the Female Body in the Writings of Julian of Norwich and Margery Kempe* (Cambridge, 1994); and '"For we be double of God's making": Writing, Gender and the Body in Julian of Norwich', in *A Companion to Julian of Norwich*, ed. Liz Herbert McAvoy (Cambridge, 2008), pp. 166–80.

12 Julian's realisation of God as divine mother is expounded in depth in *Revelation*, 52–63.

13 *Revelation*, 63. 1.

fully aware of an ethics of female bodily suffering which can act not only as textual affect but also constitute a remedy for sin, 'the sharpest scorge that ony chosen soule may be smitten with'.[14] Indeed, she readily conflates that bodily suffering and its textual representation, locating them as remedies firmly within the realm of both the medicinal and the salvific in her assertion: 'For by theyse medicins behoveth that every sinfulle soule be heled'.[15] For Julian, then, it is the medicinal script of the wounded, suffering body that God will read on the Day of Judgement. Like Christ himself: 'Though that [the sinner] be heled, his woundes be sene before God not as woundes but as wurshippes'.[16]

In her depiction of sin as physically manifesting itself as wounds, Julian is working within a tradition well established by the late fourteenth century, particularly in anchoritic and eremitic writings.[17] Within this tradition, the remedies for the wounds of sin were frequently articulated in terms of medical metaphor or allegory and, on occasion, were also allied to the nurturing ministrations of the maternal feminine. What I wish to argue in this essay, therefore, is that Julian's now renowned depiction of God-as-Mother is as much dependent upon discourses of medicinal care and cure as it is upon a feminine ethics of redemption via the abject body, and that Julian had direct access to such discourses in some of her more immediate source material.

One such likely source is the mid fourteenth-century text, *De Remediis contra Temptationes [The Remedy ayenst the troubles of temptacyons]* (c. 1352–58), originally written in Latin by the Norwich hermit William Flete, and which was translated into Middle English very soon after its inception.[18] The Middle English text begins with a statement of how Christ permits human temptation because of its profit to the soul's health:

14 *Revelation*, 39. 1.

15 *Revelation*, 39. 24–5.

16 *Revelation*, 39. 25–6.

17 On this see, for example, Joseph Ziegler, *Medicine and Religion c. 1300: The Case of Arnau de Vilanova* (Oxford, 1998), especially his Introduction, pp. 1–45.

18 The edition used here is *The Remedy ayenst the troubles of temptacyons*, in *Richard Rolle of Hampole*, ed. C. Horstmann, 2 vols (London, 1896), vol. 2, pp. 106–23. In 1964, Benedict Hackett, Edmund College and Noel Chadwick argued for this text's influence upon Julian, although Bella Millett has since advised some caution. See Benedict Hackett, Edmund Colledge and Noel Chadwick, 'William Flete's "De Remediis contra Temptaciones" in its Latin and English Recensions: The Growth of a Text', *Mediaeval Studies* 26 (1964), 210–30; and Bella Millett, *Annotated Bibliographies of Old and Middle English Literature:* Ancrene Wisse, *the Katherine Group, and the Wooing Group* (Cambridge, 1996), p. 33. But see Vincent Gillespie, '"[S]he do the police in different voices": Pastiche, Ventriloquism and Parody in Julian of Norwich', in *A Companion to Julian of Norwich*, ed. McAvoy, pp. 192–207, especially pp. 198–9.

> Our mercyfull lorde god cryst Ihesu chastyseth his children and suffreth them to be tempted for many proufytable causes to thyr soules helth & therefore sholde noo man nor woman be heuy or sory for ony temptacyon.[19]

Elsewhere in this text, God is presented explicitly as the cruel-to-be-kind 'leech' doctor who will allow putrid skin to grow on his patient's body before eventually excising it in order to restore the patient to health:

> Almyghty god werketh lyke a leche for a leche suffreth somtyme the deed flesshe to growe on hym that he hat in cure but afterward he taketh away the same and maketh the quycke flesshe to growe and soo he heleth the pacyent.[20]

Crucially, however, for the concerns of this present essay, in this same text, Flete also configures this divine healer in terms of an equally cruel-to-be-kind loving mother, a representation which may well have had a significant influence upon Julian's similar treatment of God as mother in her own writing. According to Flete:

> our lorde god dooth lyke a kynde moder; for a louynge moder that is wyse and well taught herself she wolde that her children were vertuously and well nortured; and yf she may knowe ony of theym with a defaute she wyll gyue thym a knocke on the heed; and yf the defaute be more she wyll gyue hym a buffet on the cheke; and yf he doo a grete faute she wyll sharpely lasshe hym with a rodde.[21]

For Flete, then, in terms of suffering there is little division between soul and body in this world; a chastised body equals a healthy soul. As he assures his readers: 'whyle your body and soule be togyder in this lyf they must receyue troubles as well as eases'.[22] Moreover, for Flete, such eases are 'the precious oyntement of crystes passyon',[23] which, for both Flete and Julian, is also the passion of maternal love.

These topoi also make their presence felt in the popular guidance text written for female anchorites in the early thirteenth century, *Ancrene Wisse*,[24] and, as I demonstrate below, had forged a path within anchoritic literature that had allied them to the maternal since much earlier times. *Ancrene Wisse* was a text still in circulation in various forms and recensions during the fourteenth

19 Flete, *Remedy*, p. 106.

20 Flete, *Remedy*, p. 113.

21 Flete, *Remedy*, pp. 118–19.

22 Flete, *Remedy*, p. 109.

23 Flete, *Remedy*, p. 111.

24 In *Writings*, ed. Watson and Jenkins, p. 100 n. 32, the editors argue for the influence of *Ancrene Wisse* upon Julian's writing, something that was first posited by Anna Marie Reynolds in 'Some Literary Influences in the *Revelations* of Julian of Norwich (c. 1342–post-1416)', *Leeds Studies in English* 7-8 (1952), 18–28. Again Millett points out the lack of hard evidence cited in support of this in *Annotated Bibliographies*, p. 33.

and fifteenth centuries and both Flete and Julian, as former and present recluses, were almost certainly drawing upon some version of it in their own writing.[25] Part 4 of *Ancrene Wisse*, for example, which, like Flete's text, deals protractedly with the problems of temptation, the author equates a lapsed and sinful recluse to a sick man who refuses to summon the physician:

> Sec mon haueð twa estaz swiðe dredfule. Þet an is hwen he ne feleð nawt his ahne secnesse, ant for-þi ne secheð nawt leche ne lechecreft, ne [ne] easkeð na mon read, ant asteorueð ferliche ear me least wene. Þis is þe ancre þe nat nawt hwet is fondunge.
>
> [A sick man has two very dangerous conditions. One is when he is unaware of his own illness, and so does not consult a doctor or seek treatment, or ask anyone for advice, and dies suddenly and unexpectedly. This is the anchoress who does not recognize temptation.].[26]

Elsewhere, the author embellishes this comparison in a passage which also has strong resonances with Julian's own reading of illness quoted at the start of this essay:

> Secnesse þet Godd send … is … sawlene heale, salue of hire wunden, scheld þet ha ne kecche ma. … þe mei þenne edstearten þet ilke grisliche wa, þe eateliche pinen, þurh secnesse þet agea[ð], þurh ei uuel þet her is, seliliche mei ha seggen.
>
> [Illness that God sends … is the soul's salvation, an ointment for its wounds, a shield against its receiving more [temptation] … Anyone, then, who is able to escape that terrible suffering [of damnation], those fearful torments, through a passing illness, through any suffering in this world, may count herself lucky].[27]

For the *Ancrene Wisse* author, all worldly suffering, whether physical or spiritual, literal or metaphorical, is intrinsic to life's penitential condition, and able to be healed only by the compassionate medicine of the ultimate physician, God.

The notion of confession and penance as medicine of the soul was dependent in no small measure upon the new pastoral imperative instigated by Lateran IV (1215), whose Canon 21 presented the need for annual confession by all Christians, along with a requirement for the spiritual confessor to be

25 On the literary legacy of *Ancrene Wisse*, see Catherine Innes-Parker, 'The Legacy of *Ancrene Wisse*: Translations, Adaptations, Influences and Audience, with Special Attention to Women Readers', in *A Companion to* Ancrene Wisse, ed. Yoko Wada (Cambridge, 2003), pp. 145–73. On the influence of the motherhood trope in particular, and on Flete's use of it, see pp. 158–65.

26 *Ancrene Wisse: A Corrected Edition of the Text in Cambridge, Corpus Christi College, MS 402 with variants from other manuscripts*, ed. Bella Millett, EETS o.s. 325 (Oxford, 2005). All quotations are taken from this edition. Translations are taken from *Ancrene Wisse: A Guide for Anchoresses*, ed. and trans. Bella Millett (Exeter, 2009). The page references are the same in each case (here Part 4, p. 68).

27 *Ancrene Wisse*, Part 4, pp. 69–70.

'discreet and cautious that he may pour wine and oil into the wounds of the one injured after the manner of a skilful physician'.[28] Such a conceit collapsing confession and medicine into one another, however, also reflected a much older ideal – and one which was particularly prevalent within early anchoritic writings. Within this tradition, the anchorite was exhorted to emulate Christ-the-Physician (*Christus medicus*) as part of her/his own practices of *imitatio*, drawing on a concept of the triune God as ultimate physician that can be traced back to the Old Testament, especially the Book of Ecclesiasticus. Here, the earthly physician and his medicine are presented as gifts to humankind, proffered by God as the highest physician:

> Honour the physician for the need thou hast of him: for the most High hath created him. For all healing is from God, and he shall receive gifts of the king … [I]n thy sickness neglect not thyself, but pray to the Lord, and he shall heal thee.[29]

Christ also adopts this type of rhetoric during the years of his ministry, responding to the criticism of the Pharisees at Capharnaum about his eating with sinners thus: 'They that are well have no need of a physician, but they that are sick. For I came not to call the just, but sinners.'[30] Christ's self-identification as physician here was later taken up with great enthusiasm by commentators such as Augustine (d. 430), who regarded Christ's Passion as the best medicine for restoring both physical and spiritual health.[31] Augustine was himself no stranger to ill health, as his *Confessions* clearly attest, no doubt constituting one of the reasons why, like Julian whose theodicy was also predicated on a bout of intense sickness, he devised a *dispensatio medicinalis* (or what Thomas F. Martin has termed 'a medicinal economy of salvation') with *Christus medicus* and the ointment of *caritas* at its heart.[32] In the words of Augustine:

> Medicus quis? Dominus noster Jesus Christus. Quis Dominus noster Jesus Christus? … Ille qui apprehensus, colaphizatus, flagellatus, sputis illitus, spinis coronatus, in cruce suspensus, mortuus, lancea vulneratus, de cruce depositus,

28 Fourth Lateran Council: 1215, Canon 21. Online translation at http://www.fordham.edu/halsall/basis/lateran4.asp. Accessed 15 July 2013. For a discussion of this, see also, for example, Swanson, *Religion and Devotion*, pp. 25–30.

29 Ecclesiasticus 38:1–9.

30 Mark 2:17.

31 On this see *Sources for the History of Medicine in Late Medieval England*, ed. and trans. Carole Rawcliffe (Kalamazoo, MI, 1995), p. 4. See also R. Arbesmann, 'The Concept of "*Christus Medicus*" in St Augustine', *Traditio* 10 (1954), 1–28 (p. 3).

32 Augustine, *On John's Gospel*, 36.4, cited by Thomas F. Martin in '*Christus Medicus*', Talk given at a retreat for the friars of the Province of Saint Thomas of Villanova (Villanova University, June 2005). http://www.augustinianfriends.com/readingroom/Christus_Medicus.pdf. Accessed 24 July 2013.

> in sepulcro positus. Ille ipse Dominus noster Jesus Christus; ille ipse plane, et ipse est totus medicus vulnerum nostrorum.
>
> [Who is the physician? Our Lord Jesus Christ. Who is our Lord Jesus Christ? ... He who was arrested, buffeted, scourged, spat upon, crowned with thorns, suspended on the cross, died, pierced by a spear, taken down from the cross, placed in the sepulchre. That same Jesus Christ our Lord; that same one exactly, and he is the complete physician of our wounds.].[33]

Within this economy, it is the love embodied in the Passion that comprises the primary source of healing: and, for Augustine therefore, *caritas* is *sanitas*.

The potential of the physician's curative powers to provide a *modus operandi* for the anchoritic life in particular was reflected in other early Christian writings, particularly those focusing on the solitary life. In the *Collationes* or 'Conferences' of John Cassian (d. c. 435), for example, a work detailing the exemplary lives of early desert anchorites, frequent use is made of the conceit.[34] Having lived himself as a desert recluse, Cassian was very well placed to pronounce on the hardships of this austere way of life and define its meanings.[35] The type of desert anchoritism espoused by Cassian had developed not only out of the need of early Christians to withdraw into the Egyptian desert in the face of Roman persecution, but also to enable first-hand experience of the deprivations of Christ during his ministry and his sufferings during the Passion. Austerity, bodily illness and spiritual temptation were therefore intrinsic to the early solitary life and to the economy of salvation it produced. Thus, in the *Collationes*, which feature a long series of interviews between Cassian, his friend, Germanus, and a series of experienced desert abbots, he frequently draws upon the image of God as physician to rationalise anchoritic suffering. Speaking to the abbot Theodore, for example, Germanus is informed that God is 'peritissimus medicus' ['most skilful physician'] whose 'severissima et ... caustica ignis ... medicina' ['caustic and fiery medicine'] must sometimes kill in order to cure;[36] according to Abbot Serenus, however, God is the 'clementissimoque medico' ['most merciful physician'] and 'piissimo patre' ['most kind father'];[37] similarly, Abbot Charemon sees God as 'most loving father and most gracious physician' ['piissimum patrem,

33 Augustine, *On John's Gospel*, Tractatus III, PL 35, col. 1397. My translation.

34 Sometimes also referred to as the *Conlationes*, the original text has been edited in PL 49, cols 477–1328. The modern English translation is taken from *John Cassian: The Conferences*, ed. Boniface Ramsey (New York and Mahwah, NJ, 1997). References to this translation will appear parenthetically by conference number, chapter, section and page after the citation of the Latin original.

35 For a more detailed discussion of this see Chapter 1 of my *Medieval Anchoritisms: Gender, Space and the Solitary Life* (Cambridge, 2011), pp. 11–42.

36 PL 49, col. 662A-B (*Collationes*, 6. xi, p. 230).

37 PL 49, col. 708A (*Collationes*, 7. xxviii, p. 276).

benignissimumque medicum'],[38] collapsing the patriarchal roles of physician and father into one conglomerate image of masculine salvific authority. Ultimately, therefore, Germanus is enlightened on the primary rationale behind the solitary life: self-awareness leading to the ability of the recluse to take on her or himself the role of authoritative spiritual physician: 'For there is no doubt that no one at all can recommend medicines for diseases except the person who has discovered the very origins of the illnesses' ['Nulli etenim dubium est neminem admodum posse remedia malis valetudinibus adhibere, nisi eum qui ipsas morborum origines ante praedixerit'].[39]

Such a depiction of the solitary life as shot through with the dynamics of suffering and medicinal healing through anchoritic practice is common to other early anchoritic texts preceding *Ancrene Wisse*. For example, in the tenth century, Grimlaicus of Metz adopts it as a primary hermeneutic in his *Regula solitariorum* [Rule for Solitaries],[40] the earliest known anchoritic guidance text, written at the request of a group of Benedictine anchorites to address what they saw as the lack of guidance offered to monastic anchorites by the *Rule of Saint Benedict*.[41] Taking up the conceit with some enthusiasm, Grimlaicus develops it into a much more systematic pattern of imagery, presenting God as the 'pius medicus' ['devoted physician'][42] who tends to the spiritual sickness of humanity. The recluses are exhorted to follow God's example to become expert physicians who treat the wounds caused by sin with remedies adapted to each individual case. As Grimlaicus asserts: 'Sicut enim periti medici juxta vulnerum varietates diversa adhibent medicamina, ita et solitarius singulis quibusque congruum exhortationis adhibere debet remedium.' ['Just as expert physicians use various medicines to suit the various kinds of wounds, so solitaries ought to apply to individual people an appropriate remedy of advice.'].[43] Whilst, for Grimlaicus, God is the ultimate Physician, he also explicitly casts his own authorial *self* as a physician whose *writing* provides the medicine to maintain the health of his anchoritic audience and allow his readers to become 'physicians of the soul' in their own right. As such, the passing on of health and the passing on of the written word are subsumed into the same medicinal conceit with author and physician merging in one intertextual body:

38 PL 49, col. 945C (*Collationes*, 13. xviii, p. 489–90).

39 PL 49, cols 1305B–1306A (*Collationes*, 24. xiv, p. 837).

40 *Grimlaicus: Rule for Solitaries*, ed. and trans. Andrew Thornton (Collegeville, MN, 2011). The Latin edition, *Grimlaici presbyteri regula solitariorum*, is to be found in in PL 103, cols 573–644.

41 Nevertheless, the *Regula* is strongly dependent upon Benedict's Rule, although the latter makes little recourse to medical imagery, except to present the abbot as 'prudent physician' to the excommunicated. *Rule of Saint Benedict*, ch. xxvii and ch. xxviii.

42 Grimlaicus, *Rule*, ch. 23, p. 75 (PL 103, col. 605C).

43 Grimlaicus, *Rule*, ch. 20, p. 66 (PL 103, col. 600B).

> Solent namque medici ex multorum speciebus pigmentorum in salutem poscentis quoddam genus medicamenti componere, nec seipsos praesumunt fateri creatores herbarum vel aliarum specierum, sed ministros se esse in colligendo et conficiendo asserunt. Ita et ego, non auctor hujus operis, sed minister in colligendo exstiti. Ex quarum tamen compositione specierum salus efficitur aegrotantium. Sic etiam, sic forsitan meae devotionis labor vestrae charitati, Domino opitulante, aliquid proficere valebit. Non enim, ut reor, tam sollicite mihi hanc Regulam scribere injungeretis, nisi eam diligeretis, et nisi ad propositum vitae solitariae quandoque venire voluissetis .
>
> [To heal someone who asks them, physicians prepare a medicinal compound out of many different types of herbal preparations, and they are not so presumptuous as to claim that they created the herbs or the other kinds of plants. No, they admit that they are merely assistants who collect and prepare them. That is what I am: I am not the author of this work but just the assistant who collected it. From the compound made up of these different kinds of plants, sick people will be healed. In this way then, perhaps the labour to which I have devoted myself will be able, with God's help, to be of some profit to your charity. I assume that you would not have directed me so insistently to write down this rule unless you loved it and unless you yourself desired at some time to undertake the solitary life.].[44]

For this anchoritic writer, the roles of author, physician and audience are synonymous, constituting a complex medicinal compound whose recipe will ultimately allow for the assuaging of the affliction of sin and the curing of souls.

Given that the anchoritic life was primarily monastic and male during the tenth century,[45] perhaps the most extraordinary use made by Grimlaicus of the physician motif is in Chapter 20 of the *Regula* in which he again likens the teachings of anchorites to 'periti medici' ['expert physicians'] able to treat the wounds of the sinful and tailor the medicine to suit individual circumstance. In order to embellish this image, however, he turns to the words of Saint Paul in I Corinthians 3, which configure the preacher explicitly in terms of a nursing mother, telling his audience of male anchorites: 'Non potui vobis loqui quasi spiritualibus, sed quasi carnalibus: tanquam parvulis in Christo lac vobis potum dedi, non escam.' ['I was not able to speak to you as to spiritual people, but as to carnal. As though to babies in Christ I gave you milk to drink, not solid food.'].[46] Here, whilst clearly mindful of the medieval conception of the eucharistic body of Christ as *medicina sacramentalis* (a concept focused on by Yoshikawa elsewhere in this volume), Grimlaicus is also mindful of its

44 Grimlaicus, *Rule*, 'Prologue', p. 28 (PL 103, cols 577C–578A).

45 For a recent in-depth analysis of early English anchoritism, see Tom Licence, *Hermits and Recluses in English Society 950–1200* (Oxford, 2011). On English anchoritic ideology, see Mari Hughes-Edwards, *Reading the Medieval Anchoritism: Ideology and Spiritual Practices* (Cardiff, 2012). See also McAvoy, *Medieval Anchoritisms*, as before.

46 Grimlaicus, *Rule*, ch. 20, p. 66 (PL 103, cols 600B–C).

association with the breast-milk of the Virgin and thus the inherent femininity underlying all eucharistic healing. Such an association, of course, would later become widespread within mystical and devotional works following its appropriation by Bernard of Clairvaux in the twelfth century.[47] Within this schema, having taken on human flesh from Mary and been fed by her own transmuted blood in the form of breast milk, Christ's own blood and the breast milk which fed him were ultimately one and the same.[48] The problem, here, of course, and one which was to beset Dominican thinkers such as Thomas Aquinas (d. 1244) in the thirteenth century, was that within popular medical lore breast milk and menstrual blood were also defined as essentially the same matter, albeit in different form.[49] In turn, this would suggest that all discussions and configurations of the lactating Virgin were inherently haunted by her milk's corrupt correlate, the menstruum; but, as I shall argue, this haunting was one which could just as well be read positively as negatively by those who chose to do so. Indeed, in his *Historia Ecclesiasticae*, Bede, drawing on Gregory the Great, states that 'Quae tamen mulier, dum consuetudinem menstruam patitur, prohiberi ecclesiam intrare non debet, quia ei naturae superfluitas in culpam non ualet reputari' ['a woman must not be prohibited from entering a church during her usual periods, for this natural overflowing cannot be reckoned a crime: and so it is not fair that she should be deprived from entering the church for that which she suffers unwillingly'].[50] Thus, in likening the medicine of the anchorhold to breast milk, and the physician to the mother, Grimlaicus inscribes a Marian femininity upon the curative and cleansing powers of his anchoritic audience which prefigures by some five hundred years the depictions of God as simultaneously physician and the Mother of humanity as authored by William Flete and Julian of Norwich.

A conflation between physician and mother, however, also emerges in *Ancrene Wisse*, and the centrality of blood-loss within this conflation is one which I argue had a marked influence upon Julian as she tried to grapple with

47 Bernard uses the nurturing associations of the breast-feeding mother frequently, particularly as a means of expressing the abbot's responsibility for nurturing the monastic community. On this see Caroline Walker Bynum, *Jesus as Mother: Studies in the Spirituality of the High Middle Ages* (Berkeley, CA, 1992), especially pp. 115–18.

48 For a discussion of this, see Caroline Walker Bynum, *Holy Feast and Holy Fast: The Religious Significance of Food to Medieval Women* (Los Angles and London, 1998), pp. 271–2.

49 On this see, for example, Charles C. Wood, 'The Doctor's Dilemma: Sin, Salvation and the Menstrual Cycle in Medieval Thought', *Speculum* 56, 4 (1981), 710–27. See also the discussion by Thomas Laqueur in *Making Sex: Body and Gender form the Greeks to Freud* (Cambridge, MA, 1994), pp. 35–42.

50 Bede, *Ecclesiastical History of the English People*, ed. and trans. Judith McClure and Roger Collins (Oxford, 1994), Book I, ch. 27, p. 48. Bede, *Historiam Ecclesiasticam Gentis Anglorum*. Online edition at http://www.thelatinlibrary.com/bede.html. Accessed 22 July 2013.

the full meaning of the Passion sequence she envisioned in 1373. Indeed, within the physical and metaphysical frameworks of *Ancrene Wisse*, it is the shedding of blood that is most closely associated with anchoritic cleansing and healing, both bodily and spiritual – and it is a blood-loss, moreover, which is always already feminine because of the author's relentless insistence throughout the work upon the fallen female bodies of his audience. For example, in Part 8, the author exhorts his female audience to undertake quarterly blood-lettings, a common enough medieval practice, particularly amongst religious, and a practice which, like the menses, was deemed to maintain the correct humoral balance and eliminate physical ailments from the body.[51] Indeed, as Cathy McClive has demonstrated, within certain cultural contexts, phlebotomy was actively considered to be a form of induced menstrual bleeding.[52] In the case of the female anchorites of *Ancrene Wisse*, moreover, this becomes an explicitly homosocial event, during which their normal restrictions and disciplines are to be suspended in favour of more recuperative and leisurely woman-to-woman interaction:

> Hwen ȝe beoð ilete blod, ȝe ne schule don na þing þe þreo dahes þet ow greueð, ah talkið to ower meidnes ant wið þeawfule talen schurteð ow togederes. ȝe mahen swa don ofte hwen ow þuncheð heuie, oðer beoð for sum worltlich þing sare oðer seke.
>
> [When you have been bled, you should not do anything for those three days that taxes your strength, but talk to your maids and entertain each other with improving conversation. You may do this often, when you are feeling low, or are upset about some worldly concern, or ill.][53]

Here, the healing of the female body is depicted as dependent on an elective blood-loss, perhaps associated also with menstruation, but most clearly

51 Medieval blood-letting was considered to be a way of restoring the balance of the four humours and many medical texts testify to its having been one of the most widespread of therapeutic practices, particularly in the religious Orders, for which See Angela Montford, *Health, Sickness, Medicine and the Friars in the Thirteenth and Fourteenth Centuries* (Aldershot and Burlington, VT, 2004), p. 232. For *Ancrene Wisse*'s instructions on bloodletting, see Part 8, p. 161. What is particularly interesting here, however, is that this section on blood-letting is followed by a short section added in at a later date by the author, detailing the need for the careful washing of the enclosed woman's body and clothing (p. 161), pointing towards the polluting qualities of blood. For a detailed account of the medieval practice of phlebotomy, see the introduction to *A Latin Technical Phlebotomy and Its Middle English Translation*, ed. Linda E. Voigts and Michael R. McVaughs, *Transactions of the American Philosophical Society* 74, 2 (1984), 1–69 (pp. 1–34). This text is thought to have been authored by Henry of Winchester at Montpellier in the early thirteenth century (p. 1).

52 Cathy McClive, 'Menstrual Knowledge and Medical Practice in Early Modern France c. 1555–1761', in *Menstruation: A Cultural History*, ed. Andrew Shail and Gillian Howie (Basingstoke, 2005), pp. 76–89 (p. 80).

53 *Ancrene Wisse*, Part 8, p. 161.

leading to an increased feminisation of the anchoritic space as the women converse, entertain each other and share each other's concerns.

According to medieval medical lore, as mentioned above, the menses provided a natural means for the female body to purge itself of impurities by eliminating regularly those bodily contaminants which accumulated within the womb as a result of the Fall,[54] and in this sense there are again clear correlations between both types of female blood-loss and that of Christ's salvific bleeding on the cross, which was also necessary to redeem that Fall. Indeed, in Part 2 of the text, the author actualises this connection via a specific configuration of the phlebotomised body in terms of Christ's own blood-loss. In so doing he transforms elective blood shedding from physical therapy into spiritually salvific entity:

> A mon for uuel þet he haueđ ne let him nawt blod o þe seke halue, ah deđ o þe hale, to heale þe seke. Ah in al þe world þe ewes o þe feure, nes bimong al moncun an hal dale ifunden þe mahte beon ilete blod bute Godes bodi ane, þe lette him bold o rode. Nawt o þe earm ane, ah dude o fif halue, forte healen moncun of þe secnesse þet te fif wittes hefden awakenet. Þus, lo, þe hale half ant te cwike dale droh þet uuele blod ut frommard te unhale, ant healde swa þe seke. Þurh blod is in Hali Writ sunne bitacnet.
>
> [A man who has something wrong with him does not have blood let from the part that is unhealthy, but from one that is healthy, to heal the unhealthy one. But in all the world that was suffering from fever, not one healthy part was found among the whole of humanity that could be bled other than the body of God, who had his blood let on the cross. He had this done not only from the arm, but from five parts of the body, to heal humanity of the sickness that the five senses had caused. And in this way, you see, the healthy and living part drew out that bad blood from the unhealthy one and so healed the sick part. In Holy Scripture, sin is signified by blood.'].[55]

Here God as the ultimate physician causes his son to be phlebotomised for the health of the body of humanity and, in her own regular acts of phlebotomy within the anchorhold, both elective and non-elective, the anchoritic woman is able to unite conceptually with that of the phlebotomist-Christ. Indeed, as Ziegler has demonstrated, such a configuration of a *Christus Minutor* [blood-letting Christ], whose passion was an act of altruistic phlebotomy, surfaces particularly frequently amongst the Dominican preachers of the period with whom, as Bella Millett has argued, the origins of *Ancrene Wisse* are associated.[56] Moreover, according to Thomas Aquinas, debating the Virgin's menstrual status, Mary had to furnish 'materia … sanguis mulieris' ['the

[54] See, for example, the pronouncements of Albertus Magnus in his *De Animalibus*, Liber XV, Tractatus II ('de natura spermatis'), in *Opera Omnibus*, ed. Emile Borgnet (Paris, 1891), vol. 12, especially ch. 7, pp. 117–20.

[55] *Ancrene Wisse*, Part 2, p. 45.

[56] Ziegler, *Medicine and Religion*, p. 182.

matter which is menstrual blood']57 in order to conceive and, later, feed Christ with her own breast-milk. Thus, like Gregory, even Aquinas offers a model which implicates female blood-loss as both Christic *and* Marian within the salvific schema.

Ancrene Wisse's Dominican connections are further evidenced in the associations drawn by its author between blood-letting and bathing. In Part 8, for example, just at the point where the author expounds the aforementioned need for quarterly blood-letting, he later inserts an addition to the text which emphasises the woman's need to wash regularly since, as the author adds: 'Nes neauer fulðe Godd leof' ['filth was never dear to God'].[58] Used within this context, the term *fulðe* is clearly freighted with both the blood shed from her phlebotomised body and that of her monthly menstrual flow. As Caroline Walker Bynum has demonstrated, shed blood, particularly that emanating from a woman's body, was deemed a powerful contaminant and needed to be instantly cleansed away by washing or bathing.[59] Blood loss and bathing, therefore, were frequently closely associated, both physically and metaphorically, something expressed in the writing of the thirteenth-century Parisian bishop, Ranulphe de la Houblonnière (d. 1288), who explicitly depicts the crucified Christ as undergoing phlebotomy, being washed clean by his own blood and thereby washing clean the whole of humanity.[60]

The messy business of blood-letting, therefore, was redolent with possibility when it came to articulating – and re-enacting – the complexities of sin and salvation. Indeed, in Part 7 of *Ancrene Wisse,* a section focusing on divine love, the author fully exploits this potential in his depiction of God as a mother-physician whose maternal love is so strong that she is willing to prepare for her own child a bath of blood – clearly her own – in order to save its life:

> Child þet hefde swuch uuel þet him bihofde beað of blod ear hit were ihealet, muchel þe moder luuede hit þe walde þis beað him makien. Þis dude ure Lauerd us þe weren se seke of sunne, ant swa isulet þer-wið, þet na þing ne mahte healen us ne cleansin us bute his blod ane, for swa he hit walde.
>
> [If a child had such an illness that it needed a bath of blood before it could be healed, the mother who was willing to provide this bath for it would love it very much. Our Lord did this for us – who were so infected with sin, and so polluted with it, that nothing could heal or cleanse us except for his blood … His love makes a bath of his blood – because that is what he wished.][61]

57 Thomas Aquinas, *Summa Theologiae,* 52: 26–9, 52–5 (3a, qu. 31), as cited by Wood, 'The Doctor's Dilemma', p. 720 n. 27.

58 *Ancrene Wisse*, Part 8, p. 161.

59 Caroline Walker Bynum, *Wonderful Blood: Theology and Practice in Late Medieval Germany and Beyond* (Philadelphia, 2007), pp. 18, 19, 118, 180–1.

60 On this see Ziegler, *Medicine and Religion*, p. 186.

61 *Ancrene Wisse,* Part 7, p. 149.

Here, of course we have a God who is depicted in terms of the ultimate maternal sacrifice, drawing not only upon that of the Virgin Mother who gave up her own child for human redemption, but also that of the worldly parturient mother whose life was frequently endangered by postpartum haemorrhage and other such complications. Indeed, such a reading of this episode is supported medically by the cure promoted for excessive post-partum blood flow in the so-called 'Trotula text', the popular *De Curis Mulierum* [On Treatments for Women], which prescribes that the bleeding woman be placed 'frequenter in balnis ... ad restringendum sanguinem' ['frequently in baths ... in order to restrain the blood'].[62] No doubt such a 'cure' would produce bath after bath of bloodied water in the attempts to staunch the flow and wash her clean of her own blood – certainly enough to rival the copious blood and water shed from the side-wound of Christ at the crucifixion. It is clear, therefore, that both *Ancrene Wisse* and *De Curis Mulierum* associate the curative properties of the blood-bath with a maternal blood sacrifice, offering nuance to Augustine's notion of *caritas est sanitas* and recasting it most emphatically within the feminine frame of maternal love.

The image of the divine blood-bath is rare before *Ancrene Wisse*, although it provides a dramatic episode within contemporary traditions of the Grail romance, within which it is very much associated with the feminine. For example, in one thirteenth-century tradition, Perceval's sister, Dindrane, offers her virginal blood for a leprous lady to bathe in as a cure for her affliction. In so doing, she also prevents Galahad, Perceval and Bors from having to sacrifice their own lives in an unequal battle in order to cure the same lady by means of their own male blood-shed.[63] The religious undercurrents of these episodes are clear and it is likely that the authors shared with the *Ancrene Wisse* author in drawing on the popular *Naturalis Historia* of Pliny the Elder as a source. Dating from the first century, Pliny's widely circulated work at one point expresses deep anxieties regarding Egyptian beliefs in the prophylactic properties of the human blood-bath against leprosy, writing that 'cum in reges incidisset, populis funebre, quippe in balineis solia temperabantur humano sanguine ad medicinam eam' ['When kings were attacked [by leprosy], it was a deadly thing for the inhabitants, because the tubs in the baths used to be prepared with warm human blood for its treatment.'].[64] Clearly part of an anti-

62 *De Curis Mulierum* [On Treatments for Women], in *The Trotula: An English Translation of the Medieval Compedium of Women's Medicine*, ed. and trans. Monica H. Green (Philadelphia, 2001), pp. 124–5.

63 This episode, as it appears in *La queste del saint graal*, is discussed by Peggy McCracken in *The Curse of Eve, the Wound of the Hero; Blood, Gender and Medieval Literature* (Philadelphia, 2003), pp. 8–9. McCracken reads this episode in terms of its being a Christic motif and associated with the traditions of Christian virgin martyrdom.

64 Pliny the Elder, *Naturalis Historia* VII, ed. W. H. S. Jones (London, 1956), Liber XXVI, Cap. V, pp. 270–1.

pagan propagandist enterprise, Pliny's depiction also found its way into the *vitae* of the Emperor Constantine, as recorded in the *Legenda Aurea* [*Golden Legend*] written by the Dominican Jacobus de Voragine in the mid thirteenth century (again a work which certainly drew on some of the same sources as *Ancrene Wisse*). Here Voragine recounts how, in an attempt to cure his own leprosy, the emperor was discouraged from sacrificing hundreds of small infants and bathing in their blood by the cries of three thousand distraught mothers, again allying the blood sacrifice with the maternal feminine.[65] Folkloric though these tales may be,[66] they do, however, posit what Peggy McCracken has termed 'the gendered value of blood in medieval texts'.[67] They also play most neatly into the development of a devotional hermeneutic which brings together the poetics of maternal sacrifice and the pragmatics of medicinal cure.

Such a convergence of poetics and required medical care is nowhere more evident than in the mid fourteenth-century devotional treatise written in Anglo-Norman by Henry of Lancaster (d. 1361), entitled *Le Livre de Seyntz Medicines*.[68] This text, like other contemporary Anglo-Norman treatises of its kind,[69] is also clearly indebted to *Ancrene Wisse* and the associated 'Wooing Group' texts, all of which, as mentioned, were circulating amongst the laity in various amended formats during the fourteenth and fifteenth centuries.[70] Henry, who had endured the life of a high-ranking soldier in his youth, was clearly motivated to write a devotional treatise of a penitential nature upon the urging of his friends and, most likely, his spiritual confessor, as well as responding to a deeply personal desire to expiate the excesses of his youth. *Le Livre* is a highly allegorical work dependent throughout on medical metaphor, in which Henry configures the seven deadly sins in terms of seven wounds or sores which can only be cured by the intervention of God as Divine Physician

65 See, The Life of Saint Sylvester in Jacobus de Voragine's *The Golden Legend* [*Legenda Aurea*], http://www.catholic-forum.com/saints/golden145.htm. For a Latin edition, see *Legenda Aurea: Vulgo Historia Lombardica Dicta ad Optimorum Librorum Fidem*, ed. Th. Grasse. Online edition at http://archive.org/details/jacobiavoragine00jacogoog. Accessed 22 July 2013.

66 The origins of this legendary practice have been traced back to an early Mithraic cult connected to the worship of the 'Great Mother', although the blood concerned was that of bulls, rather than children (or, in some cases, virgins). On this see Justus Friedrich Karl Hecker, 'An Historical Notice by Dr Hecker', *London Medical Gazette* 15 (1834), 813.

67 McCracken, *Curse of Eve*, p. 8.

68 For an astute treatment of this text, see Naoë Kukita Yoshikawa, 'Holy Medicine and Diseases of the Soul: Henry of Lancaster and *Le Livre de Seyntz Medicines*', *Medical History* 53, 3 (2009), 397–414.

69 See for example, the texts gathered together under the title *Cher Alme: Texts of Anglo-Norman Piety*, ed. Tony Hunt (Tempe, AZ, 2010). I am grateful to Catherine Batt for furnishing me with this reference.

70 On this, see Innes-Parker, 'The Legacy of *Ancrene Wisse*', pp. 145–73.

and his assistant the 'Douce Dame', presumably the Virgin Mary – and clearly a woman with strong maternal credentials. In the same way as Grimlaicus of Metz and the *Ancrene Wisse* author sought to feminise the role of the divine physician by attributing female characteristics to him or closely associating him with Mary, for Henry, this woman's nurse-like ministrations are necessary to supplement those of God-the-Physician since, in this author's estimation, 'un femme … toutz choses ly fait plus plesantement qe ne ferroit une homme' ['a woman … does everything more pleasantly than a man does'].[71] Most interestingly, perhaps, in Chapter 103 of this text, Henry draws explicitly upon the image of salvation as the therapeutic blood-bath, embellishing it to create a depiction that bears clear resonances with the post-partum bath of the Trotula text too. For Henry, the blood that runs from Christ's heart during the Passion merges with the 'eawe corante' ['running water'] of the spear-wound to provide a 'healthful' bath through which the patient – humankind – can be washed clean of all sin. In effect, in Henry's treatment, the blood-bath becomes a divine womb from which the Christian is to be 'reborn' as 'novels homes' [a new man]:

> Apres … si doit avoir un baigne pur tout laver et nettoier; et est une chose que moelt confort le malade et le fait legier et fresche, et luy doit sembler qu'il soit lavee de tout sa maladie et tout novels homes devenuz.
>
> [Afterwards he should have a bath to wash and clean everything; and this is something which much comforts the patient and makes him cheered and refreshed. Then it must seem to him that all his illness has been washed away and that he has become a new man].[72]

In the light of the traditions which I have been tracing in this essay, the medicinal and curative resonances between all of the texts I have been examining are startling, each having at its core a maternally-focused ideology of blood-based rebirth and salvation. Moreover, not only do these resonances demonstrate the extent to which such anchoritic discourse had broken free of the anchorhold walls and bounded and rebounded between the devout laity and back again, as Anne Savage has argued of anchoritic discourses and practices,[73] but they also clearly attest to an already inexorable proliferation of the devotional feminine, even before Julian began to perform her unique alchemy upon such ideas and sources at the end of the fourteenth century.

At an early stage in her own treatment of the Passion, Julian seems to be particularly mindful of a range of earlier treatments of such ideas in her

71 *Le Livre de Seyntz Medicines: The Unpublished Devotional Treatise of Henry of Lancaster*, ed. E. J. Arnould (Oxford, 1940), p. 233.

72 *Livre*, pp. 202–3.

73 Anne Savage, 'From Anchorhold to Cell of Self-Knowledge: Points along a History of the Human Body', in *Rhetoric of the Anchorhold: Space, Place and Body within the Discourses of Enclosure*, ed. Liz Herbert McAvoy (Cardiff, 2005), pp. 157–72.

famous description of the blood-flow emanating from Christ's scourged, crucified and wounded body. So thick and prolific is the blood that it threatens to make a veritable blood-bath of her own bed and sickroom:

> The hote blode ranne out so plentuously that ther was neither seen skinne ne wounde, but as it were al blode … And this was so plentuous to my sight that methought, if it had ben so in kinde and in substance for that time, it shulde have made the bedde all on bloude, and have passed over all about.[74]

As self-identified 'sinful wretch', Julian feels she is about to be bathed in Christ's blood which, like the waters of the earth, 'overfloweth al erth … redy to wash all creatures of sinne'. Moreover, again mindful of her sources, Julian attributes this cleansing blood-bath specifically to the 'tender love that he [Christ] hath to us',[75] a tender love that not only embellishes the qualities traditionally accorded the divine Physician whose medicine is his own blood, but also presents that blood again in terms of Augustine's tender *caritas*. For Julian, however, *caritas* in not a paternal quality but central to a maternal God who is the ultimate curer of humanity's ills by means of her own sacrificially flowing blood. Moreover, Julian categorically insists upon the centrality of such maternal femininity by casting her divine physician-phlebotomist as an explicitly breast-feeding one, thus exploiting the eucharistic associations of the bloody image pattern. In a passage reminiscent of Grimlaicus and Bernard, and almost certainly derivative of William Flete's configuration of God as the maternal physician, Julian's treatment produces what I shall term a eucharist of the feminine:

> The moder may geve her childe sucke her milk. But oure precious moder Jhesu, he may fede us with himself and doth full curtesly and full tenderly with the blessed sacrament that is precious fode of very life. … The moder may ley her childe tenderly to her brest. But oure tender mother Jhesu, he may homely lede us into his blessed brest by his swet, open side, and shewe us therein perty of the godhed and the joys of heven with gostely sekernesse of endlesse blisse.[76]

In recasting the workings of divine *caritas* and mercy within this feminine framework of unconditional, sacrificial and frequently *bloody* motherly love with which a human is fed and bathed, Julian utterly collapses into one another the figure of *Christus medicus* and that of the postpartum nursing mother freshly emerged from her own blood-bath in which her body has been washed clean. In so doing, she ultimately elides the boundaries between paternal and maternal, bringing to a complex – and unique – fruition the many uses of

[74] *Revelation*, 12. 3–8.

[75] *Revelation*, 12. 19–20; 10.

[76] *Revelation*, 60. 25–7.

these conceits that have gone before. In short, within the meditative space of her Norwich anchorhold, Julian pulls together a web of connections between the paternal Physician and the nurturing Mother in the production of a multi-gendered text and theology that are, indeed, the 'medicins [that] behoveth that every sinfulle soule be heled'.[77]

[77] *Revelation*, 39. 24.

5

'MAYBE I'M CRAZY?' DIAGNOSIS AND CONTEXTUALISATION OF MEDIEVAL FEMALE MYSTICS

Juliette Vuille

> Why do I struggle to understand this and similar episodes in Margery's life? It is because my twentieth-century psychiatry trained head tells me this should be madness, indeed others tell me this is madness.[1]

Although Alison Torn, the author of this statement, ultimately qualifies and contextualises her impressions, such remarks are symptomatic of many contemporary readers' unprompted reactions when studying late medieval mystical writings such as *The Book of Margery Kempe*, which Torn mentions here. In an age influenced by psychiatry and Freudian psychoanalysis, and when any writing, especially an autobiographical text, is automatically construed as cathartic and as revealing the author's mental pathology, there is indeed a strong compulsion to interpret and diagnose late medieval mystical accounts in order to understand them in terms and categories familiar to us. In the past twenty years, literary critics, psychologists and psychiatrists, working mostly in the field of the history of psychiatry, have attempted to pathologise visionary experience, especially in the case of the late fourteenth- and early fifteenth-century visionaries, Julian of Norwich and Margery Kempe, who will be the focus of this essay. Whilst such approaches provide an original point of entry into the works of these late medieval female mystics, this essay aims to identify and analyse the problems inherent to these pursuits. It will contend that scholars have often erred in their diagnostic undertakings by failing to take into consideration the important interconnectedness of the types of literary, religious and medical discourses which this essay collection places to the fore.

1 Alison Torn, 'Margery Kempe: Madwoman or Mystic – A Narrative Approach to the Representation of Madness and Mysticism in Medieval England', in *Narratives and Fiction: An Interdisciplinary Approach*, ed. David Robinson et al. (Huddersfield, 2008), pp. 79–89 (p. 86).

In their interpretations, psychiatrists and psychologists have often lacked the contextual knowledge of medieval medical understandings of madness, while medievalists have tended to misuse psychiatric diagnostics manuals. Further, critics have failed to take into account the socially constructed nature of most disorders that have no proven aetiology in the body, as well as the literary, religious and mystical traditions that constituted the basis for these women's re-interpretation of their visions as they dictated them or wrote them down. Julian of Norwich's and Margery Kempe's re-inscription of their visionary experiences within a conventional and culturally acceptable framework – experiences which they first interpret as madness – permitted them to conceive their altered states of consciousness as, paradoxically, an utterly sane 'divine insanity'.[2] Their re-contextualisation of an experience initially construed by them as insanity permits both mystics to use such 'going out of their mind' as a source of authority and expertise in their medieval community. Margery Kempe draws upon her first, acknowledged, bout of madness and her subsequent return to sanity to become an expert in madness, teaching and helping others who are similarly affected; in the same way, Julian initially envisions her altered state as a 'raving', but her re-interpretation of it as a heavenly vision enables her to be sought after for her abilities in *discretio spirituum* – the judgement of whether a mystical vision comes from God or the devil.[3] I therefore argue, in parallel with the other essays collected here, that one should approach late medieval mystical texts such as those by Margery and Julian from a multi-disciplinary standpoint. Only by doing so is it possible to produce a nuanced reading of these mystics' altered states of consciousness, one that takes into account not only psychiatric and medical discourses, but also literary and religious perspectives.

Julian of Norwich (c. 1343–after 1416) was an anchoress at the church of St Julian in that city. In 1373, she tells us that she contracts a 'bodelye syeknes' for a week, a sickness that would drive her to the point of death.[4] Her curate is

2 I use here the concept of 'divine insanity' developed by Elizabeth Clark in the context of female ascetics in late Antiquity. See her 'Sane Insanity: Women and Asceticism in Late Ancient Christianity', *Medieval Encounters* 3 (1997), 211–30.

3 On *discretio spirituum*, or the discernment of spirits, see Rosalynn Voaden, *God's Words, Women's Voices: The Discernment of Spirits in the Writing of Late-Medieval Women Visionaries* (York, 1999). While I do not contend that Margery ever became an authority on matters of *discretio spirituum* for her contemporaries, it is my belief that her re-interpretation of her altered state of consciousness as a sort of sane, divine insanity enabled her to a certain extent to effect her own *discretio spirituum* and thus lend authority to her visions. On *discretio spirituum* in the context of Margery Kempe, and especially Julian's advice to her, see Naoë Kukita Yoshikawa, *Margery Kempe's Meditations: The Context of Medieval Devotional Literature, Liturgy and Iconography* (Cardiff, 2007), pp. 62–73.

4 Julian of Norwich, *Vision*, ch. 2, lines 1–2, in *The Writings of Julian of Norwich: A Vision Showed to a Devout Woman and A Revelation of Love*, Medieval Women: Texts and Contexts 5, ed. Nicholas Watson and Jacqueline Jenkins (Turnhout, 2006). All further

sent for to give her the last rites, and as she fastens her eyes upon the crucifix he presents her, her pain abates and she experiences visions, mainly centred on the Passion. When she regains consciousness, she explicitly links her visionary experience to madness, telling a religious man at her bedside that she had been mad that day: 'then cam a religious person to me and asked me how I fared, and I saide I had raved to day'.[5] When the man interprets her altered state as a divine revelation, she is greatly ashamed to have doubted her mental health. She is then visited by devils in her sleep in punishment for her unbelief, and when she wakes up, she is given a last vision of God who confirms that her mystical experience did not arise from madness: 'witte it welle, it was na ravinge that thowe sawe today'.[6] Julian is thus comforted in her sanity through a threefold validation of her mystical experience, the *probatio* given by authorities in heaven (God), earth (the religious man) and hell (the tormenting devils). With such universal support, soon afterwards she transcribes this experience in a short text, *A Vision Showed to a Devout Woman*. Later, she undergoes further revelations and writes a longer text, *A Revelation of Love*, in the 1390s.[7]

Margery Kempe (c. 1373–after 1439) was a prosperous laywoman of King's Lynn – then Bishop's Lynn – in East Anglia. She was the daughter and wife of merchants and a mother of fourteen children, as well as a contemporary of Julian of Norwich, whom she recounts visiting in her *Book*. The *Book* tells us

references to Julian's works will be made to this edition, adopting the editors' titles (*Vision* for the short text and *Revelation* for the long text). References will be given by section/chapter and line number. Scholars have speculated on the nature of this physical illness. James McIlwain considers different possibilities, such as diphtheria, Guillain-Barre syndrome, tick paralysis and botulism, arguing in favour of the latter. Richard Lawes suggests on his part pneumonia as a more likely suspect. See McIlwain, 'The "bodelye sykenes" of Julian of Norwich', *Journal of Medieval History* 10 (1984), 167–79 and Lawes, 'Psychological Disorder and Autobiographical Impulse in Julian of Norwich, Margery Kempe and Thomas Hoccleve', in *Writing Religious Women: Female Spiritual and Textual Practices in Late Medieval England*, ed. Denis Renevey and Christiania Whitehead (Cardiff, 2000), pp. 217–43 (pp. 235–8).

5 *Revelation*, 66. 12–13. According to the *Middle English Dictionary*, the main meanings of 'raven' are 'to be or become mad' and 'to be delirious (from a fever, wound, etc.)'. Julian may be playing here on a secondary meaning of 'raven' – 'to experience religious ecstasy; see a vision' – in order to already point her audience toward the correct interpretation of her altered state of consciousness.

6 *Vision*, 22. 22–3.

7 Nicholas Watson posits a later date for the redaction of both works. He considers the possibility that the *Vision* was written ten to fifteen years later than the date hitherto accepted by scholars, and that *Revelation*, which he argues was begun as soon as the *Vision* was completed, long occupied Julian, perhaps even until her death after 1416. On this, see Watson, 'The Composition of Julian of Norwich's *Revelation of Love*', *Speculum* 68 (1993), 637–83. Whether or not such a later date of composition is accepted, it is important, in the context of this article, to note that Julian's works were the result of a long enterprise of formulation and re-interpretation of her visionary experience.

that, as a result of the birth of her first child, she becomes seriously ill, often despairing for her life. Believing she will die, she sends for a priest to hear her confession and administer extreme unction. As the priest is 'a lytyl to hastye' and does not let her finish recounting the sin she intended to confess, she goes 'owt of hir mende' and is assaulted by devils for more than eight months.[8] She verbally attacks her family and friends, attempts to injure herself and for this reason is tied to her bed. Subsequently, she has a vision of Christ who at once heals her of her madness. After this initial vision, she often 'dallies' with Christ and different saints, and has visual, olfactory and auditory visionary experiences. From this point onward, her unusual displays of devotion are marked by her gift of tears and a gift of crying out and roaring, received initially during her pilgrimage to Jerusalem.[9] This behaviour often leads to her being slandered by her contemporaries, who rebuke her for her disruptive conduct. However, her problematic actions are never interpreted by them as madness; instead, they prefer to ascribe it to a possession by the devil, a physical illness or even heresy.[10]

In this way, when Julian of Norwich and Margery Kempe suffer the physical illnesses that lead to their first visionary encounter with the divine, they initially believe themselves to be mad but, after this first experience, both women recover and never fear madness again, nor do their contemporaries suspect them of madness. Their subsequent altered states of consciousness are interpreted variously as mystical experience, possession by the devil, heresy, or as having a physical origin. Divine insanity and demonic possession are therefore seen by their contemporaries as separate from a madness rooted in the body, even if the manifestations or symptoms are similar, making it difficult especially for Margery's peers to decide between a spiritual or a physical aetiology for her behaviour. Julian, after her first doubts, and Margery, after her first bout of madness, strive to present their altered states of consciousness as arising from a spiritual, mystical experience, rather than madness, a term which, alongside the more common 'woodness', was in the medieval period more generally reserved for the medical conditions of mania or melancholia, and was rooted in the body.

8 *The Book of Margery Kempe* (henceforth *BMK*), Book I, ch. 1, p. 7, in *The Book of Margery Kempe*, ed. Sanford Brown Meech and Hope Emily Allen, EETS o.s. 212 (London, 1940). All further references will be to this edition, by book, chapter and page number.

9 '& sche had so gret compassyon & so gret peyn to se owyr Lordys peyn þat sche myt not kepe hir-self fro krying & roryng þow sche xuld a be ded þerfor. And þis was þe first cry þat euyr sche cryed in any contemplacyon.' *BMK*, I, 28, 68.

10 Some say, due to her relentless screaming, that she has contracted the 'fallyng euyl' (*BMK*, I, 44, 105), an illness nowadays associated with *grand-mal* epilepsy, or a 'cardiakyl er sum oþer sekenesse' (*BMK*, I, 61, 151), the 'cardiakyl' being characterised by pain in the heart, palpitation, feebleness, profuse sweating and excess of emotions (MED s.v. 'cardiacle').

Indeed, our notion of how medieval medicine understood and dealt with mental disorders has evolved greatly in the past few decades. The different Greek theories of the body and the soul trickled down to the later medieval period by way of Latin compilations and Arabic medical writers, such as Haly Abbas, Rhazes and Avicenna, who endorsed and reformulated the medical theories of their Greek forefathers.[11] Medieval medical writers were thus knowledgeable in Hippocratic, Aristotelian and Galenic views of mental disorders. Although medieval theorists saw the soul as immortal and immaterial, it was not unusual for them to think that it could be cured by treating its main functioning organ, the brain, or more generally the body.[12] When a mental disorder manifested itself, it was believed to originate from an imbalance in the humours (for example, an excess of black bile in the case of melancholia), and treated accordingly by acting upon the body. Treatments included medication, a particular diet and regimen of exercise and rest, dry cupping, bloodletting or baths.[13] Hildegard of Bingen, for instance, saw madness as being caused by an excessive coldness of the brain, and advised it be treated with the application of a *deich*/paste containing laurel powder, blessed-thistle water, and wheat flour on the patient's head in order to bring warmth to the brain.[14] Medieval scholars therefore believed in a strong connection between physical illness and mental illness, be it mania or melancholia, and conversely conceived that spiritual diseases of the soul, linked with sin and vices, could have an effect on the body.[15] Leprosy, for example, was often believed to arise from a tendency to lechery.[16] For this

11 Stanley W. Jackson, *Melancholia and Depression: From Hippocratic Times to Modern Times* (New Haven, CT and London, 1986), p. 48.

12 Ángel González De Pablo and N. J. R. Evans, 'The Medicine of the Soul: The Origin and Development of Thought on the Soul, Diseases of the Soul and their Treatment in Medieval and Renaissance Medicine', *History of Psychiatry* 5 (1994), 483–516 (p. 489).

13 De Pablo and Evans, 'The Medicine of the Soul', p. 504. See also Naoë Kukita Yoshikawa, 'Holy Medicine and Diseases of the Soul: Henry of Lancaster and *Le Livre de Seyntz Medicines*', *Medical History* 53, 3 (2009), 397–414. Yoshikawa notably mentions the fact that Henry prescribes the topical application of a freshly killed cockerel to cure his own delirium (pp. 408–9).

14 Hildegard of Bingen, *Liber subtilitatum diuersarum naturarum creaturarum*, trans. on the basis of Copenhagen, Royal Library, MS Ny Kongelige Samling 90b by Margaret Berger, in her *Hildegard of Bingen: On Natural Philosophy and Medicine, Selections from* Cause et cure (Cambridge, 1999), p. 106.

15 On the interconnectedness between physical and mental illness, soul and the body, see also Muriel Laharie, *La folie au Moyen Âge: xie-xiiie siècles* (Paris, 1991).

16 On this, see Saul Nathaniel Brody, *The Disease of the Soul: Leprosy in Medieval Literature* (Ithaca, NY and London, 1974), pp. 101–6, and Carole Rawcliffe, *Leprosy in Medieval England* (Woodbridge, 2006). The link between lechery and leprosy can be exemplified, for instance, in the lecherous behaviour of Margery's son and his subsequent punishment with a disease resembling leprosy.

reason, the physical treatment for both mental and physical illnesses was sometimes complemented by a 'religious therapy' that involved confession and penance.[17]

This brief overview informs us of a few of the interpretations and reactions that the mystics and the people they encountered formulated for their visionary experiences. This, for instance, explains why Margery's contemporaries always posited a physical, not a mental, illness to explain her peculiar behaviour. Further, Julian interprets the visions experienced during her physical illness as madness as soon as she regains consciousness, due to the strong interconnectedness between mental and physical illness. Finally, as mentioned elsewhere in this volume, the link made between sin and imbalance of the body and mind elucidates why Margery interprets her failed confession as the initial cause for her madness.[18]

In this context, one can understand why neither the religious man at Julian's bedside nor the witnesses of Margery's roaring and crying ever believe them to be mad in the medieval understanding of madness, that is to say, manic or melancholic. It is only in the twentieth century that scholars have attempted to ascribe a psychiatric diagnosis to the mystical experiences of both Julian of Norwich and Margery Kempe. Robert Thouless posits that Julian's visions were hallucinations showing a precarious mental balance.[19] Richard Lawes agrees with Thouless's assersion that Julian experienced hallucinations, which, according to him, were the 'psychological effects of physical illness'.[20] Conrad Pepler, on his part, thinks that Julian's visions arose from an 'extreme pathological state' which caused her to be 'delirious' and to suffer an 'acute neurosis induced perhaps by an over-enthusiastic life of penance and solitude'.[21] As early as 1671, Julian's visionary experience had been linked with hysteria: Edward Stillingfleet termed her a '*Hysterical* Gossip' whose text was but 'blasphemous and senseless tittle tattle'.[22] Later critics have considered such a diagnosis for Julian of Norwich, but have more often than not rejected it: for George Tyrrell, the 'unity and coherence' of her texts demonstrates a 'life-long habit of active mental control, such as excludes the supposition of an hysterical temperament',[23] while Paul Molinari, who carries out a sort of modern, rationalist *discretio spirituum* with regard to Julian's showings, rejects neurosis and hysteria as diagnoses, since these would depreciate her visions,

17 De Pablo and Evans, 'The Medicine of the Soul', p. 510.

18 *BMK*, I, 1, 7.

19 Robert H. Thouless, *The Lady Julian: A Psychological Study* (London, 1924).

20 Lawes, 'Psychological Disorder', p. 239.

21 Conrad Pepler, *The English Religious Heritage* (London, 1958), p. 312.

22 Edward Stillingfleet, *A Discourse Concerning the Idolatry…* (London, 1671), p. 260, cited in *The Writings of Julian of Norwich*, p. 453.

23 George Tyrrell, 'Julian of Norwich', *The Faith of the Millions* (London, 1901), http://www.gutenberg.org/files/10139/10139.txt [accessed 15 March 2014].

and attempts to prove that they had a divine aetiology.[24] Scholars, therefore, have recently considered that diagnosing Julian with a mental illness would diminish the value of her teachings, and have thus rejected such readings on the basis of authenticity, structure or clarity. Only Stillingfleet could deem Julian a hysteric, as his rejection of Roman Catholicism led him to discredit Julian's visions too, thereby revealing one of the reasons behind scholars' impulse to diagnose Julian and Margery: if one rejects the tenets of Roman Catholicism, or even the existence of a Christian God, one is only left with science and medicine to rationalise these women's mystical states.

Furthermore, while recent scholarship has claimed to move away from an often-deemed antiquated qualitative criticism of literary works, some academics' decision to avoid attempting to symptomatise Julian of Norwich's visions because of their respect for the originality, structure or clarity of her prose indicates that they are still very much guided in their criticism by aesthetic considerations: good literature cannot have been produced by a madwoman. This state of affairs is offset by the very different treatment several contemporary critics have reserved for Margery Kempe. Margery, whose intelligence and education have often been disparaged and belittled, and in whose *Book* they have failed to tease out any structure or clarity of thought, has not escaped recent attempts at diagnosis. Margery has therefore repeatedly been categorised as a hysteric.[25] Edmund Colledge calls her a 'morbid neurotic' and an 'incurable hysteric with a large paranoid trend' whose contemporaries dismissed her as a 'hysterical epileptic',[26] and Nancy Partner adopts a Freudian reading of the *Book* whereby her hysteria is the expression of her alleged incestuous love for her father.[27] Other scholars following this trend include Hope Emily Allen, William Ober, Hope Weissman and Julia Long, among others.[28] With the advent of the

24 Paul Molinari, *Julian of Norwich: The Teaching of a 14th-Century English Mystic* (London, 1958).

25 The popularity of this interpretation can to some extent be explained by the fact that the *Book of Margery Kempe* was rediscovered in 1934, when psychoanalytic literary criticism was most fashionable.

26 Eric Colledge, 'Margery Kempe', in *Pre-Reformation English Spirituality*, ed. James Walsh (New York, 1966), pp. 210–23 (214–15).

27 Nancy Partner, 'Reading the *Book of Margery Kempe*', *Exemplaria* 3 (1991), 29–66.

28 See Hope Emily Allen's 'Introduction' in *The Book of Margery Kempe*; David Knowles, *The English Mystical Tradition* (London, 1964), pp. 147–9; Justin McCann, 'The Book of Margery Kempe', *The Dublin Review* 200 (1937), 103–16 (pp. 110–13); William Ober, 'Margery Kempe: Hysteria and Mysticism Reconciled', *Literature and Medicine* 4 (1985), 24–40; Hope Weissman, 'Margery Kempe in Jerusalem: *Hysterica Compassio* in the Late Middle Ages', in *Acts of Interpretation: The Text and its Contexts, 700–1600*, ed. Mary J. Carruthers and Elizabeth D. Kirk (Norman, OK, 1982), pp. 201–17; Trudi Drucker, 'The Malaise of Margery Kempe', *New York State Journal of Medicine* 72 (1972), 2911–16; Julia Long, 'Mysticism and Hysteria: The Histories of Margery Kempe and Anna O.', in *Feminist Readings in Middle English Literature: The Wife of Bath and All Her Sect*,

Diagnostic and Statistical Manual of Mental Disorders III (DSM III) in 1980, the clinical manifestations that had until then been subsumed under the hysteria label developed by Charcot and Freud were assigned to different 'disorders': somatisation, conversion, dissociative and histrionic personality disorders, the latter corresponding best, according to critics, to Margery Kempe's experience.[29] Other diagnoses range from mental illnesses such as neurosis, bipolar disorder, puerperial psychosis or depressive psychosis of the puerperium, and schizoaffective psychosis,[30] to physical illnesses which have an effect on the mind: Tourette's syndrome or temporal lobe epilepsy.[31] Such a plethora of diagnoses not only reflects the difficulty of using a mystical treatise as the basis for a psychiatric evaluation, but also suggests that such an undertaking may lead to a variety of results depending on the approach selected.

It is not within the purview of this essay to argue whether or not Margery Kempe suffered from temporal lobe epilepsy, or if Julian of Norwich's visions were caused by her fever. The goal is rather to foreground and critique the different approaches selected by scholars who attempt to pathologise Julian and Margery, in order to highlight the potential problems inherent in such undertakings. First and foremost, it is important to note that the division of hysteria into the aforementioned four disorders is a testimony to the fact

ed. Ruth Evans and Lesley Johnson (New York and London, 1994), pp. 88–111. For a useful summary of these diagnoses, see David Aers, 'The Making of Margery Kempe: Individual and Community', in *The Book of Margery Kempe*, ed. and trans. Lynn Staley (New York and London, 2001), pp. 256–64.

29 American Psychiatric Association, *Diagnostic and Statistical Manual of Mental Disorders* DSM-V (Washington, DC, 2013), dsm.psychiatryonline.org [accessed 15 March 2014]. For Margery as suffering from histrionic personality disorder, see notably Mary Farley, 'Her Own Creature: Religion, Feminist Criticism, and the Functional Eccentricity of Margery Kempe', *Exemplaria* 11 (1999), 1–21. Richard Lawes also considers this diagnosis, only to reject it: see his 'The Madness of Margery Kempe', in *The Medieval Mystical Tradition, England, Ireland and Wales*, ed. Marion Glasscoe (Cambridge, 1999), pp. 147–68 (pp. 150–2).

30 For neurosis, see Sheila Delany, 'Sexual Economics, Chaucer's Wife of Bath and *The Book of Margery Kempe*', in *Feminist Readings in Middle English Literature,* pp. 72–87. Phyllis R. Freeman, Carley R. Bogarad and Diane E. Sholomskas argue that she suffered from bipolar disorder and post-partum psychosis: see their essay 'Margery Kempe, a New Theory: The Inadequacy of Hysteria and Postpartum Psychosis as Diagnostic Categories', *History of Psychiatry* 1 (1990), 169–90. Lawes, in 'The Madness of Margery Kempe', argues for a depressive psychosis of the puerperium. Gordon Claridge, Ruth Pryor and Gwen Watkins make use of the SADSL-L (Schedule for Affective Disorders and Schizophrenia-Lifetime Version) in order to diagnose Margery with schizoaffective psychosis: see their volume *Sounds From the Bell Jar: Ten Psychotic Authors* (Basingstoke, 1990).

31 For Tourette's Syndrome, see Nancy Stork, 'Did Margery Kempe Suffer from Tourette's Syndrome?', *Mediaeval Studies* 59 (1997), 261–300. For temporal lobe epilepsy, see Lawes, 'The Madness of Margery Kempe', and his 'Psychological Disorder'.

that psychiatric discourse is an ever-evolving one.[32] Further, the meaning of hysteria itself has evolved and continues to change, from that posited by the Greeks in Antiquity to definitions of the present day by way of Charcot and Freud. In this way, diagnosing a medieval mystic with 'current' mental disorders is of little use, since such categorisation is an epistemological one often pertinent to a specific moment and therefore tells us much less about late medieval mystics' madness than it does about psychiatric advances at the time of the scholar's interpretation. Lawes, for instance, criticises his predecessors for 'invoking outdated psychiatric concepts', contrasting their method with his, based on 'current psychiatric practice'.[33] This represents a Whig interpretation of psychiatric history, which, according to Peter Sedgwick, is a 'liberal, evolutionist and sympathetic [perspective on] modern diagnostic categories as the criterion of reality against which earlier discoveries are to be tested and found wanting'.[34] Phyllis Freeman, Carley Bogarad and Diane Sholomskas have attempted to bypass such a pitfall by pathologising Margery's visionary experience through medieval medicine, arguing she suffered from episodes of both mania and melancholia, only then equating these medieval concepts with the modern notion of bipolar cyclical disorder. However, they have failed to recognise the fact that *The Book of Margery Kempe* is not written as a chronological narrative, but rather adopts the structure of a conversion narrative, which renders difficult their evaluation of melancholic and manic cycles.[35] Further, their evidence appears inadequate, notably for their diagnosis of mania. For instance, they mention Margery's successful business venture as a brewer for three to four years, and the 'self-inflated manner' with which she boasts of her success, as evidence of 'mania-like behaviour'.[36] Were she truly manic, it is doubtful her business would have lasted so long, and attracted such success.[37]

Not only is the nomenclature used by these critics dependent on time, it is also dependent on the culture or locale that formulates them. For instance, the terminology of disorders previously associated with hysteria in the *Diagnostic and Statistical Manual of Mental Disorders V* (DSM V) issued by

32 Indeed, psychiatry itself is a relatively new term, coined only in 1808 by the German physician Johann Christian Reil. On this, see Andreas Marneros, 'Psychiatry's 200th Birthday', *The British Journal of Psychiatry* 193 (2008), 1–3.

33 Lawes, 'The Madness of Margery Kempe', p. 147.

34 Peter Sedgwick, *Psycho Politics* (London, 1982), p. 129.

35 For *The Book of Margery Kempe* as a conversion narrative, see Juliette Vuille, '"I wolde I wer as worthy to ben sekyr of thy lofe as Mary Mawdelyn was": The Magdalene as an Authorizing Tool in the *Book of Margery Kempe*', in *Mary Magdalene in Medieval Culture: Conflicted Roles*, ed. Peter Loewen and Robin Waugh (London, 2014), pp. 208–25 (pp. 211–12). For a good case of the *Book* being structured to highlight Margery's development as a *sponsa Christi*, see Yoshikawa, *Margery Kempe's Meditations*.

36 Freeman, Bogarad and Sholomskas, 'Margery Kempe: A New Theory', p. 186.

37 For a similar criticism, see Stork, 'Tourette's Syndrome?', p. 276.

the American Psychiatric Association, is different from that found in ICD 10, the *International Statistical Classification of Diseases: Classification of Mental and Behavioural Disorders*, published by the World Health Organisation and primarily used in Europe.[38] These cultural and historical factors, and the concomitant changes in nomenclature, are particularly important when the disorders have – at least as yet – no provable cause in the body, as is the case for most of the mental illnesses attributed by critics to Julian and Margery. A good example of this is the contemporary notion of 'anorexia nervosa', often paralleled with medieval anorexia, or 'holy anorexia',[39] a phenomenon which diametrically differs from its modern counterpart: medieval anorexia was not considered an illness, although it was sometimes frowned upon by male clerics, and was often used by late medieval women as a way to express their sainthood or the validity of their visionary experience.

Only two scholars, among those who have attempted to diagnose Julian and Margery, have found a biological aetiology to the mystics' visionary experience, thus ascribing to them pathologies which must have existed in much the same form in the medieval period as now, although the expression and interpretation of similar symptoms may be very different depending on the period, and must be culturally informed. For instance, Stork offers an interesting reading of Margery Kempe's behaviour, arguing that she suffered from Tourette's syndrome.[40] While this diagnosis would neatly 'explain' Margery's inability to refrain from expressing her devotion through the body, notably when she screams,[41] Stork's interpretation that Margery's unconfessed sin at the beginning of the *Book* might have been coprolalia, that is, the compulsion to repeat expressions, often obscene in nature, is rather far-fetched.[42] Further, her decision to undertake a

38 World Health Organization, *ICD 10: International Statistical Classification of Diseases and Related Health Problems: Classification of Mental and Behavioural Disorders* (Geneva, 1992–94). The main difference between the DSM V and the ICD 10 is that in the latter dissociative and conversion disorders are classified together, with dissociation being conceived as the primary phenomenon.

39 The problematic term 'holy anorexia' was coined by Rudolph Bell, in his *Holy Anorexia* (Chicago, IL and London, 1985). See also Caroline Walker Bynum, *Holy Feast and Holy Fast: The Religious Significance of Food to Medieval Women* (Los Angeles and London, 1987).

40 Stork, 'Tourette's Syndrome?', 261–300. For a criticism of Stork's diagnosis, see Lawes, 'Psychological Disorder', p. 242 n. 32.

41 For an interpretation of the expression of Kempe's devotion through the body in the context of late medieval mysticism, see Denis Renevey, 'Margery's Performing Body: The Translation of Late Medieval Discursive Religious Practices', in *Writing Religious Women*, ed. Renevey and Whitehead, pp. 197–216.

42 A more likely interpretation of the nature of Margery's unconfessed sin is that it was heretical in content, something that is supported by the priest's reluctance to let Margery finish her confession. Private communication with Sarah Salih and Jocelyn Wogan-Browne, 30 May 2013.

quantitative rather than a qualitative survey of contemporary mystical sources in order to define which traits of Margery's behaviour were 'normal' or 'abnormal' is misguided due to the fragmentary nature of the evidence available to us for this period. Finally, Stork succumbs to one of the most widespread failings of studies attempting to pathologise medieval mystics, that is in only considering the parts of the texts that best 'fit' a diagnosis, silencing other textual moments which would serve to invalidate it. In the case of *The Book of Margery Kempe*, for instance, Margery describes the evolution of the physical manifestations of her affective devotion, from her gift of tears to her unrestrained crying and roaring. Stork's decision to consider Margery's loud fits of crying as the main expression of Tourette's syndrome fails to acknowledge such a development.

Richard Lawes also offers an interpretation of Julian and Margery's visions as being caused by physical illnesses, probably pneumonia in Julian's case, and post-partum psychosis as well as temporal lobe epilepsy in Margery's.[43] Lawes offers a thoughtful medical interpretation of the two mystics, aware and careful of the dangers such analyses pose. In particular, he reflects on the impact of cultural and historical changes, and discusses the fact that the texts studied are not even remotely intended for a diagnosis and that the symptoms described constitute interpretations after the fact within a conventional and recognisable mould of the medieval mystical tradition.

The main reservation one can have with regard to Lawes' approach is his choice to enlist the help of contemporary psychiatric statistical manuals, such as the DSM and the SADSL-L, in order to formulate a diagnosis.[44] This is a problematic endeavour, as the *caveat* in the introduction to the DSM-IV (used by Lawes and Farley) points out that it should only be used in a clinical context, by trained professionals:

> DSM-IV is a classification of mental disorders that was developed for use in clinical, educational, and research settings. The diagnostic categories, criteria, and textual descriptions are meant to be employed by individuals with appropriate clinical training and experience in diagnosis. It is important that DSM-IV not be employed mechanically by untrained individuals. The specific diagnostic criteria included in DSM-IV are meant to serve as guidelines to be informed by clinical judgment and are not to be used in a cookbook fashion.[45]

In this context, Lawes's remark that the terms Hoccleve uses to describe his mental state in the Prologue to the *Regiment of Princes* 'fit very well with

43 Lawes, 'Psychological Disorder'.

44 Such manuals are used by Lawes in his 'Psychological Disorder' and his 'The Madness of Margery Kempe', as well as by Farley, in 'Her Own Creature' and by Claridge, Pryor and Watkins in *Sounds from the Bell Jar*.

45 American Psychiatric Association, *Diagnostic and Statistical Manual of Mental Disorders* (Washington, D.C, 2000), p. xxiii.

modern diagnostic manuals'[46] presents a problematic, 'cookbook' desire to arrange medieval manifestations into more or less corresponding categories in the DSM-IV. One may remark, in addition, that the DSM-IV precludes diagnosing a mental illness when the behaviour of the subject is considered habitual or acceptable in his or her culture:

> A clinician who is unfamiliar with the nuances of an individual's cultural frame of reference may incorrectly judge as psychopathology those normal variations in behavior, belief, or experience that are particular to the individual's culture. For example, certain religious practices or beliefs ... may be misdiagnosed as manifestations of a Psychotic Disorder.[47]

In this way, although Margery's behaviour sometimes irritated her contemporaries, both Julian and Margery's visionary experiences were accepted by the majority, and understood by many to fall within an established tradition of mystical visions and revelations, and thus would simply not be recognised as mental disorders by the DSM-IV.

Indeed, most critics disregard the literary genre from which they draw the symptoms that will eventually help them form a diagnosis. Julian and Margery are influenced in their accounts of their altered states of consciousness by the traditional way of representing such visions and revelations within the genre of the medieval mystical tradition.[48] The fact that Margery's detractors often tend to refer to her *Book* as the first autobiography in the English language rather than as the work of a mystic is perhaps symptomatic of their reluctance to consider her writing in the light of other mystical works, preferring to associate it with a genre linked, at least since Freud, with madness and the cathartic impulse to self-medicate through one's autobiographical writing.[49] A good instance of this is Lawes, who privileges the genre of autobiography over that of the mystical treatise in his 1999 article, revealingly entitled 'Psychological Disorder and Autobiographical Impulse'. While he notes the importance of literary genre on the portrayal of symptoms, and mentions the

46 Lawes, 'Psychological Disorder', pp. 224–5.

47 DSM-IV, p. xxiv.

48 Many critics have considered these visionaries, notably Margery, in the context of late medieval mystical writings. See, for instance, Allen's notes to her edition of *The Book* and her introduction, pp. lviii–lix; Susan Dickman, 'Margery Kempe and the Continental Tradition of the Pious Woman', in *The Medieval Mystical Tradition in England*, ed. Marion Glasscoe (Cambridge, 1984), pp. 150–68; and Janette Dillon, 'Holy Women and their Confessors or Confessors and their Holy Women? Margery Kempe and Continental Tradition', in *Prophets Abroad: The Reception of Continental Holy Women in Late-Medieval England*, ed. Rosalynn Voaden (Cambridge, 1996), pp. 115–40.

49 On the opposition between mystical and autobiographical, and the gendered bias that leads some critics to associate women with the latter genre, see Karma Lochrie, *Margery Kempe and Translations of the Flesh* (Philadelphia, PA, 1991), pp. 61, 226.

influence of the mystical tradition on his sources, he defends his diagnostic approach by stating that 'cultural contexts and conventions are always involved in mediating accounts of psychiatric symptoms ... in all ages and societies, whether the accounts are oral or written'.[50] However, his defence does not seem sufficient. The mediation that can be observed between a psychiatrist and his patient is not at all comparable to the mediation that is involved in the recovery of symptoms in treatises such as that of Julian or Margery, who follow different conventions and aims, for instance, those of presenting their visions as acceptable and authoritative. For this purpose, they structure and interpret the memory of their visionary experiences alongside cultural and literary guidelines that encourage them to emphasise certain aspects or manifestations of their altered state.[51]

In this context, Margery's tendency to tears, sobbing and crying out loud is explained by Lawes as an indication that she suffered from temporal lobe epilepsy, corresponding to the seventh of the eight main symptoms he retains as indicators of this illness: 'People may laugh or cry during a seizure'.[52] However, notwithstanding the fact that Margery only cries, and never laughs, during her altered state experiences, the recurrence of the topos in her *Book* is highly unusual: she is said to weep more than 200 times and to cry loudly not less than 180 times.[53] Even if these emotional outbursts had been triggered by temporal lobe epilepsy, such emphasis can only be explained through Margery's conscious imitation of the gift of tears given to continental mystics such as Marie d'Oignies and Elizabeth of Hungary, who are both explicitly mentioned by her amanuensis as precedents and validations for her displays of emotion:

> he louyd hir more & trustyd more to hir wepyng & hir crying þan euyr he ded be-forn, for aftyrward he red of a woman clepyd Maria de Oegines & ... & of þe plentyuows teerys þat sche wept, þe which made hir so febyl & so weyke þat sche myth not endur to beheldyn þe Crosse, ne heryn owr Lordys Passyon rehersyd, so sche was resoluyd in-to terys of pyte & compassion. ... Also, Elizabeth of Hungry cryed wyth lowed voys, as is wretyn in hir tretys.[54]

50 Lawes, 'Psychological Disorder', p. 223.

51 On Margery Kempe and her use of memory in the process of composition of the *Book*, see Yoshikawa, *Margery Kempe's Meditations*, notably p. 1, where she argues that 'the *Book* unfolds to the reader a creative experience of memory in which meditation functions as a spiritual mnemonic'.

52 Lawes, 'The Madness of Margery Kempe', p. 158.

53 Stork, 'Tourette's Syndrome?', p. 283.

54 *BMK*, I, 62, 152–4. For Margery's gift of tears as *imitatio* of earlier saints than Marie d'Oignies and Elizabeth of Hungary, notably Mary Magdalene and the Virgin Mary, see Susan Eberly, 'Margery Kempe, St. Mary Magdalene, and Patterns of Contemplation', *The Downside Review* 368 (1989), 209–23; Vuille, '"I wolde I wer"', pp. 216–17 and Liz Herbert McAvoy, *The Book of Margery Kempe: An Abridged Translation, Translated from the Middle English with Introduction, Notes, and Interpretive Essay* (Cambridge, 2003), pp. 105–26.

Margery's irrepressible weeping and loud crying, seen by Lawes and Stork as evidence of epilepsy or Tourette's syndrome, seem indeed quite conventional when paralleled with Marie d'Oignies and her own gift of tears. Both the *Life of Marie d'Oignies* and *The Book of Margery Kempe* echo each other by presenting their tears in the same terms: while Margery feels 'compunccyon wyth gret plenté of teerys', Marie is said to be blessed with 'so mykel grace of compunxyone, so grete plente of terys'.[55] Furthermore, neither Margery nor Marie is able to restrain her weeping, which increases if they attempt to do so. Criticised for their unbecoming behaviour, both prove that they cannot help their outcries by means of a miracle: others are temporarily gifted with their *gratia lacrimarum*, and find themselves unable to restrain their tears in the same way as the mystics. This validates Margery's and Marie's outbursts.[56]

Other visionary experiences which scholars have often interpreted as symptoms of mental illness may have been brought about by a fashion for a certain type of vision, such as Margery's vision of the Eucharist shaking and flickering in the hands of the priest in the manner of a dove:

> On a day as this creatur was heryng hir messe, a yong man and a good prest heldyng up the sacrament in hys handys ovyr hys hed, the sacrament schok and flekeryd to and fro as a dowe flekeryth wyth hir wengys. And, whan he held up the chalys wyth the precyows sacrament, the chalys mevyd to and fro as it schuld a fallyn owt of hys handys ... Than seyd owyr Lord Jhesu Crist to the creatur, 'Thow schalt no mor sen it in this maner, therfor thank God that thow hast seyn. My dowtyr, Bryde, say me nevyr in this wyse.'[57]

55 *BMK*, I, 32, 80. *Life of Marie d'Oignies* I, ch. 5, in *Three Women of Liège: A Critical Edition of and Commentary on the Middle English Lives of Elizabeth of Spalbeek, Christina Mirabilis, and Marie d'Oignies*, ed. Jennifer Brown (Turnhout, 2008), p. 92. Oxford, Bodleian Library, MS Douce 114, the manuscript containing the lives of Marie d'Oignies, Elizabeth of Spalbeek and Christina Mirabilis, is dated c. 1420–50. It is therefore possible to evoke the intriguing likelihood that these lives circulated at a time when Julian of Norwich and Margery Kempe were still alive, and perhaps that Margery had access to the *Life of Marie d'Oignies* and was able to reproduce the conventional formulation of Marie's gift of tears to describe her own weeping in *The Book*.

56 Compare, for instance, both women's inability to abstain from weeping in *BMK*, I, 78, 185 and *Three Women*, p. 93. Similarly, the two mystics imbue others with the grace of weeping in *BMK*, I, 45, 108 and *Three Women*, p. 93. A miracle similar to that effected by Marie and Margery is also mentioned in *BMK*, I, 68, 165–6, and in the 'Lyf of Saint Katherin of Senis', ed. Carl Horstmann, *Archiv für das Studium der neueren Sprachen und Litteraturen* 76 (1886), 33–112, 265–314 and 353–91 (p. 266). Elizabeth of Hungary cannot hold back her tears and her loud crying either: 'soo bytterly she weped that she myght not wyth-holde her from vtterly sobbynges and cryenges wyth voyce'. See Horstmann (ed.), 'The Reuelacions of Saynt Elysabeth of Hungary', *Archiv für das Studium der neueren Sprachen und Litteraturen* 76 (1886), 392–400.

57 *BMK*, I, 20, 47.

This episode is interpreted by Lawes as being caused by the distorted perception that often accompanies epilepsy.[58] However, Caroline Walker Bynum has demonstrated that the rise of eucharistic devotion from the thirteenth century onward went hand in hand with an increase in the number of eucharistic miracles, and that female mystics were most often the recipients of such miracles. The tradition of hanging a pyx in the shape of a dove above the altar caused, she explains, 'some mystics to think they saw the Holy Spirit winging toward them, the wafer in his beak'.[59] Margery Kempe's gift of tears and her inability to restrain her crying, as well as the eucharistic vision often cited by critics to support diverse diagnoses, therefore appear to be utterly conventional when paralleled with contemporary mystical literature.

As already noted, Stork and others often fail to consider Julian's and Margery's visionary experiences as a whole, preferring to fragment them into short passages which illustrate the symptoms which they wish to categorise. However, such an approach does not reflect the fact that any account of a visionary experience in late medieval mystical writings follows a strict pattern of development that needs to be considered in its entirety. Only by so doing is it possible to realise that what these critics see as disconnected 'symptoms' actually changes over time to represent the spiritual growth of Julian and Margery as mystics. For instance, Margery's gift of tears does not transform into loud cries until her pilgrimage to Jerusalem. Julian's and Margery's first visionary experiences echo each other and follow a conventional and well-rehearsed pattern that can be teased out of other accounts of female mystics across the Channel. Julian and Margery first experience an altered state of consciousness and go 'out of their minds', when they are physically ill, to the point of death:

> And when I was thirty yere old and a halfe, God sent me a *bodily sickness* in the which I ley three days and three nightes, and on the fourth night I toke all my rightes of holy church, *and wened not to have liven till day*. And after this I langorid forth two days and two nightes, and on the third night *I wened oftentimes to have passed, and so wened they that were with me.*[60]
>
> And, aftyr that sche had conceyved, sche was labowrd wyth grett accessys tyl the chyld was born, and than, what for labowr sche had in chyldyng and for sekenesse goyng beforn, *sche dyspered of hyr lyfe, wenyng sche mygth not levyn.*[61]

Such a state was virtually a prerequisite for visionary experience as it is seen in the conventional accounts of nuns' ecstatic and visionary experiences of the late thirteenth and early fourteenth century, known as *nonnenbücher*[62] and in the

58 Lawes, 'The Madness of Margery Kempe', p. 160.

59 Bynum, *Holy Feast*, p. 60.

60 *Revelation*, 3, 1–5, my emphasis.

61 *BMK*, I, 1, 6, my emphasis.

62 On *nonnenbücher*, see notably Gertrud Jaron Lewis, *By Women, For Women, About*

popular lives of Elizabeth of Spalbeek or Christina Mirabilis.[63] Although Julian tells us that she 'desired never no bodily sight ne no maner shewing of God',[64] she expresses a desire for a bodily sickness before it occurs, and places emphasis on the fact that this illness should be accompanied by a near-death experience, requesting that she and others believe herself to be dying.[65] This leads us to the interesting hypothesis that she may in fact have desired this particular type of bodily sickness to the point of death, knowing that such an experience was usually conducive to a visionary experience in mystical literature.

Julian of Norwich's slowly spreading paralysis during her illness is another symptom which has led critics to shed much ink in their effort to reach a diagnosis: 'thus I indured till day, and by then was my body dead from the middes downward, as to my feeling … After this the over part of my body began to die, so farforth that unneth I had any feeling.'[66] This can be paralleled with the experiences of countless other late medieval mystics: Elizabeth of Spalbeek, for example, 'is raueshed or sche ryse fro hir bedde, and sche abydeth in the same staat that sche is rauisched in a good while alle starke as an ymage of tree or stoon withouten felynge or mouynge and brethe'.[67] Julian and Elizabeth also make use of iconographical representations of the Passion – a crucifix for Julian, and a 'tabil ful wele depeynte with an ymage of oure Lorde crucifyed' for Elizabeth,[68] as the springboard for their visionary experiences.

The resolution of Margery's and Julian's illnesses, and the end of their mystical encounter with the divine, also share the same pattern as other visionary accounts. Julian and Elizabeth of Spalbeek experience alongside their visions a very sudden abating of their physical pain, while Margery is suddenly made whole by her vision of Christ. Both Julian and Margery share with other mystics, for instance Catherine of Siena, the pattern of having visions of God and then visions of fiends or demonic temptations in order

Women: The Sister-Books of Fourteenth-Century Germany (Toronto, 1996). On the conventions of female mystics' *vitae*, especially in the *nonnenbücher*, see Bynum, *Holy Feast*, pp. 83–4.

63 For Elizabeth of Spalbeek and Christina Mirabilis, whose near-death experience is so extreme that her friends actually believe her dead and take her body to the church before she comes back from her vision, see *Three Women*, pp. 32–3, 57. Christina Mirabilis, like Margery Kempe, is believed mad and possessed by devils, and bound with 'chaynes of yren' (p. 57). Catherine of Siena tells her confessor that 'the hyghest comfort that I haue, is whan I suffre ony dysease: for that I shall haue the perfyte vysyon of god': see 'The Lyf of Katheryn of Senis', p. 279.

64 *Revelation*, 3, 41.

65 'Wenande myselfe that I shulde die, and that alle creatures that sawe me might wene the same': *Vision*, 1, 24–5.

66 *Revelation*, 3, 14–29.

67 *Three Women*, p. 29. See also 'Lyf of Katheryn of Senis', pp. 88, 265.

68 *Three Women*, p. 33.

to prove the authenticity of their first encounter with the divine.[69] While I do not contend that Julian and Margery had knowledge of all of these lives, the motif of a near-death experience due to an illness, paralysis or stiffness in the body while the mind is ravished by visions, followed by complete recovery and further visions of devils, is so recurrent in late medieval mystics' lives that the parallel between this traditional motif and their own experience could hardly have escaped them. While their actual experience might not have fit this mould perfectly, they quite naturally made use of available conventions when re-interpreting their illnesses in the specific context of late medieval mystical writings about women. In this way, Julian and Margery conceived their visions alongside the conventions of medieval mystical tradition, and it will be apparent that they were similarly understood in this way by contemporaries.

Julian and Margery both recognise that their experience is very close to medieval understandings of madness. Julian fears she has raved when she wakes up, and Margery compares her conduct on several occasions to that of a madwoman. In a vision, she runs to and fro 'as it had ben a mad woman, crying and roryng', 'as it had be a woman wythowtyn reson'.[70] However, this appearance of insanity actually reveals and proves the authenticity of the visionary experience and of the mystic's behaviour, as Margery's amanuensis shows by quoting from the Middle English version of the Pseudo-Bonaventurean *Stimulus amoris*, the *Prick of Love*, when he attempts to show that Margery's loud cries belong to the mystical tradition:

> Bone-auentur wrot of hym-selfe þes wordys folwyng, 'A, Lord, what xal I more noysen er cryen? þu lettyst & þu comyst not, & I, wery & ouyrcome thorw desyr, begynne for to maddyn, for lofe gouernyth me & not reson ... I bowe, Lord, þei þat se me irkyn and rewyn, not knowyng me drunkyn wyth þi lofe. Lord, þei seyn "Lo, ȝen wood man cryeth in þe stretys," but how meche is þe desyr of myn hert þei parceyue not.'[71]

In this passage, the amanuensis evokes the possibility of interpreting Margery's fits of roaring and crying as the symptoms of madness, only to frame this possibility within a quotation from an authoritative mystical source. Margery is not insane, or rather, her insanity is a divine insanity, which authenticates her visions and validates her behaviour. Such a notion of 'divine insanity' is also developed, for instance, by Walter Hilton when he describes the grace brought about by contemplation as causing the body of the mystic to move around like that of a madman: 'it maketh the bodi, yif grace come myghtili, for to stire and turne heer and theer as a man that were mad or dronken and can have noo reste'.[72] Such a notion is similar to that developed by Elizabeth Clark in the

[69] See, for instance, 'Lyf of Katheryn of Senis', pp. 79, 81.

[70] *BMK*, I, 80, 193.

[71] *BMK*, I, 63, 154.

[72] Walter Hilton, *The Scale of Perfection*, ed. Thomas H. Bestul (Kalamazoo, MI, 2000),

context of female ascetics in late ancient Christianity, who 'recast their alleged "insanity" as a supreme form of sanity'.[73] Margery's and Julian's experiences, being interpreted through the lens of the mystical tradition, were therefore seen as a 'sane', or holy, form of insanity by their contemporaries, notably the 'religious person' at Julian's bedside and Margery's scribe. A further witness of this is the early sixteenth-century annotator of the only extant manuscript of Margery's *Book*. The commentator, writing in red ink in the manuscript's margins, associates Margery's crying, fainting and auditory or olfactory 'hallucinations' with the experience reported by such respected names as Richard Rolle and the later Carthusian monks Richard Methley and John Norton. Karma Lochrie, remarking on this, notes that 'these comments together point to one disturbing conclusion, that two Carthusian monks engaged in the same mystical practice of falling down and crying loudly – what some have called "morbid enthusiasm" and hysteria – that Kempe describes'.[74] In this way, the annotator 'clearly found Kempe's roaring to be a legitimate expression of religious devotion, and one with which he was familiar'.[75]

Julian of Norwich and Margery Kempe therefore use the conventions and traditions of mystical texts to recast their visionary experiences into the mould of a holy, or 'sane', insanity, an accepted, authorising, divine insanity. In the religious and mystical context of the medieval period, their altered state of consciousness was not considered as a mental disorder, nor is it believed to be so in such contemporary manuals as the DSM-IV and V. Margery's first bout of madness and Julian's short-lived belief that she is mad paradoxically enable them to become experts on madness, sanity and, in the case of Julian, *discretio spirituum*. In their experiential knowledge of what is madness and what is a vision from the devil, both mystics are not only able to validate their own visionary experience as acceptable and truthful, but they can also help others: by virtue of her experiential authority on madness, Margery cures a mad woman whose symptoms echo her own post-partum depression,[76] while Julian is cited by Margery as an 'expert' in *discretio spirituum*.[77]

I, ch. 30, lines 760–2. Female mystics' behaviour often causes them to be seen as mad by onlookers. See, for instance, the 'Life of Christina Mirabilis', in *Three Women*, pp. 114–15: 'supposynge hir wode and ful of fendes – atte laste with grete laboure toke hir and bonde hir with chaynes of yren'.

73 Clark, 'Sane Insanity', 211.

74 Lochrie, *Translations of the Flesh*, p. 210. On John Norton and Richard Methley, see James Hogg, 'Mount Grace Charterhouse and Late Medieval English Spirituality', *Analecta Cartusiana* 82 (1980), 1–43.

75 Lochrie, *Translations of the Flesh*, p. 211.

76 This episode is recounted in chapters 74–5 of *BMK*, pp. 176–9.

77 'Sche was bodyn be owyr Lord for to gon to an ankres in þe same cyte whych hyte Dame Ielyan.' She shows her 'many wondirful reuelacyons … to wetyn yf þer wer any deceyte in hem, for þe ankres was expert in swech thyngys and good cownsel cowd ȝeuyn' (*BMK*, I, 18, 42).

PART III

FIFTEENTH-CENTURY POETRY AND THEOLOGICAL PROSE

6

PURGATORY AND SPIRITUAL HEALING IN JOHN AUDELAY'S POEMS

Takami Matsuda

All the extant writings of John Audelay are preserved in Oxford, Bodleian Library, MS Douce 302, compiled c. 1426–31, which, according to Susanna Fein, 'consists of four genre-based mini-anthologies, each with its own internal arrangement in planned sequence'.[1] The four sections are, respectively: a series of didactic and meditative poems entitled the 'Counsel of Conscience', a series of salutations, a sequence of religious carols, and a small section consisting of devotional prose and verse at the end of the codex.[2] It has been pointed out that Audelay's poems abound in references to illness and its cure, and do so with personal urgency.[3] Admonition or counsel to the readers often ends with what is called the 'signature stanza' in which the author names himself almost obsessively as the blind Audelay. In addition to loss of eyesight, he seems to have been suffering from prolonged sickness with no immediate cure as he was assembling his book. He explains in the 'Epilogue to the Counsel of Conscience' that he was called to write this book as he lay sick, dreaming.[4] In view of this apparently terminal condition, it is understandable that the corpus of his writing is characterised by the close link between physical and spiritual illness at both literal and metaphorical levels and that Audelay often refers to Purgatory when he speaks of remedy against spiritual illness.[5]

1 John the Blind Audelay, *Poems and Carols (Oxford, Bodleian Library MS Douce 302)*, ed. Susanna Fein, TEAMS Middle English Texts Series (Kalamazoo, MI, 2009), p. 5. All quotations from and references to Audelay's poems are from this edition.

2 Susanna Fein, 'John Audelay and His Book: Critical Overview and Major Issues', in *My Wyl and My Wrytyng: Essays on John the Blind Audelay*, ed. Susanna Fein (Kalamazoo, MI, 2009), pp. 3–29, especially p. 9.

3 Cf. Jeremy J. Citrome, *The Surgeon in Medieval English Literature* (New York, 2006), pp. 83–111.

4 'Audelay's Epilogue to the Counsel of Conscience', lines 27–34, 482–5.

5 Robert J. Meyer-Lee counts nineteen references to Purgatory in the poems. See 'The Vatic Penitent: John Audelay's Self-Representation', in *My Wyl and My Wrytyng*, ed. Fein, pp. 54–85, especially p. 84 n. 47.

Purgatory for him is both his next destination and a metaphor for penitential process, and by analysing the contexts in which this word is used, we can see how he understood the illness of the soul and its cure.

Fashioning himself as a sick and blind man at the end of his life, Audelay employs the whole spectrum of themes and motifs of death in his codex, including a vision of the afterlife (a version of the *Visio S. Pauli*), the Three Living and the Three Dead, 'visitatio infirmorum' as well as lyrics and carols on approaching death and Marian intercession. Sudden death is a repeated theme which he sometimes evokes in a plain didactic manner, or with reference to recent plague, or to a historical figure such as King Robert of Sicily.[6] The immanent danger of sudden death, combined with his bodily affliction, leads him to despise his flesh, claiming, in the 'Timor mortis' carol', that 'Of myselfe nothyng I se, / Save filth, unclennes, vile styng'.[7] This 'contemptus mundi' attitude is, however, what made it possible for him to purchase heaven in the end, as he says at the end of the codex.[8] Audelay apparently seeks no cure for his bodily illness and blindness, but while resigning himself to this physical condition, he transforms bodily illness to a means to heal the spiritual, both for himself and for the readers.

The link between physical and spiritual illness is more than just metaphorical. Illness can literally be regarded as a visual manifestation of sin, because the illness of the body is said to come from that of the soul. Metaphors of spiritual illness are quite common in Middle English, and as Jeremy Citrome pointed out, there is a surgical link between moral laxity and the formation of wounds.[9] The fifteenth-century *Boke of the Craft of Dying* speaks disapprovingly of the current tendency to readily seek a physical cure without first resorting to a spiritual one, making an implicit reference to Canon 22 of the Fourth Lateran Council (*Cum infirmitas* [or *Quum infirmitas*]) which imposed confession on the sick before medical or surgical treatment could take place:

> For oftetymes, as a certeyne decretall seyth, bodyly syknes co*m*myth of the siknes of the soule; and therfor þe pope in the same decretall chargith streiȝtly eu*er*y bodyly lech þat he ȝeue no sekman no bodyly medicyn, vnto þe tyme þat he haue warned & inducid hym to sech his sp*irit*uall lech. But þis cou*n*cell ys now for-slewthed almost of all men, & is turned in to þe contrary; ffor men seken so*n*ner & besilier aft*er* medicyns for þe body, þan for þe soule.[10]

6 'The Remedy of Nine Virtues', lines 94–8; 'On the World's Folly', lines 37–42; 'Song of the Magnificat', lines 49–52.

7 'Dread of Death', lines 7–16, 25–8.

8 'Audelay's Conclusion', lines 27–33.

9 Citrome, *The Surgeon*, pp. 88–9.

10 *Yorkshire Writers: Richard Rolle and His Followers*, ed. C. Horstmann, 2 vols (London, 1895–96), vol. 2, p. 416.

Illness can also literally be a messenger of death and damnation. The *Pricke of Conscience* says that sickness makes man lose sight of everything else but pain, so that when the moment of death comes, he cannot think of God nor of himself:

> His mensangere may be called sekenes
> Þat comes byfor als ofte felled es;
> For sekenes ofte a man swa pynes
> Þat thurgh þat payn hys mynd tynes,
> For he may than thynk on noght elles
> Bot of þe payn þat with hym duelles.
> Bot when þe ded comes aftirward
> And hym byhoves fele mare hard,
> Þan sal he be in swylk drede sette
> Þat he sal God and hymself forget,[11]

The price of this oblivion is, needless to say, hell. Sickness, however, does not always have this damning consequence. Audelay says sickness gives us a foretaste of the pain of death, and because this experience can effectively turn the sinner to repentance out of fear, God sometimes uses sickness for that purpose:

> I come not to cal ryghtwys men
> To penans, as I you say,
> Bot thos that in erth synful bene —
> Hem I clepe, both nyght and day! —
> With disese and sekenes, yif that I may
> Make ham to mend thai done amys.[12]

Audelay likens a sinful man to 'a seke mon / That is yschakyd and schent with the aksis'[13] and calls sin the wound of the soul. Even though he does not develop a complex metaphorical programme for spiritual cure as does Henry of Lancaster,[14] this is a sustained metaphor in Audelay. To treat this wound, one needs a surgeon who can provide the 'salve' of confession and contrition:

> Dredles, uche dedly sunne Y declare a wounde,
> That when the Fynd hath foght with youe, and hath the maystré
> Then most ye seche a surgoun yif ye wyl be save and sound,

11 *Richard Morris's Prick of Conscience: A Corrected and Amplified Reading Text*, ed. Ralph Hanna and Sarah Wood, EETS o.s. 342 (Oxford, 2013), lines 2024–33.

12 'God's Address to Sinful Men', lines 25–30. Also cf. 'Visiting the Sick and Consoling the Needy', lines 55–60.

13 'Marcolf and Solomon', lines 910–11.

14 Cf. Naoë Kukita Yoshikawa, 'Holy Medicine and Diseases of the Soul: Henry of Lancaster and *Le Livre de Seyntz Medicines*', *Medical History* 53, 3 (2009), 397–414.

That con sothlé serche your sore and make youe hole.
Confession and contresion, thi salve schal hit be,
The penans of thi penetawnsere, thi satisfaccion;[15]

The basic assumption behind such a claim is that spiritual illness, unlike bodily illness, is never without a cure because the medicine is ultimately provided by Christ or Mary. As Diane Watt argues, the Virgin Mary's role as physician is comparable to that of Christ.[16] In Audelay's salutations, Mary is especially hailed as the medicine for our sin or the soul's physician.[17]

The cure, however, may not be complete before death and it may continue into Purgatory. Purgatory is an intermediary place unlike heaven or hell, but it is different from the Earthly Paradise (or the older Abraham's bosom) where the purged soul awaits entry into heaven, in that Purgatory is not so much a static waiting room as a process. As a process, however, it is unlike this world which is also often regarded as a process of a journey, in which people go about in various directions, as Egeus describes in Chaucer's *Knight's Tale*.[18] Purgatory is a process that has a single direction, with the eventual release promised at the end.

The promise of release does not make Purgatory itself less fearful nor its pains easier to bear. When Purgatory refers literally to a place in the afterlife, the association is often more penal than purgative. When Audelay claims that 'uche syn eponyst, truly, / In erth, in purgatoré, or ellis in helle' or 'To purgatoré or to hel ye most nede go' unless your penance is complete, the penal aspect of Purgatory is highlighted.[19] The idea that pains of Purgatory and hell, despite their difference in function, are little different in terms of harshness, is not uncommon.[20] There is an example of the 'infernalised' Purgatory in some visions of the afterlife, especially in the *Vision of William of Stranton*, a fifteenth-century English version of *St Patrick's Purgatory*, whose account of its pains actually comes closer to the *Vision of St Paul* also retold by Audelay.[21] The idea appears in another vision, that of the *Revelation of Purgatory* shown to a woman in 1422, which explains the presence of three purgatories, that of

15 'Marcolf and Solomon', lines 897–902.

16 Cf. Diane Watt, 'Mary the Physician: Women, Religion, and Medicine in the Middle Ages', pp. 27–44 in this collection of essays.

17 'Salutation to Jesus for Mary's Love', line 62; 'Salutation to Mary', line 101; 'Gabriel's Salutation to the Virgin', line 12; 'Carol 16. Saint Anne Mother of Mary', line 3.

18 'The Knight's Tale', I, 2847–9, in *The Riverside Chaucer*, ed. Larry D. Benson, 3rd edn (Oxford, 2008).

19 'Visiting the Sick', lines 142–3; 'God's Address to Sinful Men', lines 115–19.

20 *The Pricke of Conscience*, lines 2739–49; *Middle English Sermons, edited from British Museum MS. Royal 18 B. xxiii*, ed. W. O. Ross, EETS o.s. 209 (Oxford, 1940), pp. 41–2.

21 Cf. *St Patrick's Purgatory: Two Versions of Owayne Miles and the Vision of William of Stranton, Together with the Long Text of the Tractatus de Purgatorio Sancti Patricii*, ed. Robert Easting, EETS o.s. 298 (Oxford, 1991), p. lxxxi.

righteousness, mercy and grace. This tripartite scheme, probably conceived under the influence of the vision of Bridget of Sweden,[22] is useful in clarifying the idea of Purgatory in Audelay. The Purgatory in which the sinner is justly punished, is what the *Revelation of Purgatory* calls the 'purgatorye of right-wisenes' whose fire is 'an instrument of Goddis ryȝtwisnesse to purge ȝow of ȝour syn'.[23] Even if admittance to Purgatory is the manifestation of divine mercy, once in Purgatory, God can be a stern judge in exacting penance due. Of the punishments there, we find a graphic description reminiscent of the *Vision of St Paul*:

> And for þis foule mystrust and foule disvse of ȝour body, tak her [þese] bittyr peynes in purgatory and þese addres and þese snakes euer to gnaw on ȝow til our bandes of syn be wasted away and til God have shewed on ȝow his mercy. Ffor wit ȝe welle þis is noȝt helle – þis is an instrument of Goddis ryȝtwisnesse to purge ȝow of ȝour syn in purgatory. And for ȝe wold noȝt vse penaunce in ȝour lyfes and ar ȝe came her.[24]

The harshness bears some resemblance to a vision of Bridget of Sweden, to whom Audelay also dedicated a carol.[25] Bridget of Sweden's *Revelations*, assembled and published by Alphonse of Pecha shortly after Bridget's death in 1373, includes a vision of three purgatories: that of severe purgation in which the souls are tormented by alternating heat and cold and sights of demons,[26] the purgatory in which pain is alleviated by intercessory masses and works of charity, and the purgatory of peaceful waiting, that is the Earthly Paradise, where the only pain is the lack of the vision of God.[27] In Bridget's first purgatory, which hovers darkly above hell, the greatest torment comes from the fact that the souls are not allowed to know of their release.[28] In both cases, punishment appears more penal than remedial or purgative.

The most frequent references to Purgatory in Audelay, however, carry a metaphorical association as he stresses, in one way or another, that 'Better hit

22 Mary C. Erler, '"A Revelation of Purgatory" (1422): Reform and the Politics of Female Visions', *Viator* 38 (2007), 321–47, especially pp. 335–7.

23 References are to *A Revelation of Purgatory by an Unknown, Fifteenth-century Woman Visionary*, ed. and trans. Martha P. Harley (Lewiston, NY, 1985), pp. 83 (line 790), 76 (lines 575–6).

24 *A Revelation of Purgatory*, p. 76 (lines 569–78).

25 Cf. Susanna Fein, 'Mary to Veronica: John Audelay's Sequence of Salutations to God-Bearing Women', *Speculum* 86(2011), 964–1009, especially pp. 989–92.

26 *The Revelations of Saint Birgitta*, ed. W. P. Cumming, EETS o.s. 178 (Oxford, 1929), p. 48 (lines 24–31).

27 Cf. *The Liber Celestis of St Bridget of Sweden*, ed. Roger Ellis, EETS o.s. 291 (Oxford, 1987), vol. 1, p. 260.

28 'it vnder-stondyth nott wheder it shall come to reste after purgacion, or ells be dampned': *The Revelations of Saint Birgitta*, p. 50 (lines 7–8). Cf. *Liber Celestis*, vol. 1, p. 261 (lines 3–6).

is now fore thee / To wenche the fuyre of purgatoré'.[29] In 'Visiting the Sick and Consoling the Needy', the reader is told to scrutinise his conscience to become aware of sin and know objectively what penance is due:

> Then mesoure thi wynd with repentans,
> And schryve thee clene of alle thi synne.
> Then wey the fouyre with trew balans —
> What purgatoré thou schuldist have then.[30]

Here, 'purgatoré' signifies penance one should do, either in this world or in Purgatory. Penance is indeed the medicine for those sick in soul – 'Fore hom ned is heren oune medsyn, / Bot thai that beth seke in soule, iwys' – as Audelay concludes in the following stanza.[31]

The more penance is done in this world, the less is left to be fulfilled in Purgatory, so that the link between the two is direct, rather than metaphorical. The idea that prolonged sickness may be purgatorial and can exempt the dead from post-mortem purgation is also seen in one of the visions of Bridget of Sweden, which speaks of a woman who 'fell seke that endured all the tyme of hir lyfe, tyll she was purged and wyth ryg[ht] grete deuocyon yaue vp the spritte'; after death, she was immediately taken to heaven by Peter.[32] Similarly, Audelay ends 'Epilogue to the Counsel of Conscience' with a prayer for purgatory here in this world:

> And to the Holé Gost foregete I noght,
> Fore him I thonke specialy,
> That wit and wysdam to me hath broght
> To foresake my syn and my foly.
>   In this word here levyng,
>   To have my payne, my purgatory,
>   Out of this word or that I dy,
>   A, gracyus God, gramarsy,
>   To grawnt me grace of good endyng![33]

A similar prayer is also found in Richard Rolle:

> Now, swete Jhesu, graunt me here wilfully to suffre deseises and tribulacions for þy sake, and nevyr to gurche for sekenesse ne for wronges of man, bot ever to þank þe of al þy sondes. And graunt me, Lord Jhesu, purgatory for my synnes er I deye, and hertely, Lord, continuely hit to pray; and when hit

29 'Visiting the Sick and Consoling the Needy', lines 100–13, 126–30, 144–56; cf. 'Marcolf and Solomon', lines 931–5; 'God's Address to Sinful Men', lines 153–9.

30 'Visiting the Sick and Consoling the Needy', lines 135–8.

31 'Visiting the Sick and Consoling the Needy', lines 163–4.

32 *The Revelations of Saint Birgitta*, p. 41 (lines 32–4).

33 'Audelay's Epilogue to the Counsel of Conscience', lines 473–81.

cometh, Lord, yif me pacience and hert hooly to þank þe of þy blesful and gracious sond.[34]

Such prayers presuppose that it is the manifestation of divine mercy and grace that tribulation in this world is made purgatorial. To be afflicted in this world may itself be a sign of divine favour, as was believed to be true of lepers.[35] When their suffering is elevated to the proof of divine attention, they paradoxically become the elect few, and this logic presupposes that they are exempt, or have much greater chance to be exempted, from penance in Purgatory which is much harsher by comparison. In this respect, the *Revelation of Purgatory* speaks of 'sekenesse and grete tribulacions in þis wor[l]de' as 'þe purgatory of mercy',[36] conferring a special purgatorial status on physical illness. This direct link between this world and the next is important. However hard one may strive to do penance in this world, the crucial thing is to be admitted into Purgatory, not to fail at the moment of death through despair or over-confidence. For all the preparations and help rendered by the *ars moriendi* manuals, indulgences, prayers and charms against sudden death, and promised intercessions by living friends and relatives, one must pass the final test alone at the threshold of death. To avoid the crucial failure, the message Audelay repeats throughout the codex is that God grants remission of sin if you have contrition.[37] *Contritio*, as opposed to *attritio*, can function as a sort of a panacea which brings about an instant cure to the sinful soul because it is achieved with divine infusion of grace, not by free will alone.[38] But Audelay uses contrition in a less restricted sense of 'sorrow of heart and detestation of sin committed, with the purpose of not sinning in future' (MED), that is, as a feeling and resolution of human free will which remains precarious without divine grace. The identification of penance as a purgatory can reassure the sinner against this anxiety. Focussed on the future, worldly penance becomes the beginning of a process which, passing through confession and absolution, ends with the satisfaction of penance due, which in turn may continue until after death, that is, to Purgatory. To call worldly penance a purgatory is to see the suffering in this world as the beginning of this process, identifying it as the one-way process that will not fail at death because, once in Purgatory, there is no turning back. No matter how harsh the punishment is, even to the extent one is no longer certain of release, as in Bridget of Sweden's first Purgatory, one will be released sooner or later. The mere fact that you are

34 *English Writings of Richard Rolle*, ed. Hope Emily Allen (Oxford, 1931), p. 34 (lines 211–19).

35 Carole Rawcliffe, *Leprosy in Medieval England* (Woodbridge, 2006), pp. 57–9.

36 *A Revelation of Purgatory*, p. 82 (lines 765–73).

37 'Virtues of the Mass', lines 73–8, 151–6.

38 H. Dondaine, *L'Attrition suffisante* (Paris, 1943), pp. 7–8.

allowed to enter Purgatory 'means you have already chosen right and are en route to heaven';[39] in other words, a patient is admitted to the care of the divine surgeon and will be treated with the only medicine that promises cure, unlike the case of bodily sickness. When identified as a purgatorial process, penance is transformed into a long-term medical treatment that begins in this life as earthly purgatory and, continuing over the threshold of death, ends in Purgatory in the afterlife. To speak of a cure for spiritual sickness by calling it a purgatory is to encourage the sinner to look beyond the threshold of death toward this vision of the Purgatory from which one will be ultimately released.

This otherworldliness of the healing process is readily seen in Audelay's attitude to the religious who has the authority to enjoin penance on the laity. Throughout the codex, Audelay addresses both the laity and the religious, sometimes simultaneously in such poems as 'Visiting the Sick and Consoling the Needy' and 'Malcolf and Solomon'. As a chantry priest of Haughmond abbey and before that a chaplain to Lord Lestrange of Knockin, Shropshire,[40] Audelay is conscious of the duty of the clergy to intercede for souls of the dead and repeatedly admonishes his fellow clergymen to that end:

> Ye prestis, I pray youe take good kepe,
> That mas ne matens nyl say ne syng:
> Ye deprevyn the Trenetė of his worchip,
> And al sayntis in heven with him dwellyng,
> And al Cristin soulis in payne bydyng
> Affter your prayors in purgatory,
> And al your god-doers of here helpyng.[41]

While there was a Lollard criticism regarding whether sacraments administered by bad priests were valid or not, Audelay is quite orthodox in defending the role priests are authorised to play.[42] He claims that God has granted the

39 Robert Easting, '"Choose Yourselves Whither to Go": John Audelay's *Vision of Saint Paul*', in *My Wyl and My Wrytyng*, ed. Fein, pp. 170–90, especially p. 183.

40 On the event in his life that may have led to his penitence, see, most recently, Michael J. Bennett, 'John Audelay: Life Records and Heaven's Ladder', in *My Wyl and My Wrytyng*, ed. Fein, pp. 30–53.

41 'Epilogue to the Counsel of Conscience', lines 326-32; cf. 'Virtues of the Mass', lines 245–52.

42 Alastair Minnis, *Fallible Authors: Chaucer's Pardoner and Wife of Bath* (Philadelphia, 2008), pp. 54–74. On Audelay's possible criticism of ecclesiastical practice in 'Marcol and Solomon' and Arundel's *Constitutions*, see James Simpson, 'Saving Satire after Arundel's *Constitutions*: John Audelay's "Marcol and Solomon"', in *Text and Controversy from Wyclif to Bale: Essays in Honour of Anne Hudson*, ed. Helen Barr and Ann M. Hutchison (Turnhout, 2005), pp. 387–404; Richard Firth Green, 'Marcolf the Fool and Blind John Audelay', in *Speaking Images: Essays in Honor of V. A. Kolve*, ed. R. F. Yeager and Charlotte C. Morse (Asheville, NC, 2001), pp. 559–76.

power of sacramental forgiveness of sin to priests, even if they themselves are immoral:

> Fore God hath graunt of his grace to curatis his pouere —
> Thagh thai ben synful men — to asoyle youe of your synne,
> Thorgh vertu of the sacrementte, sothlé I yowe enseure;
> No mon mese in this matere yif he wyl savyd bene.[43]

On that assumption, he tells the clergy more than once to moderate the penance they impose, bearing the future Purgatory in mind, lest too strict penance might make sinners despair.[44] Assuming that penance is autonomous, Audelay sees the cure for the sickness of the soul pragmatically from the standpoint of a doctor overseeing the whole process of treatment.[45] A medicine prescribed by an immoral doctor works just as effectively. As Jeremy Citrome has pointed out, Audelay compares the urgency of confession to surgical treatment, assuming that a priest is absolutely necessary as a surgeon of the soul.[46]

One effective medicine that works to alleviate pain and shorten the process of healing is the indulgence. One of Audelay's salutations is to Bridget of Sweden, who was 'an eminent propagandist for indulgences, especially for pardons for the dead', according to Martha Driver.[47] It gives the account of her acquisition of a jubilee indulgence in 1350 as well as the grant of pardon to Syon abbey by Henry V. Audelay actually attaches indulgences to the text of some other prayers as well, such as those granted by Pope Gregory and Pope John XXII,[48] as well as to the image of the Holy Face on fol. 27v. Such devotional pardons attached to prayers and images were common both as accessory texts in manuscript Books of Hours and as standard contents of the early sixteenth-century printed Book of Hours.[49] Indulgence is called a fruit of

43 'Marcolf and Solomon', lines 806–9.

44 'Marcolf and Solomon', lines 923–30; 'God's Address to Sinful Men', lines 137–44.

45 'Marcolf and Solomon', lines 897–922.

46 Citrome, *The Surgeon*, p. 109.

47 Martha W. Driver, 'John Audelay and the Bridgettines', in *My Wyl and My Wrytyng*, ed. Fein, pp. 191–217, especially p. 203.

48 'Instruction for Prayer 5' (before 'Prayer for Pardon after the Levation' (p.79); 'Virtues of the Mass' lines 409–11 (before 'Saint Gregory's Indulgence' (p. 91); 'Pope John's Passion of Our Lord', lines 1–8.

49 Robert N. Swanson, 'Praying for Pardon: Devotional Indulgences in Late Medieval England', in *Promissory Notes on the Treasury of Merits: Indulgences in Late Medieval Europe*, ed. R. N. Swanson (Leiden, 2006), pp. 215–40. Susanna Fein also notes that some of Audelay's prayers are based on septenaries that are commonly found in the Books of Hours: see 'English Devotions for a Noble Household: The Long Passion in Audelay's *Counsel of Conscience*', in *After Arundel: Religious Writing in Fifteenth-Century England*, ed. Vincent Gillespie and Kantik Ghosh (Turnhout, 2011), pp. 325–42, especially p. 336.

divine mercy[50] or identified as 'a purgatory of mercy', along with sickness and tribulations in this world, in the *Revelation of Purgatory* (765–73). However, the mere acquisition of pardons offered no guarantees and there was always the chance that they may be wasted due to the fault of the recipient.[51] Even though the treasury of merits of the Holy Church is large enough to pay all the debts of all Christians,[52] to benefit from it, one must be contrite and be admitted to Purgatory in the first place. Indulgences can work only if this is a part of the healing process that begins with penance identified as earthly purgatory. One can then be assured that, with this optional medicine, pain will gradually but steadily diminish, just as one's physical wound gradually heals.

Audelay's two voices, to the laity and to fellow clergy, both deal with Purgatory in the context of spiritual healing that is ultimately completed in the afterlife. However, there is also a third voice, which is the voice of Audelay himself asking for intercession. The act of writing the codex on his deathbed for the salvation of readers becomes a self-reflexive act of confession and petition to readers to intercede for him. Audelay is requesting in reciprocity prayer for his soul by the readers, who can be healed through his book:

> Yef ye wil have any copi,
> Askus leeve and ye shul have,
> To pray for hym specialy
> That hyt made your soules to save,
>   Jon the Blynde Awdelay.[53]

As both Robert Meyer-Lee and Susanna Fein have pointed out, Audelay the chantry priest in turn becomes a founder of the chantry chapel where readers come to pray for him as successive chaplains. As he asks the readers to pray for his soul, the codex is transformed into a (perpetual) chantry for him in which the act of reading functions as intercessory prayers.[54] We may say that the reading of 'indulgenced' poems works to redeem the author's life.[55] In the matter of death and Purgatory, the motive is never purely altruistic. Those who pray for the dead will be justly rewarded in return. There is a rather literal illustration of this reciprocal merit in the All Souls Day legend in the *Legenda aurea*, in which the dead rise from their graves to save from an enemy the one

50 *The Book of Vices and Virtues*, ed. W. N. Francis, EETS o.s. 217 (Oxford, 1942), p. 195.

51 R. N. Swanson, *Indulgences in Late Medieval England: Passport to Paradise?* (Cambridge, 2007), p. 17.

52 *The Pricke of Conscience*, lines 3922–5.

53 'Audelay's Conclusion', lines 44–8; also cf. 'The Remedy of Nine Virtues', lines 99–102.

54 Meyer-Lee, 'The Vatic Penitent', pp. 67–8; Susanna Fein, 'Death and the Colophon in the Audelay Manuscript', in *My Wyl and My Wrytyng*, ed. Fein, pp. 294–306, especially p. 296.

55 Driver, 'John Audelay and the Bridgettines', p. 208.

who habitually prayed for them.[56] Audelay emphasises this reciprocity with respect to his readers, as well as those whose duty is to do service to the dead, including executors.[57]

Reciprocity is also the main theme in Audelay's rendering of the popular Three Living and Three Dead narrative. The tie between the dead and the living is strengthened when they are made fathers and sons, and the narrative ends not only with the living reforming their lives but literally with the building of a chantry chapel.[58] Audelay envisages his future self and stands on the side of the dead, as one of the Three Dead, warning and urging readers to pray for him at the same time.

After the admonitory Three Living and Three Dead, there is a popular Latin poem on mutability, 'Cur mundus militat', which introduces the theme of vanity and mutability. Audelay's concluding verse begins by reaffirming the theme of mutability, repeating that all earthly joys vanish and man dies suddenly. Audelay then speaks of how he succeeded in despising this false world, before concluding with the admonition to fellow Christians to be aware of his example:

> Herfore Y have dyspysed this worlde,
> And have overcomen alle erthely thyng.
> My ryches in heven with dede and worde
> I have ypurchest in my levyng,
> With good ensampul to odur gefyng.
> Loke in this book; here may ye se
> Hwatt ys my wyl and my wrytyng.
> All odur by me war for to be!
>   Bewarre, brether, Y yow pray,
>   Yowre mysdeds that ye amende
>   Owte of thys worlde or that ye wende,[59]

Susanna Fein suggests that Audelay 'talks about his life in the past tense, and thus speaks virtually as if he were one of the Dead'.[60] Although the end of 'Audelay's Conclusion' appears as admonitory as 'Three Dead Kings', here it is mixed with and mitigated by the sad awareness of mutability. The subtle change of tone may be related to the fact that the final two items are by the second scribe, added after some interval.[61] In this sense, one may say that

56 The scene is used as the illustration of the Office of the Dead for the *Très riches heures de duc de Berry* (fol. 90v).

57 'Visiting the Sick and Consoling the Needy', lines 339–59.

58 'Three Dead Kings', lines 93–4, 138–40.

59 'Audelay's Conclusion', lines 27–37.

60 Fein, 'Death and the Colophon', p. 302

61 Susanna Fein, 'Good Ends in the Audelay Manuscript', *The Yearbook of English Studies* 33 (2003), 97–119 (p. 108).

Audelay speaks as if he were already in Purgatory, undergoing purgation and waiting for intercession. The ending of the 'Book of Conscience' can be interpreted in a similar manner:

> God hath me chastyst fore my levyng;
> I thong my God, my Grace, treuly,
> Fore his gracious vesityng.
>   Beware, seris, I youe pray,
> Fore I mad this with good entent,
> In the reverens of God Omnipotent.
> Pray fore me that beth present —
>   My name is Jon the Blynd Awdlay.[62]

Also using the past tense, Audelay thanks God for 'his gracious vesityng', that is, for allowing his earthly tribulation to have a purgative function. Again, this sounds as if he were already in Purgatory and asking for intercessory prayer.

Thus Audelay appropriates the figure of the 'revenant' from Purgatory in addressing the readers. In the 'revenant' narrative, such as the *Gast of Gy*, the *Revelation of Purgatory*, or the *Awntyrs of Arthure*, the torment of the revenant is emphasised graphically, after the tradition of the visions of the afterlife, but unlike the souls tormented in such visions, the revenants betray that they are aware of their eventual release while they often play the role of the propagandist of Purgatory, offering detailed instructions concerning intercessory mass and prayers.[63] They are the privileged dead who are allowed to return as ghosts by special permission. In this respect, it is perhaps no coincidence that Audelay refers more than once to the Dives and Lazarus episode.[64] This is not only to emphasise the importance of works of mercy, especially the merit of charity to the poor, which is a recurrent theme,[65] but Audelay also seems to be identifying himself with the Lazarus figure who is allowed to return from Purgatory with a warning. It is perhaps for the same reason that he includes the *Vision of St Paul*, in which Paul prays for the Sunday respite from tortures, or for that matter, mentions how God granted St Francis special grace to fetch his brother from Purgatory, in one of the carols:

> Crist he grawnt thee, specialy,
> Fore on his Passion thou hadist peté,
> To feche thi breder out of purgatori,

62 'Epilogue to the Counsel of Conscience', lines 500–7.

63 Harley, *A Revelation of Purgatory*, pp. 61 (lines 85–7), 63 (lines 129–31); 'The Gast of Gy', lines 423–35 in *Three Purgatory Poems: The Gast of Gy, Sir Owain, The Vision of Tundale*, ed. Edward E. Foster (Kalamazoo, MI, 2004), pp. 37–8; *The Awntyrs off Arthure*, ed. Ralph Hanna, III (Manchester, 1974), lines 140–1, 319–23.

64 'Marcolf and Solomon', lines 536–9; 'God's Address to Sinful Men', lines 241–6.

65 'Visiting the Sick and Consoling the Needy', lines 79–86; 'God's Address to Sinful Man', lines 197–232; 'Carol 3: Seven Works of Mercy', lines 15–35.

That ly in ther in rewful aray.
  Saynt Frances, to thee I say,
  Save thi breder both nyght and day![66]

Like Lazarus or St Paul, Audelay is also sent back to warn people, as he lay dreaming in his illness.[67]

It has been pointed out that blindness gave Audelay a 'vatic' power of spiritual insight,[68] but it can also be said that he acquired this privileged status because of his illness. Serious illness can sometimes lead to a visionary experience, as in the fifteenth-century *Vision of Edmund Leversedge*,[69] so that his status as a gravely ill old man who stands at the threshold of death makes him a more appropriate candidate for a visionary or a prophet. Audelay is both a revenant from Purgatory asking for intercession and a prophetic figure of authority sent back to warn people. As one of the elect, he experiences Purgatory as a purgatorial process of healing leading to the promised cure, in which his pain can gradually diminish, with the intercession of the living. This understanding of Purgatory may be compared to Catherine of Genoa's idea of Purgatory as found in *Trattato sul Purgatorio,* first published in 1522. Catherine of Genoa speaks of Purgatory in terms of daily increase of joy rather than of diminishing pain;[70] there, suffering is no longer associated with cleansing of sin nor with penance but with joy of healing. Behind Audelay's cautionary voice, there is the same belief in healing that this continuous process of Purgatory brings to the repentant dead.

As we have seen, Audelay's intention in compiling the codex is to talk about spiritual healing as a single process that begins in this world and is completed after death in Purgatory. As long as tribulation in this world can be regarded as purgatorial with the grace of God, the process is that of healing, of gradual relieving of pain. The fact that this is a continuous process is strengthened by the fact that 'purgatory on earth' is not necessarily a figurative expression but conveys the sense of a specific locale where purgation is actually carried out. In this sense, Purgatory is both a place and

66 'Saint Francis', lines 25–30.

67 'Epilogue to the Counsel of Conscience', lines 27–41.

68 Susan Powell, 'John Audelay and John Mirk: Comparisons and Contrasts', in *My Wyl and My Wrytyng*, ed. Fein, pp. 86–111, especially p. 97; Meyer-Lee, 'The Vatic Penitent', p. 76. Audelay also merges himself with John the Evangelist, the archetypal visionary: see Fein, 'English Devotions for a Noble Household'.

69 *The Vision of Edmund Leversedge: A Fifteenth-Century Account of a Visit to the Otherworld edited from BL MS Additional 14193*, ed. Wiesje F. Nijenhuis (Nijmegen, 1991).

70 Caterina da Genova, *Vita Mirabile / Dialogo / Trattato sul Purgatorio*, ed. Filippo Lovison (Rome, 2004), p. 248.

a process at the same time.[71] It is also important to realise that there is no clear-cut dividing line between literal and metaphorical purgatories, owing to the very nature of Purgatory itself. Because the biblical foundation for the existence of Purgatory was a figurative one, being based on 'ipse autem salvus erit sic tamen quasi per ignem' ['he himself shall be saved; yet so as by fire'] (I Corinthians 3:15), there continued to be several possibilities for the place where purgative punishment is carried out, both on earth and in the otherworld, even after the idea of Purgatory as a specific locale was fairly well established in the twelfth century, as one may see in the legend for All Souls Day in the *Legenda aurea*.[72] Purgatory was both a specific locale and a metaphor for penance or prolonged suffering, and this means in turn that even when it refers metaphorically to tribulation in this world, the allusion to a specific locale is not absent. In this respect, the *Revelation of Purgatory* speaks of the third purgatory, that of grace:

> a man or a woman hase maste contenede his synnes and moste vsede þam, þare he sall be puneschede if God will gyfe hym grace and come noghte in þe generalle paynes of purgatorye.[73]

This seems to refer to the kind of situation in which the soul is allowed to do penance at the place where a particular sin was committed, the classic case of this being the episode of the dead serving as a bath attendant at the place where he indulged himself while alive, recorded first in Gregory's *Dialogues*.[74] A similar idea is found in the *Pricke of Conscience* which speaks of a special Purgatory in contrast to the common one.[75] It is the purgatory of grace, because when purged in this way somewhere on earth, the soul may be allowed to appear to the living to ask for intercession.

If we see this idea of Purgatory at the place of sin as being reflected also in Audelay, his Purgatory gains another dimension. Because Purgatory can be appointed as a specific locale both in this world and the next, it is literally one continuous process of cure for the soul. Spiritual healing, unlike physical healing, always finds a cure. That process of healing is the process not only of diminishing pain but also of growing hope and, while one needs to fix one's eye firmly on the place beyond the threshold of death – that is, Purgatory – to complete it, the process begins in this world. To identify penance as Purgatory is to offer the ultimate healing to the sickness

71 Liz Herbert McAvoy, 'Envisioning Reform: *A Revelation of Purgatory* and Anchoritic *Compassioun* in the Later Middle Ages', in *The Medieval Mystical Tradition in England: Exeter Symposium VIII*, ed. E. A. Jones (Cambridge, 2013), pp. 141–55, especially p. 142.

72 Cf. Takami Matsuda, *Death and Purgatory in Middle English Didactic Poetry* (Cambridge, 1997), pp. 19–21, 56–9.

73 *A Revelation of Purgatory*, p. 82 (lines 775–8).

74 Gregory, *Dialogorum Libri IV*, IV. 55, PL 77, cols 417A–C.

75 *The Pricke of Conscience,* lines 2872–89.

of the soul, the promise of cure and the gradual alleviation of pain. The identification implies that the medicine is not in any way thwarted by the condition of this world; rather one is filled with the hope that the process of healing transforms itself, once in Purgatory after death, into the gradual increase of joy. By repeatedly referring to penance in this world as Purgatory, Audelay asserts that there is an ultimate medicine for spiritual illness that will promise recovery and cure.

7

REGINALD PECOCK'S READING HEART AND THE HEALTH OF BODY AND SOUL

Louise M. Bishop

During the tumultuous fifteenth century in England, the vernacular English writings of the bishop of Chichester, Reginald Pecock (c. 1395–c. 1461), unnerved some readers, eventually to a lethal degree for the prelate.[1] In a 1457 letter that precipitated legal action, the Viscount Beaumont (1409–60) – one of the strongest supporters of the Lancastrian cause, remaining unusually loyal during the War of the Roses – expressed his concerns to his monarch, King Henry VI (1421–71). Beaumont's worry centres on Pecock because the bishop, 'thurgh presumpcioun and curiosite demed by hym in his owne wytte',[2] has threatened the realm's Christian orthodoxy. Beaumont writes that a multiplicity of opinions, including Pecock's, verges towards heresy:

> And yt ys so now þat grete noyse rennyth that þer shuld be diuerse conclusyons labored and subtilly entended to be enprented in mennes hertis, by pryvy, by also vnherd, meenes, to the most pernicyous and next to peruercyoun of our faith.[3]

Beaumont fears that a 'great noise', a cacophony of conclusions that he considers deadly and destructive ('pernicious', with a sense of disease pervading the word) as well as dangerously inverted and false ('perversion', with a sense of reversal), spells danger to Christian orthodoxy. Not only

1 Wendy Scase, 'Reginald Pecock', *English Writers of the Middle Ages*, ed. M. C. Seymour, Authors of the Middle Ages 3 (Aldershot, 1996), pp. 69–146: this essay provides the biographical details of Pecock's life, as well as a selection of edited documents relating to Pecock.

2 Scase edits a letter of approximately 24 June 1457, from the register of Richard Ashton, abbot of Peterborough, preserved in Cambridge, University Library, MS 2, fols 43r, 43v (copyright of the Dean and Chapter of Peterborough Cathedral), from Viscount Beaumont to Henry VI: it urges the king to take action against Pecock: see 'Pecock', p. 121.

3 Scase, 'Pecock', p. 121.

does Beaumont express his anxiety in terms of bodily health and healing: he adds to his expression of anxiety a noisy labour couched in terms of intent ('entended'), print ('enprented'), and secrecy ('pryvy' and 'unherd'). Beaumont suggests that the goal of heresy's words – the ground on which the controversy rests, and on which Henry's reputation lies – is the heart. Beaumont portrays the individual subject's heart – the healthy body's centre, home of intent, hidden yet printable, affected by sound as well as silence – as material and secret, a potentially dangerous seat of words heard, read, kept and efficacious. A simplified Middle English translation of a Latin original – for example, the Middle English *Doctrine of the Hert*, manuscripts of which passed between religious and lay women – could only partially meet such concerns.[4] On the other hand, Beaumont addresses his sovereign king and his royal heart in a different manner. Beaumont implores King Henry to let his heart continue to act differently from the hearts of his subjects. Henry is to 'lete passe out into lyght the grete flames of faith kept and myghtly brennyng euer in your brest, I dar say fro so yonge age þat yt myght be mervayled in that tyme so yonge, the fervence þeroff, and blyssed be God, so contynued and encresed to this day'.[5] The royal heart is imaginatively localised as central, 'kept', yet powerfully effective; its metaphoric flames burn in, and then out of, the chest. The faithful flames of the king's heart have continually increased presumably since his infancy: Henry VI was crowned king at the age of nine months. These flames, unlike the secret words Pecock has put in men's hearts, ought – and do – come to light. Beaumont's letter makes hearts and words visible.

Bishop Pecock paid for his opinions with recantation, burned books, and a lonely end of life, but his fall from grace may have been prompted, as Wendy Scase and others suggest, less because of his ostensible unorthodoxy than in order to consolidate besieged Lancastrian power.[6] That Beaumont's charges against Pecock as well as his adulation of King Henry come wrapped in hearts both literal and metaphorical prompts an analysis that examines the overlapping meanings these instances raise. Literal and metaphoric hearts intertwine with medieval ideas about the heart as seat of understanding, the role of the passions concerning health, the effects of reading, and the reach of English politics in the fifteenth century. Interpretations of a reading heart

4 See *The Doctrine of the Hert: A Critical Edition with Introduction and Commentary*, ed. Denis Renevey, Christiania Whitehead and Anne Mouron (Exeter, 2009), the introduction to which explains the simplifications the translation's intended female audience ostensibly prompted. See also *A Companion to* The Doctrine of the Hert*: The Middle English Translation and Its Latin and European Contexts*, ed. Denis Renevey and Christiania Whitehead (Exeter, 2009).

5 Scase, 'Pecock', p. 121.

6 Scase, 'Pecock', pp. 103–18; R. M. Ball, 'The Opponents of Bishop Pecok', *Journal of Ecclesiastical History* 48, 2 (1997), 230–62; Roy Martin Haines, 'Reginald Pecock: A Tolerant Man in an Age of Intolerance', *Studies in Church History* 21 (1984), 125–37.

benefit from historical analysis of reading's material effects understood philosophically, theologically and medically.

To treat this metaphoric and literal heart, the following analysis compares two groups of Middle English texts that exemplify several discursive meanings of the heart in late medieval England. The first is the *oeuvre* of Bishop Reginald Pecock, a fifteenth-century proponent of Middle English prose and vernacular readers. The other, the Middle English *The Doctrine of the Hert*, an apparently sanctioned fifteenth-century translation of *De doctrina cordis*, a popular and much-translated thirteenth-century devotional tract for both religious and lay audiences. Pecock's works[7] got him in trouble, while *The Doctrine of the Hert* enjoyed wide popularity.[8] These Middle English texts show complex intersections between bodily health and bodily knowledge for which reading, as Beaumont's condemnation indicates, is a key and contested activity. Foregrounded are the dangers Beaumont recognised in Pecock's writings. Attention to the heart unearths layers of administrative terror, educated trust, and passionate orthodoxy that animate these and other Middle English texts. Eventually – and past the era with which this essay is concerned – the location of self-understanding moves from the contested heart to a rational head. English institutions continued, ideologically as well as scientifically, to handle the kinds of problems Beaumont raised at the same time that they furthered English monarchs' consolidation of royal power. A Cartesian understanding of the human body as a machine helped to externalise the danger of seditious reading so that Tudors and Stuarts administered surveillance through bureaucracies like the Stationers' Register. But the medical and metaphoric origins of these efforts to understand reading and control readers lie in the heart.

A WORD ABOUT VERNACULARITY

Evidence for later medieval literature that treats intersections between health, hearts, minds and words appears, naturally enough, in Latin texts. But vernacular textuality is what got Pecock into trouble. The conscious treatment of vernacular production apparent in Pecock's prologues to his works suggests this essay's focus on the vernacular. As Pecock writes in his prologue to the *Donet*:

[7] Edited works by Pecock include; Reginald Pecock, *The Repressor of Over Much Blaming of the Clergy*, ed. Babington Churchill (London, 1860); *The Reule of Crysten Religioun*, ed. Reginald Greet and William Cabell (London, 1927); *The Donet*, ed. Elsie Vaughan Hitchcock, EETS o.s. 117 (London, 1921); *The Folewer to the Donet*, ed. Elsie Vaughan Hitchcock, EETS o.s. 164 (London, 1924); *Reginald Pecock's Book of Faith: A Fifteenth Century Theological Tractate*, ed. J. L. Morison (Glasgow, 1909), available on the Internet at http://name.umdl.umich.edu/AJH1649.0001.001.

[8] As mentioned above, *The Doctrine of the Hert*, along with the companion volume, provides a counterpoint to Pecock's work for this essay.

> For God knowith that for helthe of Christen peplis soulis, and for noon victorie to be woone by me in my side, neithir for envy glorie or rewarde to be had a this side god, I sette me into the labour of my bokis making.[9]

The abundance of pious vernacular texts like *The Doctrine of the Hert* indicates the vigour of vernacular translation in the late Middle Ages and the benefits of literary attention to English vernacular literature. Although there are dangers to treating 'vernacularity' as a monolith, its different iterations help us understand Beaumont's condemnation of Pecock and the language he uses for it. For Pecock and others – but not for all – life-and-death stakes were involved in the production and reading of Middle English works in the fifteenth century.[10]

The last twenty years' research on vernacular reading in late medieval England has focused on vernacular theology, thanks to Nicholas Watson's *Speculum* essay from the early 1990s.[11] Several critics' works have added to Watson's outline and complicated the picture of fifteenth-century reading and, through analyses of book ownership and book sharing, have deepened Watson's outline of a readerly self conditioned by vernacularity. Readers' varied activities, and the alliances between and among readers initially suggested by Watson's article, animate the work of Mary Erler, who has explored the networks of affinity and vernacular book-sharing and book-giving between women who were often, but not exclusively, in religious orders.[12] While Erler concentrates on women's active book-sharing networks, Andrew Cole, also in the wake of Watson's article, historicises Pecock's texts. Cole recasts the seemingly inflammatory nature of Pecock's prose to show, as a paradox, its unoriginal defence of the vernacular. Cole reads Pecock as nostalgic, rather than timely, in his condemnation of John Wyclif and the Lollards.[13] Cole implies that Pecock's vernacular works are not revolutionary, but pull from a forty-year-old discourse that found its origin, and its energy,

9 Pecock, *The Donet*, p. 5; also reproduced in *The Idea of the Vernacular: An Anthology of Middle English Literary Theory, 1280–1520*, ed. Jocelyn Wogan-Browne and Ian R. Johnson (University Park, PA, 1999), p. 99.

10 Among recent essay collections treating at large the dynamism of late fourteenth- and early fifteenth-century theological literary controversies deeply enmeshed in questions of vernacular English are *Wycliffite Controversies*, ed. Mishtooni Bose and J. P. Hornbeck (Turnhout, 2011); *After Arundel: Religious Writing in Fifteenth-Century England*, ed. Vincent Gillespie and Kantik Ghosh (Turnhout, 2011) and *Form and Reform: Reading across the Fifteenth Century*, ed. Shannon Gayk and Kathleen Tonry (Columbus, OH, 2011).

11 Nicholas Watson, 'Censorship and Cultural Change in Late-Medieval England: Vernacular Theology, the Oxford Translation Debate, and Arundel's Constitutions of 1409', *Speculum* 70 (1995), 822–64.

12 Mary C. Erler, *Women, Reading, and Piety in Late Medieval England* (Cambridge, 2002).

13 Andrew Cole, 'Heresy and Humanism', in *Oxford Twenty-First Century Approaches to Literature: Middle English*, ed. Paul Strohm (Oxford, 2007), pp. 421–37.

in the last part of the fourteenth century and the beginning of the fifteenth. Justifications like the one with which Pecock introduces his *Donet*, arguing for vernacular books' importance to their medieval audiences and cited above, have a pedigree that precedes the fifteenth century. A version of such a justification appears, for instance, in the entertaining 'Dialogue Between the Lord and the Clerk on Translation', apparently produced by John Trevisa circa 1390.[14] According to Cole, vernacular texts from the first part of the fifteenth century, like their immediate predecessors in the late fourteenth century, aimed at religious orthodoxy and remained aloof from the Lancastrian regnal politics. In Pecock's case, not aloof enough: the Viscount Beaumont, in the fifteenth century, takes pains to condemn Bishop Pecock's heart-imprinting vernacular writings.

The Middle English translation of *De doctrina cordis* and the manuscripts that remain of many other translated and original Middle English works make clear late medieval England's growing appetite for vernacular reading. The modern edition of *The Doctrine of the Hert*, by citing contemporary pietistic Middle English prose texts that resonate with themes, words, and meanings woven into that text, exemplifies this active vernacular milieu.[15] The edition's citations include Middle English works like the *Ancrene Wisse*, *The Book of Vices and Virtues*, *Sawles Warde*, *The Book for a Simple and Devout Woman*, *The Desert of Religion*, and *Speculum Vitae* (also known as 'A Mirror for Lewde Men and Women'). These texts demonstrate deep cultural interest in vernacular English theological prose, exactly that with which Pecock was 'imprinting men's hearts by secret and unheard means'. The question remains why Pecock's condemnation was so complete and absolute.

THE HEALTHY HEART AND ITS PASSIONS

Medieval concepts of the heart's functions differ from modern ones in two significant ways. The first is that the heart was considered the centre of both the literal body and the metaphorical self. Unlike the modern idiom of brain-centredness, medieval concepts put the heart at the centre of self-understanding.[16] The second is that the heart's action was considered to be not only distributive within the body, but propulsive outside of it.[17] Because

14 *Idea of the Vernacular*, ed. Wogan-Brown and Johnson, pp. 130–4.

15 The sixty pages of introduction to the edition demonstrate the breadth of the text's reach, its popularity, and the differences between versions that indicate translators' different audiences and their attempts to reach them: see *The Doctrine of the Hert*, especially pp. xxii–xxiii, xxxvii–xxxviii.

16 See Michael Frampton, *Embodiments of Will: Anatomical and Physiological Theories of Voluntary Animal Motion from Greek Antiquity to the Latin Middle Ages, 400 B.C.–A.D. 1300* (Saarbrücken, 2008), especially pp. 31–56 for a history of the heart/brain controversy.

17 Heather Webb, *The Medieval Heart* (New Haven, CT, 2010), especially ch. 2.

of medieval medical and philosophical understandings of spirits and spiritual exchange, the medieval semiotic heart was not limited to an individual body.[18] Such ideas about the heart's spirits and their exchange between inside and outside match theories of intromission and extromission that characterise medieval analyses of sight, another instance of spirit-based exchange.[19] Taken together, they demonstrate ideas about spiritual materiality and the heart's role that are very different from those of today.

University-oriented analyses of the heart, reflecting features of Aristotelian natural philosophy, appear in many places in late medieval thought and literature.[20] According to Latin university texts like *Anatomia Vivorum*, 'spirit', a combination of blood and air, is made in the heart. *Pneuma* – Aristotle's word for spirit – makes for the matter of the heart, insofar as the spirits in the heart are both made in, and also simultaneously inhabit, the heart. As a mixture of blood and air, spirit is unlike any other material substance. But spirit, like the heart and even the soul, is still considered to have a material substantiality. Light as air, extant in the heart and moved by the soul, spirits work throughout the body. Just as important as a concept of spirit, movement is key to a medieval understanding of the heart and its spirits. Aquinas's *De motu cordis* ('On the motion of the heart') figures all bodily motion as coming from the heart:

> Dico autem motum naturalem animalis eum qui est cordis: quia, ut Philosophus dicit in liber De motu Animalium, 'existimandum est constare animal quemadmodum civitatem bene ac legitime rectam. In civitate enim quando semel stabilitus fuerit ordo, nihil est opus separato monarcha quem oporteat adesse ad singula eorum quae fiunt, sed quilibet facit quae ipsius sunt ut ordinatum est, et fit hoc post hoc propter consuetudinem … in quodam principio corporis existente alia quidem vivere, eo quod apta nata sunt facere proprium opus propter naturam. Sic igitur motus cordis est naturalis quasi consequens animam, inquantum est forma talis corporis, et principaliter cordis'.
>
> [I myself say that the motion of the heart is a natural motion of the animal. As the Philosopher says in On the Motion of Animals, 'We should consider the animal as if it was a city under good and legitimate governance. For in a city with this kind of stability of order, there is no need for a separate ruler for each and every event, but instead everyone does everything as planned, and things proceed according to custom … with the soul present in the principle of the body, the other parts live and perform their own special work as nature made them. Thus, the motion of the heart is a natural result of the soul, the form of the living body and principally of the heart'.][21]

18 Eric Jager, *The Book of the Heart* (Chicago, 2000), especially ch. 1.

19 An informative analysis of medieval theories of intromission and extromission can be found in Suzannah Biernoff, *Sight and Embodiment in the Middle Ages* (Basingstoke, 2002), especially ch. 1.

20 A foundational study of early anatomy is George W. Corner, *Anatomical Texts of the Earlier Middle Ages: A Study in the Transmission of Culture* (Washington, DC, 1927).

21 Gregory Froehlich, *De motu cordis*, DeSales University Aquinas Translation Project,

Movement is thus effected by the material movement of spirits from the heart into the rest of the body.

Modern religious idioms may cater to concepts of spirit that, in order to answer contemporary science's definition of materiality, do not invest the spirit with 'matter'. But a medieval conception of spirit always considers it to be material substance. Perhaps a helpful way to understand the medieval idea of 'spirit' used to describe bodily workings is to consider the modern phrase 'spirits of turpentine'.[22] The phrase refers to the substance, and also to its effects. Turpentine's strong odour is invisible yet real, and its 'spirits' do its work of dissolving things like paint. Turpentine's spirits are simultaneously always contained in the turpentine at the same time that they, as smell, are continually emitted.

Even more challenging to a modern audience is the medieval idea that the heart is propulsive and sends spirit outside of the body. As Heather Webb puts it in her book, *The Medieval Heart*, 'the medieval heart was as respiratory organ, open and porous, radically available to the outside world and host to various incorporeal circulations'.[23] The medieval heart is propulsive; it makes spirits, and it contains the soul.[24] In this trio of propulsion, spirits and soul we grasp how different from a modern idiom medieval concepts of materiality were; at the same time we recognise the beating heart's centrality to these discourses. Essentially, medically-inflected concepts of the heart depended on material exchanges in their articulation of human physiognomy. At the same time, material spirit is essential to medieval concepts of the heart's function: the heart is home to a 'cardiocentric system of spirits'.[25] The heart's porosity fitted hand-in-glove with understandings of material external spirits moving through the five senses into the brain, and then moving from the brain into the heart as seat of understanding, after which the heart's material spirits move outward to effect motion in the body and outside of it. Porosity and movement – material being and exchange – is everything, both for good and for bad.

This material heart and material spirit also inflect medieval understandings of the human frame and human experience. A tradition dating to Aristotle's *Posterior Analytics* and explored by medieval philosophers like Aquinas, Duns Scotus and Ockham locates in the heart, not the brain, a uniquely human

http://www4.desales.edu/~philtheo/loughlin/ATP/De_Motu_Cordis/De_Motu_Cordis.html. See also M. O. R. Boyle, 'Aquinas's Natural Heart', *Early Science and Medicine* 18, 3 (2013), 266–90.

22 See, in the *Middle English Dictionary*, the entry for 'terebentine', which yields modern English turpentine. The medieval substance was made from the terebinth tree, of which 'the whole plant emits a strong smell: bitter, resinous or medicinal' (http://quod.lib.umich.edu.libproxy.uoregon.edu/cgi/m/mec/med-idx?type=id&id=MED44882&egs=all&egdisplay=compact).

23 Webb, *Medieval Heart*, p. 20.

24 Webb, *Medieval Heart*, p. 20, p. 20 n.15.

25 Webb, *Medieval Heart*, p. 27.

understanding that combines will, intellect and affect. Augustine figured the heart as 'the inner self and the inward life'[26] and, as such, the heart is invested metaphorically and materially with the Christian idiom of self. Margaret Bridges writes, 'At its best, the heart figures the stable centre of the self, the steadfast locus of secular and religious values such as constancy, pity, mercy, faith, hope or charity'.[27] As historian of science Peter Biller notes, 'A dictum found in Henry of Susa's *Lectura* on the section on reasonable suppositions in the *Five Books of the Decretals* (pre-1271) was that one grasps interior matters through external things: *per exteriora comprehenduntur interior*'.[28] The heart is the seat of human understanding; it is the site of imagination and engagement[29] but it is also a *heart*, a recognisable material organ in the centre of individual bodies.

Vivid metaphors figure the heart's combination of materiality and spirituality. *The Doctrine of the Hert* recommends flaying the heart to make it receptive to ecstatic union with the divine: 'Thou must nedis flee þin hert from þe old skynne of his own wille, and also þi body from þe skynne of temporal goodes, þat þou mow to þi lord be made able for to be receyvid.'[30] The heart's skin – which, in this reading, because it is the obstinate will, requires violent discipline – is metaphoric and literal at the same time. The spirits that traverse heart and body consort simultaneously with both will and heart. Will resides in – it *is* – the heart's skin.

The route to the interior heart is the five senses or, in Middle English, 'the five wittes': their sensory information goes from brain (simple understanding) to heart (deep re-*cor*-ding that informs the soul's choice to move). Sensory experience moves to the heart – the seat of the soul – and effects human understanding, although we ought to remember that this material movement is *spiritual* and not *mechanical* in a Cartesian sense. How like other skin is the heart's? *The Doctrine of the Hert* does not answer that question. Instead, it point outs that the skin of the head houses the five senses and notes that sensory deception harms the individual. Led by her senses to consider herself 'more discrete, more witty, and more kunnyng þan oþer',[31] an individual might suffer a deception that endangers her soul's health:

26 Jager, *Book of the Heart*, p. 29.

27 Margaret Bridges, 'Ubi Est Thesaurus Tuus, Ibi Est Cor Tuum: Towards a History of the Displaced Heart in Medieval English', *Micrologus: Natura, Scienze e Societa Medievali/ Nature, Sciences and Medieval Societies* 11 (2003), 501–19 (p. 506).

28 Peter Biller, '"Deep Is the Heart of Man, and Inscrutable": Signs of Heresy in Medieval Languedoc', in *Text and Controversy from Wyclif to Bale: Essays in Honour of Anne Hudson*, ed. Helen Barr and Ann M. Hutchison (Turnhout, 2005), pp. 267–80 (p. 277).

29 Frampton, *Embodiments of Will*; Jager, *Book of the Heart*.

30 *Doctrine of the Hert*, p. 22.

31 *Doctrine of the Hert*, p. 23.

> But now take hede þat a skynne, þe more sotil it is and þynne, þe worse it is, and þe harder for to be flayn from þe body. Right so, because þat þe proper willes of a soule is more sotil, in as much as it is withinforth, þan temporal goodes, þe wiche ben oughtward, therefore it is moche more harder a cloystrer to spoyle himself from his own willes þan from temporal possessiouns ... Do away, sister, yif þou wil not so be trobled, þe skynne of þin own wille, and þan make redy þin hert for be receyvid of oure lord.[32]

In both instances – in the heart-centred one, to discipline the will; in the head-centred one, to discipline the senses' appetites – flaying the *material* and *metaphoric* skin profoundly combines the spiritual, metaphoric and literal to train the soul. The heart is both figure and organ, home of the will, centre of being. The heart joins substance and meaning, and its porous nature, co-terminus with the will, receives and transmits *nearly*-immaterial understandings. Yet, according to Viscount Beaumont, it is 'printable' – like the skin of parchment. Since the royal heart escaped dangerous imprinting with Pecock's diverse conclusions, Henry VI's seemingly-porous breast will burn ever brighter.

Exchange inflects the micro-macrocosmic position of the porous heart in human health. Aquinas figured all bodily motion as coming from the heart, casting its movement as original; he then analogises the heart's motion in the body to the stars' motions in the cosmos. His analogy shows that heart health is tied to the macrocosm. Astrological medicine was part and parcel of university medical training. Allied with Aquinas, Latin academic medicine and its Middle English translations tied human health to the planets and astrology. The heart's health reflects a macro-microcosmic intersection beyond the heavens' respective motion that makes the heart reflect the cosmos. '*The Eleccioun of Times*', a Middle English translation of an unidentified Latin original extant in six fifteenth-century manuscripts and given its title by Lister Matheson, presents the planets and signs and also identifies propitious times for various activities. It includes this bit of information for the correct timing for medicine aimed at the heart:

> Whan þe Mone is in Leone, than is goode to speke to kyngis or to potestatis of the reme, & to sett an house or a castell or to entire into an house, & for to by or to chang goold & all thingis þat are yelow or safferan hewid in coloure, & for to do a medyson to þe hert or to þe Iyuer or to þe stomak or ony of þe inwarde thingis to be don with[in]forth.
>
> But it is perilous than to begin a long werk, or to kut in ony cloth or to clothe [f. 17] þe new, for owder he shal be smyten with a swerd or he shal be seke with that clothe. And also take non medicions nor drynk inward, for he shall cast hit out ayen with bloode. And witt it well, it is perilous þat time but if a man can goveryn himselue wethinforthe.[33]

32 *Doctrine of the Hert*, pp. 22–3.

33 'A Treatise on the Elections of Times', in *Popular and Practical Science of Medieval England*, ed. Lister Matheson (Ann Arbor, MI, 1994), p. 55.

The heart effects these inner and outer transactions because of its spirits: it has also been frequently conceived as the body's sovereign.[34] The medical advice that *The Eleccioun of Times* presupposed for its readers understands the heart's sovereign position and the power of its spirits. The text reflects features of Aristotelian natural philosophy that include the porous workings of the heart. Note that the time for medicines for the heart and inward things is the same as the time to speak to kings, and the text counsels internal self-discipline. Moreover, just as the heart rules the inward life, so kings rule the outward life – although Viscount Beaumont wishes it were otherwise as far as Pecock's heart imprinting goes.

Another important feature of the Middle Ages' registers of materiality appears in a consideration of material effusions of the heart called *passions* in Middle English. Pecock, in his *Reule of Christian Religion*, lists a series of substances, the forbidding of which is meant to control lust:

> þe seid fervent appetite or lust may come by pricking fumys or stemys gendering in þe privei fleisch by eeting of hoote and kene spicis or sawcis, or by garlijk or oynouns or oþer such hoot and kene þingis, and by habundauns of wijnd filling þe privey fleisch and by hoot humouris coming fro þe liver and from þe hert into þe priuey fleisch, bi hoot diet in ouer greet mesure and haunte or by talking or seeyng or heering or touching or þenking willfully wiþoute neede vpon þe fleischly deed or vpon ny3e purtenauncis þerto þou3 noon habundaunce or replecioun of þe seid mater be wiþynneforþ in þe vessels of þe seede.[35]

Notice the lack of differentiation between things material and 'worded' – thoughts – which modern audiences would distinguish as material and non-material. An over-hot diet works in the same way that wilful thoughts do to inflame desire. The fumes and steams engendered in the loins come from garlic, onions and spices; gas from hot humours in the liver and heart inflates the privates. The humours that come from the liver and the heart are themselves the 'hot and keen things' that result from using the senses – seeing, hearing, touching. They bring into the heart – without apparent need but with the very wilfulness of human thought and human hearts in tandem – impressions of the 'fleshly deed'. Yet, even though food and thoughts in equal measure affect the privy flesh, they do not necessarily force too much 'seed' to be produced in the 'vessels'. The strata of materiality that put thoughts and onions into the same sentence exemplify medieval understandings of *material* spirits and passions – what we would call emotions – having their seat, along with the will and vital spirit, in the heart and moving throughout the body.

Not only does Pecock's list refuse to hierarchise material or spiritual things, with wilful thoughts working like onions and garlic to inflame the flesh; the

34 Webb, *The Medieval Heart*, ch. 1, 'The Sovereign Heart': this chapter explains this ample metaphor.

35 Pecock, *Reule of Crysten Religioun*, p. 348.

passions – material in substance, affected by food as much as by thought – are, as Pecock tells us, unavoidable: 'Thou maiste neuer putte vttirli aside fro thee the seid natural passions from the lou3er appetites and from thi wil'.[36] The human frame, with the heart at the centre, cannot help but have its passions: 'Neuer of eny wijs sect it was holde that moral virtues schulden not stonde with passions, or that a man owith or my3te bi strength of moral vertues delyuer him from alle passions.'[37] Unavoidable natural passions nevertheless play integral roles in making moral choices:

> Fferþirmore, eche of þo seid passions had helpiþ and forþeriþ us, namelich at sum while into deedis of moral vertue to be gendrid, and eche of þo passions in sum maner had and kept lettiþ vs þerfro, as also vpon euer eiþir parti now seid we haue oft experience. Wherfore by good resoun þo passions whiche conforten oure kynd mowe be liknyd to mete and drynk, and þo passions whiche hurten oure kynde mowe be liknyd to venym and poysoun.[38]

We see in the way Pecock uses an analogy of passions to food, thoughts and moral choices the real aim of his vernacular writing: moral considerations. *The Doctrine of the Hert* makes a similar analogy for the ultimate heart-felt divine love, using food and the tasting of the divine.

> Þou shalt undirstond in þis place wisdom þat I take for þe knowleche of þe swetnes of God, had, as may be in þis life, bi experience. To þe wiche experientale swetnes enduceth us þe prophere, whan he seith þus: *Gustate, et videte quoniam suavis et Dominus*. 'Tastith' he seth, 'and seeth how swete oure lord Jhesu is'. First he sayth 'tastith' and afterward he seith 'seeth', for þe tast of God bringeþ a soule to þe knowleche of God.[39]

Again we see the easy overlap between senses and intellect, the literal and metaphorical. But a materiality of spirit combined with the heart's porosity suggests a sense of literal, material taste remaining in the admonition to 'taste'. We might read these passages as simply metaphoric. But our understanding of a material soul inflects these lines aimed at medieval readers with a heart-centred sense of divine taste and passion imbued with moral considerations.

The taste of the heart and its central moral role are at the centre of the idiom of lovesickness that unfolded during the thirteenth century.[40] Constantine the African's eleventh-century *Viaticum*, foundational in bringing Arabic medical sources to the medical school at Salerno, began in the thirteenth century to include Peter of Spain's *Commentary* on it. The *Commentary* of Peter, who

36 Pecock, *Folower to the Donet*, p. 112.

37 Pecock, *Folower to the Donet*, p. 114.

38 Pecock, *Reule of Crysten Religioun*, p. 112.

39 *Doctrine of the Hert*, p. 86.

40 Mary Wack, *Lovesickness in the Middle Ages: The Viaticum and Its Commentaries* (Philadelphia, 1990), provides this history of Constantine and the commentaries cited.

later became Pope John XXI (1276), reflects his practice in teaching the *Viaticum*; in that fashion, Peter's text helped to disseminate Constantine the African's text. Peter's analysis of lovesickness, however, changes between the first and second versions. In the first version, Peter analyses lovesickness in terms of the brain, heart and testes (a masculine audience is assumed). Peter divides the emotion of love in two: he comes to the conclusion that when love is an *appropriate* emotion it is located in the heart, while its morbid condition – lovesickness – is located in the brain. Peter's second version revises this trio. Peter removes the heart to make lovesickness spring from a duet: the brain and testes become the sites of consideration. 'Mind and body collaborate in the lover's decline.'[41] But, unlike the first version's tripartite division that includes, unsurprisingly, the testes along with heart and brain, the later version treats only the brain and testes.

One might read the change to indicate that the heart is losing its place in the intellectual, if not the popular, conversation of the day: not only is the heart taken out of a university-oriented conversation about lovesickness, but dropping it from the picture diminishes the heart's role in understanding the self – which is, following Augustine, the topic for academic and intellectual inquiry. The removal of the heart in the second version could reflect an impulse to distinguish popular definitions of lovesickness from academic ones. It could also reveal another step on the road of the scientific-medical-imaginative understanding of the brain's function: could Peter's change show an early iteration of a discourse that makes the brain, rather than the heart, the seat of the self and self-understanding? As such, it would presage modern senses of self and consciousness. However, another way to read Peter's elision of the heart emphasises the legitimacy of the heart as the seat of *appropriate*, God-centred love. Removing the heart from the trio of lovesickness-affected organs to make lovesickness a brain-testes system fits Peter's larger, theologically-inflected purpose of dividing romantic love from divine love. This move further legitimates the heart's place as centre of the self. Keeping the heart out of the lovesickness equation lets it remain the locus for a theologically and ethically approved, legitimate, even orthodox love focused on the divine, yet still reflective of the self. These are the senses on which Pecock and *The Doctrine of the Hert* depend. For the interplay of moral considerations, spirit and *soma*, the heart is key. Available for theologically-inflected vernacular writing, the heart is the centre of the self somatically, metaphorically and medically. But, for Viscount Beaumont, that self-centred heart is subject to pernicious imprints.

The heart is the seat of being and understanding in *both* a material *and* a metaphoric fashion. To use another of Webb's formulations, the heart does not have the limits of function, meaning or effect that a division between

41 Wack, *Lovesickness*, p. 97.

materiality and metaphor – the modern idiom – would give it. Instead, the heart is protean. The existence of lay understanding of different routes into the heart, and the fact that some things – like words[42] – stay there, certainly worried Viscount Beaumont. Beaumont's description of people's reading hearts, with their hidden vernacular words, along with his paean to the king's flaming chest, exemplify these attitudes toward, and understandings of, the heart and its porous nature.

THE HEART IS WHERE IT'S AT: THE EFFECTS OF READING

The heart, organ of life and death, is a persistent metaphor for the self, central to Western conceptions of being and consciousness for millennia. Milad Douiehi, assessing appearances of the heart as trope, asserts that, for Aristotle, the heart 'provides the support and founding analogue for life in general, both biological and political'; it is the 'biological and mythological, political and physiological' centre.[43] Aristotle noticed that what forms first in an egg is the chick's heart. For him, this observation gives evidence of the heart's literal, medical and metaphorical centrality. What may start with Aristotle's chicken continues in the Christian tradition, *pace* Augustine followed by Aquinas, Scotus and Ockham. Analogically, materially, as well as experientially, the heart is the *primum mobile*.

The *primum mobile*, in its actions, combines inside with outside macro-microcosmically in every possible sense. Inside and outside constantly mesh, and the path to understanding is simultaneously material and spiritual. *The Doctrine of the Hert*'s description of the heart's subtle 'skin', the will, exemplifies an understanding of its audience's 'inside' and 'outside' being simultaneously discreet, intimately connected, and redolent of moral considerations, materially and spiritually. Inside and outside are not indistinguishable, but both are intimately connected to moral equations and moral action. Both inside and outside, and their confluence, are needed to effect human understanding. The heart – semiotic and literal site of emotion or, more properly, of 'passions' both spiritual and secular – is at one and the same time the stable healthy self, the metaphoric as well as literal centre, seat of understanding, porous and emanating, and the *primum mobile*. The heart intimately ties together morality with materiality even as it moves and exudes spirit.

The conscience, a fundamental concept for this interplay of materiality and spirituality, is, according to the *Middle English Dictionary*, 'The mind or heart as the seat of thought, feeling, and desire; attitude of mind, feelings. … The faculty of knowing what is right, esp. with reference to Christian ethics;

42 Jager analyses the word-based heart: see *Book of the Heart*, ch. 3, 'The Scriptorium of the Heart'.

43 Milad Douiehi, *A Perverse History of the Human Heart* (Cambridge, MA, 1997), p. 4.

the moral sense … solicitude, anxiety'.[44] The word derives from Latin and Old French, and the Church's engine of confession and penance made conscience a familiar term and concept.[45] Following along from the pious traditions of academic Christian orthodoxy, the conscience becomes an explicit, named target of many Middle English poetic and pious texts, including the *Prick of Conscience* and *Piers Plowman*. For a medieval audience, however, neither the words nor the concepts of 'conscience' – sense of right and wrong – and 'conscious' – individual wakefulness – have been distinguished. Modern English 'conscious' means a 'witness to oneself, inwardly sensible or aware'. It derives from Latin 'conscio', which denotes being aware of a wrong, while Latin 'conscius' is a 'knowing in common, conscious with, witnessing (the guilty)'.[46] The Latin roots of the modern English word 'conscious' reveal the deep, even foundational resonance of self/other connection at the beginning of Western thought. These words show *being* as a *joining* rather than a *separation*. The use, in Middle English, of the word 'conscience', along with an understanding of hearts and their porosity, reminds us to meld modern English 'conscience' and modern English 'conscious' in contexts that consider the material heart. King Henry's shining chest exemplifies this jointure of spirit, material and morality, all centred on the royal heart. 'Conscience', tied to morals and ethics, is community oriented, but what trumps that community orientation today is the modern, individual 'consciousness'. After the medieval period, concepts of 'conscience' and 'conscious' separate on the basis of a new kind of existential self-understanding. The intellectual currents of the Renaissance era, as well as its scientific developments, establish a bottom line of human experience that erodes a prior sense of universal, spiritual participation.[47] Following the principle of *cogito ergo sum*, seventeenth-century English began to divorce the state of self-awareness from the state of 'other awareness' that the Latin roots of 'conscious' as well as 'conscience' invoked for a medieval audience.

The medieval conscience was a target not only of poets but of preachers. The sermon was considered a vital route to the conscience, its words affecting its hearers and their hearts. Preaching was a primary purpose of the cleric's vocation. Sermons were considered to be pedagogic and their instruction

44 *The Middle English Dictionary* is part of *The Middle English Compendium*, ed. Frances Ann McSparran (Ann Arbor, MI, 1998: Internet resource).

45 Thomas J. Tobin, '"He made his confession and told all his misdeeds": The Rise of the Internal Consciousness between 1100 and 1500', *Janus Head* (Summer 1998), internet resource, http://www.janushead.org/JHSummer98/ThomasTobin.cfm.

46 See the *Oxford English Dictionary* definition of 'conscious', http://www.oed.com.libproxy.uoregon.edu/view/Entry/39475?redirectedFrom=conscious&, accessed online 9 March 2014.

47 The literary critic Owen Barfield posited a sense of participation as signal for premodern self-consciousness: see *Saving the Appearances: A Study in Idolatry* (Middletown, CT, 1988).

ideally moved their audiences.[48] Late fourteenth-century prelates like John Mirk translated Latin sermons into English to serve as handy compendia for preachers. The vast critical literature on medieval sermons establishes their central role and their ubiquity. Publicly-preached sermons were ubiquitous and Pecock's contemporary notoriety included his sermons.[49]

Although a prelate and, seemingly, a gifted preacher, Pecock favoured the *read* over the *preached*, the *expository* over the *hortatory*: 'A curat mai not neither ou3te forto alwey rynge at the eeris of hise suggettis.'[50] But are *read* words effective? Since the target of both reading and hearing is the understanding central heart, the heart plays a role in the question of effectiveness. The amount of time thought necessary for reading to affect an individual developed in the cloister and emphasised long-term repetitive practice centred on prayerful rumination; later, more 'modern' idiom foregrounds intellection and individual understanding over liturgically-apt repetition.[51] *The Doctrine of the Heart* exemplifies these values directed at a reader's heart. The text was popular in Latin; it enjoyed broad popularity in its vernacular translations in Dutch, French, German, Italian and Spanish,[52] of which *The Doctrine of the Hert* is the Middle English instantiation. The Middle English text's modern editors assert that, while the translation seems to have been aimed at female religious, one of its manuscripts was owned by a laywoman whose sisters were nuns.[53] *The Doctrine of the Hert* in its very title indicates its dependence on, as well as its revealing of, concepts of what the heart meant to readers. Rather than ringing ears, the reading heart can be, like Henry VI's, a porous yet orthodox beacon.

The seven books in the Middle English *Doctrine of the Hert* may shorten and often eliminate parts that could be considered more esoteric or learned, but the text's goal is clear: affecting the hearts of its ostensibly non-Latin-literate female readers. The reader, 'Good sister', is advised to 'take hertly heede to þees comfortable wordis'.[54] The text notes the way reading marks the

48 On rhetoric, see Martin Camargo, 'Defining Medieval Rhetoric', in *Rhetoric and Renewal in the Latin West 1100–1540*, ed. Constant Mews, Cary Nederman and Rod M. Thomson (Turnhout, 2003), pp. 21–34; on sermons, see *John Mirk's Festial: Edited from British Library MS Cotton Claudius A.II*, ed. Susan Powell, EETS o.s. 334 (Oxford, 2009); *A Macaronic Sermon Collection from Late Medieval England: Oxford: Bodley MS 649*, ed. and trans. Patrick J. Horner, Studies and Texts 153 (Toronto, 2006); Siegfried Wenzel, *Latin Sermon Collections from Later Medieval England: Orthodox Preaching in the Age of Wyclif* (Cambridge, 2005).

49 See Scase, 'Pecock', pp. 95–9 for details about Pecock's problematic sermons.

50 Pecock, *The Repressor*, vol. 1, p. 219.

51 See Duncan Robinson, *Lectio Divina: The Medieval Experience of Reading*, Cistercian Studies 238 (Collegeville, MN, 2011), for a history of reading practice begun through repetition in the cloister.

52 *Doctrine of the Hert*, p. xvii.

53 *Doctrine of the Hert*, pp. liii–lv.

54 *Doctrine of the Hert*, p. 35.

heart: 'Thou puttiest wel oure lord as a mark upon þin hert, whan þour servist him with devocioun in redyng, praying, and contemplacioun'.[55] The *Doctrine* considers thoughts as emanating from, as well as protecting, the heart: lusty thoughts 'defendyn not thin hert from þe fende, but raþer bring in þe fende'.[56] Advice includes avoiding lusty thoughts in order to fortify the heart:

> Therfor, sister, put away such lusty þoughtes and lift up þin hert in holy þoughtes, þat it fall not from þe hert to þe flesh, but þat it abyde in þe hert with þe herte, þat þou mow sey as Davyth seyth: *Meditatus sum cum corde meo*. 'I have beþought me with myn hert'.[57]

As noted previously, *The Doctrine of the Hert* uses food to metaphorise ultimate heart-felt divine love, through the vehicle of taste, with the biblical '*Gustate, et videte quoniam suavis et Dominus*' glossed to make knowledge the combined senses of taste and seeing.[58] Knowledge happens in the heart, and *The Doctrine of the Hert* illustrates sympathies among hearts, thoughts and food that, as Pecock's work illustrates, define a medieval understanding of how words, like spirits, work materially in the reading heart.

The nature of language itself was an issue animating scholastic analysis. A scholastic etymological habit of mind recognises difference and development in individual languages as it simultaneously posits Augustinian identity between word and thing.[59] Such scholastic understanding supports translation. Vernacular language will affect the heart in the same way that another language will. Although words exist in the heart – imprinted on it, written on it – these words transcend language limitation while the heart bears a material imprint. That material imprint leads to books shaped as hearts and other kinds of medieval reading's *realia*.[60]

Are vernacular readers given to the same sense of absolute understanding the scholastic etymological frame asserts? Not exactly. Pecock asserts – not uniquely – that higher animals as well as human beings follow syllogistic reasoning of a formally logical sort.[61] Thus, it is not logical thinking – not

55 *Doctrine of the Hert*, p. 43.

56 *Doctrine of the Hert*, p. 50.

57 *Doctrine of the Hert*, p. 81.

58 *Doctrine of the Hert*, p. 86.

59 Robert Pasnau, *The Cambridge History of Medieval Philosophy*, 1st edn, vol. 1 (Cambridge, 2009), especially John Marenbon, 'The Emergence of Medieval Latin Philosophy', pp. 26–38; Steven P. Marrone, 'The Rise of the Universities', pp. 50–62; and Dag Nikolaus Hasse, 'The Soul's Faculties', pp. 305–19. See also Wack, *Lovesickness*, pp. 60–3.

60 Jager, *Book of the Heart*, includes illustrations of heart-shaped books on pp. 123, 127, 129.

61 Pecock, *Folower to the Donet*, ch. 8: he defends his assertion of this similarity between animals and people in the 'wirchyngis of eny powers' (p. 35) and asserts that both he and 'clerkis … knowlechen an Ape and a foxe to knowe all þe same þingis which y holde and seie þe ape and þe foxe to knowe' (p. 38).

reason alone – that can suffice to distinguish the human. What differentiates human understanding from animal reason is, for Pecock, a unique feature of the human being that he terms the 'doom of reason'. 'Doom' means 'judgment'; 'reason', *ratio*, is the rational soul. The 'doom of reason' is Pecock's term for the unique combination of will, intellect and affect that signally marks human consciousness apart from animal nature.

In his *Reule of Christian Religion* Pecock points to his understanding of an individual's 'doom of reason' and asserts his trust in this unique feature of the human frame:

> Wherefore folewith that men forto lyue in this now seid wise in her fre wil and in alle her othere powers thoru3 alle her dedis aftir the doom of resoun, is the service and lawe by which men owen to serue thee, lord, as bi to hem according service divers and different from the service of beestis.[62]

The 'doom of reason', a kind of writing inherent in the human heart, activates human understanding in men's souls, as Pecock reaffirms in his introduction to 'The Repressor':

> alle the trouthis of lawe of kinde which Crist and hise Apostlis taughten and wroten were bifor her teching and writing and were written bifore in thilk solempnest inward book or inward writing of resounis doom, passing alle outward bookis in profite to men for to serve God. ... the seid inward preciose book and writing buried in mannis soule ... mowe be taken bi labour and studiyng of clerkis mo conclusiouns and treuthis and governauncis of lawe of kinde and Goddis moral lawe and service.[63]

The 'doom of reason' is not the conscience, despite that particular feature's long pedigree; it is conceived as a 'pre-book' written in men's souls. The heart as the seat of the soul becomes its seat of words. Pecock leaves poetry and allegory to others; for his analysis of moral action, he invests trust in a reader's 'doom of reason'. The doom of reason governs a man within; in the complex of heart, spirit and soul, the doom of reason defines Pecock's trust in his readers.

Pecock's 'doom of reason' allows him to trust vernacular readers. The sixth chapter of his *Repressor* asserts that the 'outwardli ... writing of penne and ynke' matches 'the inward book of lawe of kinde, biried in mannis soule and herte'. In his *The Book of Faith*, Pecock values the material word alongside the word in the heart through a quotation from the Book of Deuteronomy 11:18–19:

> Putte ȝe these wordis in ȝoure hertis and soulis, and hange ȝe tho wordis for a signe in hondis, and sette ȝe bitwixe ȝoure iȝen; teche ȝoure sones that thei

62 Pecock, *Reule of Crysten Religioun*, p. 228.

63 Pecock, *The Repressor*, ed. Babington, vol. 1, pp. 30–2. Also reproduced in *Idea of the Vernacular*, ed. Wogan-Browne and Johnson, pp. 101–2.

> thenke in tho wordis, whanne thou sittist in thin house, and goist in the wey, and liggist doun and risist.[64]

Just as onions, garlic and thoughts affect individual health in equal measure, so the ubiquitous word of thought and re-readable *written* word stand as sign of the material and active conscience-oriented heart-bound soul, governed by the 'doom of reason'. Etymological habits of mind conceived in an Augustinian framework certify the absolute transparency of language; the heart-centred 'doom of reason' supports vernacular translation. Even though the reading heart is not literally transparent, Pecock trusts it, and the doom of reason.

Both Pecock's work and *The Doctrine of the Hert* are in accord in their heart-centred and heart-active understanding of meditative reading as cure. Both know that reading marks the heart. Pecock's theory of an individual 'doom of reason' located in the heart accords well with the effects the *Doctrine* wishes for its audience: 'abide in the heart with the heart' makes thinking and the heart one and the same. Still, the marking of the heart that the popular and seemingly authoritative *Doctrine* outlines passed muster and inspired no witchhunts; the printing of readers' hearts that Pecock entrusts to the doom of reason brought him to ruin. Pecock's error is to formalise his trust in readers via the heart-centred 'doom of reason'. While the *Doctrine* escaped condemnation for its passionately reading hearts, those same hearts, despite Pecock's articulation of a trustworthy 'doom of reason', contributed to Beaumont's condemnation of the prelate's heart-printing and its ostensible secrecy. As an exceptionally cruel blow to Pecock, Beaumont constructed the now-disgraced prelate's sentence to specify not only his removal from his bishopric of Chichester but that he 'haue no bookis to look on but oonly a portuos, a masse book, a saulter, a legende and a bible [and] haue nothing to write with, ne stuff to write vpon'.[65] Beaumont's need to ban Pecock's *writing* shadows the interior place where writing exists: the heart. As much as Pecock trusted readers, Beaumont mistrusted Pecock. Pecock was forbidden to create new books – and, in the event, he never did, but died shortly after arriving in his cell.

ENGLISH POLITICS IN THE FIFTEENTH CENTURY

The heart is a scholastically-legitimised, theologically-appropriate, individual health-oriented centre of understanding. The complex of *soma*, love and

64 Reginald Pecock, *Book of Faith: A Fifteenth Century Theological Tractate*, ed. J. L. Morison (Glasgow, 1909), p. 240. Internet resource: http://name.umdl.umich.edu/AJH1649.0001.001.

65 Scase edits Oxford, Bodleian Library, MS Ashmole 789, fol. 326r, which is a letter from Thomas Bourgchier, archbishop of Canterbury, to the abbot of Thorney abbey, giving instructions for Pecock's confinement; Scase asserts that the undated letter was 'probably written in early 1459, at the latest shortly after 7 April 1459': see *Reginald Pecock*, pp. 139–40.

lovesickness that animates poets throughout the medieval period could conceivably contest Christian orthodoxy. While parody may be one way to meet the challenge inherent in discursive and material connections between health and reading,[66] another that removes the heart from illicit love can turn it towards licit divine love (as Peter of Spain argues in the *Commentary*),[67] which opens the door for Pecock's 'doom of reason'. Insofar as the heart's love participates in the theologically sound act of reading via the 'doom of reason', and the theologically sound ecstasy described for the cloistered sister in *The Doctrine of the Hert*, the 'doom of reason' operates within the confines of orthodoxy. The mind is, for Pecock as well as for others like Peter of Spain, always in a body in need of health, and its place is actually *in*, and propelled *out* of, the porous heart.

At the same time that reciprocal ideas about embodiment and subjectivity, which have changed over time, colour a reader's understanding of his reading heart, the heart can be figured as materially tough and difficult to affect materially and symbolically. Pecock laments the features that make his detractors such a problem for him, asking God to 'amende' those infected by 'detraccioun and diffame, pride, sturdy herte, and envie spoken and written'.[68] Note that the 'sturdy heart' inhabits the same referential stream as less material but nonetheless problematic actions: detraction, defamation and, the deadliest sin of all, pride. Note too that all these features are both spoken and written, another example of Pecock's devotion to written words, including vernacular words. Beaumont, too, believes in the heart's centrality and effectiveness. But the viscount did not trust readers. That a 'sturdy heart' can be conceived as a *negative* feature for an individual may surprise a modern reader who expects 'good' hearts to be strong. But the medieval reader, understanding hearts as porous and ubiquitous, as well as being a habitation of shared spirits, could celebrate a heart-centred but infinitely sharable 'doom of reason' – or, like Beaumont, fear it. Such concerns, like Beaumont's, could take the form of debate about print and about secrecy, which was exactly what Beaumont worried about. What may, in the earlier Middle Ages, have stood as a constant and easy interplay between the literally material and the ethical and attitudinal – food and thought – cannot exist in tandem forever. By the sixteenth century, modernity wields the knife of reason and rationality. Material, ethical, and attitudinal spirits lose their places in a heart that previously, overflowing with spirit, propelled fire from Henry VI's chest.

It is true that understandings about the act of reading changed over the course of the Middle Ages. By the fifteenth century, as battles raged between Lancaster and York on the English countryside, battles – intellectual,

66 Julie Orlemanski, 'Jargon and the Matter of Medicine in Middle English', *Journal of Medieval and Early Modern Studies* 42, 2 (2012), 395–420.

67 Wack, *Lovesickness*, pp. 83–125, especially pp. 92–4.

68 Pecock, *The Donet*, p. 8.

philosophical, theological – raged also over the heart. What got reading into trouble was its effectiveness. What got Pecock into trouble was his trust. Reading imprints people's hearts. That it does so secretly, despite the factor of the heart's porosity, worried Beaumont. Porosity cannot match the problem of administrative control. Indeed, a deep suspicion of the effects of vernacular reading on individual hearts that inspired Beaumont to forbid Pecock to write *anything* underscores not only the vitality of the vernacular book but the material bases of reading, writing, thinking and feeling. Whether or not Pecock, by using others' arguments rather than inventing his own to support vernacular reading, was unoriginal in his defence of vernacularity mattered little to Beaumont.[69] A sentence that removes from Pecock's hands writing implements, if not prescribed books, indicates a fear of readers' independent thought. It was his explicit trust in congregants' and readers' hearts, and not suspect theological opinions, that ultimately doomed Pecock, condemned by the *secular* authorities beyond the religious authorities' expectations.[70] The bottom line for evaluating Pecock and Beaumont is that, when read, books work. They have an effect on the heart, an effect that Pecock trusted and believed in. Beaumont knew it too. Books signal the complicated and, as Beaumont noticed, *secret* effect that the practice of reading has on an individual heart. The porosity of the heart could spell danger on its own; only flaming royal hearts are to be trusted. Modernity will eliminate those flames, too.

Expressions of anxiety about heart-imprinted secrecy and worrying about the invisibility of heart writing use now-lost understandings of the human heart that trade upon the heart's health and effectiveness. Beaumont's sentence makes visible the powerful imaginative and literal hold vernacular English was thought to have on a newly-reading public, and presages later censorship born of a mistrust that Pecock's 'doom of reason' could not fathom.

69 Cole is interested in a momentary, mid-century efflorescence of bishops aiming for literary careers, 'Heresy and Humanism', pp. 435–7.

70 Scase, *Reginald Pecock*, pp. 111–17: 'By exerting their authority against Pecock, the crown could hope to harness and redirect to their own ends the powerful anticlerical feeling which was too often associated with the failure of the monarchy's authority, with unrest, lawlessness and sedition' (p. 117).

PART IV

DISFIGUREMENT AND DISABILITY

8

DISABLED CHILDREN: BIRTH DEFECTS, CAUSALITY AND GUILT

Irina Metzler

Medieval causalities of birth defects interconnect medical and literary texts, which in turn reflect religious attitudes. Arguably religious or philosophical notions influenced, and in many cases predated, the medical discourse,[1] all of which notions fed into literary texts – as many of the essays included in this volume similarly attest. The modern separation of religion from science, the spiritual from the secular, would have been nonsensical to the medieval mind.

How, then, did medieval normative texts – texts such as theological, philosophical or medical tracts, which reflect and reinforce commonly-held beliefs and cultural norms – explain the existence of congenital disability, that is, disability present from birth? In short, medieval texts tried to solve these problems by looking at sexuality, sin and conception. Conception here is meant in a dual sense, with concept as intellectual notion, and conception as physical begetting, in other words, a medieval aetiology of congenital disability. Previous research has more or less completely neglected the topic of congenitally disabled children, with the notable exception of John Boswell on the abandonment of children, and, in an oblique way, John Block Friedman on the monstrous races, but neither of these focuses on disability as the primary research question.[2] This essay therefore traces the 'absent presence' in history of congenitally disabled people, who, in some ways, have been continuously present within history – all societies at all times have had disabled people – but whose history is not part of the mainstream and needs to be reconstructed from scattered, random references.

1 See Paul Diepgen, 'Der Einfluß der autoritativen Theologie auf die Medizin des Mittelalters', *Akademie der Wissenschaften und der Literatur*, Abhandlungen der geistes- und sozialwissenschaftlichen Klasse 1 (Mainz, 1958), pp. 1–20.

2 John Boswell, *The Kindness of Strangers: The Abandonment of Children in Western Europe from Late Antiquity to the Renaissance* (New York, 1988); John Block Friedman, *The Monstrous Races in Medieval Art and Thought* (Cambridge, MA, 1981).

By way of introduction it is apposite to make a comparison with modern definitions and statistics. In 2012 the World Health Organisation (WHO) defined birth defects, or congenital anomalies, as 'structural or functional anomalies, including metabolic disorders, which are present at the time of birth'.[3] In terms of causality, however, the WHO estimates that approximately half of all cases of congenital anomalies cannot be assigned to a specific cause. What makes definition even more difficult, for the modern as much as for the medieval incidence of congenital impairment, is the continuum-like nature: as Judy Sture asks, 'When is a condition a defect, and when is it an extreme of normal development?'[4] For the majority of what we term 'developmental defects', modern science postulates an origin during the early stages of embryonic development. Such developmental abnormalities may occur in both the skeleton and the soft tissues, and may range from anomalies so minor that they are asymptomatic, to such severity as to be incompatible with sustained life.[5] Some modern statistics place the matter in perspective. It is estimated that around 2% of babies are born today with a major birth defect, a figure rising to 7% if minor defects are included; babies born before 37 weeks gestation are more likely to be affected, as are babies considered 'small for gestational age' including low birth weight. Genetic defects, passed on to the foetus via the parents' chromosomes, *and* environmental factors acting on genes or chromosomes in the foetus, can cause mutations. However, as Sture also asserts, 'most authorities are agreed that the majority of birth defects are most likely the result of a combination of genetic and environmental factors, interacting in some complex manner which is yet to be identified'.[6] According to a study published in 1993, it was estimated that 20% of defects were of genetic origin alone, 2–3% were due to environmental causes including maternal infection, another 2–3% due to drugs and chemicals, and 1–2% due to maternal metabolic disease; with the remainder assumed to be multifactorial, i.e., a combination of both genetic and environmental causes.[7]

We thus encounter cross-cultural concern with providing aetiologies for congenital impairment – the search for a reason, an explanation, anything that helps make sense of a senseless event, seems to be a common human impulse. The perceived normal course of events is the birth of a regular, healthy child,

[3] WHO Fact sheet no. 370, October 2012. http://www.who.int/mediacentre/factsheets/fs370/en/ (accessed 21 June 2013).

[4] Judi Sture, 'Congenital and Developmental Conditions', in *'Lepers outside the Gate': Excavations at the Cemetery of the Hospital of St James and St Mary Magdalene, Chichester, 1986-87 and 1993*, ed. John Magilton, Frances Lee and Anthea Boylston, Chichester Excavations 10, CBA Research Report 158 (York, 2008), pp. 157–63 (p. 157).

[5] Sture, 'Congenital and Developmental Conditions', p. 157.

[6] Sture, 'Congenital and Developmental Conditions', p. 157.

[7] Sture, 'Congenital and Developmental Conditions', p. 157, referring to M. I. Levene and D. Tudehope, *Essentials of Neonatal Medicine*, 2nd edn (Oxford, 1993), p. 194.

and parents worldwide and in all epochs struggle to come to terms with what is an abnormal event, regardless of how much love, care and attention the child does or does not receive later in life. A modern anthropological example is provided by Harlan Lane in connection with congenital deafness:

> Mothers in one central African nation report that on discovering that their child was deaf, their first thought was to verify that their ancestors had been properly buried. Mothers in many societies consider the cause of their child's deafness to be spirit aggression. We are fragile and dependent beings, they seem to imply, and deafness can be retribution for a moral failing.[8]

In his book on intellectual disabilities, Chris Goodey draws illuminating parallels between the medical and psychological description of modern 'coping strategy'. Parents in the contemporary Western world are informed by the experts (obstetricians, paediatricians and so forth) that their child is disabled. Almost as a reciprocal gesture, those experts expect parents to demonstrate a ritualised hierarchy of reactions (among others initial shock, followed by rejection of the child, leading to acceptance of the diagnosis). This is termed the 'coping strategy', and is comparable to the pre-modern version of such a 'desanctification ritual', in which supernatural agents such as devils, witches or fairies were blamed for producing the 'wrong' child.[9]

So, what caused the 'wrong' child according to medieval notions? Medieval thought has commonly used the imagery of the microcosmos,[10] whereby the human body represents on the small scale the ordering and hierarchy of the wider world on the large scale. William of Conches (c.1090–c.1160) stated in his *Sacramentarium* that the body from head to foot is likened to all of creation.[11] By analogy, what can go wrong with the macrocosmos, i.e., the corruption of the world through sin, can also go wrong with the microcosmos, i.e., the corruption of the body through illness. Refinements and additions were made throughout the high Middle Ages to this basic notion. In particular, the entire business of engendering children was focused upon in terms of the analogy of

8 Harlan Lane, *The Mask of Benevolence: Disabling the Deaf Community*, 2nd edn (San Diego, CA, 1999), p. 11.

9 Chris Goodey, *A History of Intelligence and 'Intellectual Disability'* (Farnham, 2011), p. 260.

10 Cf. Rudolph Allers, 'Microcosmos: From Anaximandros to Paracelsus', *Traditio* 2 (1944), 319–407.

11 William of Conches' text is attributed to Honorius Augustoniensis in the only current edition available, in PL 172, cols 738–806, especially col. 758, where the human body is described in quadripartite terms of four humours, seasons and elements. See also M. Goodich, *From Birth to Old Age: The Human Life Cycle in Medieval Thought, 1250–1350* (Lanham, MD and London, 1989), p. 65. The Venerable Bede wrote in *De temporum ratione*, ch. XXXV, on the four seasons, elements and humours, that 'homo ipse, qui a sapientibus microcosmos, id est, minor mundus appellatur' ('man himself was by the ancient philosophers called a microcosm, that is a miniature world'), in PL 90, col. 458B.

the corporeal and the spiritual. Of fundamental importance was the notion of sin, especially Original Sin. Augustine, writing in the late fourth century, had set the tone: though God had given humans the capability for sexual intercourse, and in essence the act was good, in practice every concrete act of intercourse was evil and therefore every child could literally be said to have been conceived in the sin of its parents.[12] Such ideas went a long way. By the thirteenth century a bestiary compiler could say that all new-borns, of all species, are 'dirty': 'In fact, all recently born creatures are called "pulli", because they are born dirty or polluted',[13] and only the act of baptism both metaphorically and literally cleans the infant. Given the fact that human beings only enter this world by procreation, one may then ask how, in medieval aetiologies, temporal factors and the actual practices of intercourse determined the appearance and character of the child.

In a series of translations of writings known as the *Pseudo-Clementines* from Greek into Latin as *The Recognitions* around AD 410 by Rufinus, texts which were very popular in the Middle Ages and survive in numerous manuscripts,[14] a passage states that sexual incontinence is accompanied by demons whose 'noxious breath' produces an 'intemperate and vicious progeny ... And therefore parents are responsible for their children's defects of this sort, because they have not observed the law of intercourse'.[15] Here, in late Antiquity, we already have the main line of argument that was to be pursued throughout the Middle Ages, which can be summed up as follows: intercourse at the wrong time and in the wrong way will result in the birth of defective children.[16] The *Chronicon Salernitanum* (chapter 14), written in

[12] Augustine, *De peccatorium meretis et remissione*, cap. 57 (XXIX), *The Works of St Augustine*, trans. Marcus Dodd (Edinburgh, 1885), vol. 2, referenced in Vern L. Bullough, *Sexual Variance in Society and History* (New York, 1976), p. 193.

[13] Oxford, Bodleian Library, MS Bodley 764, quoted by M. J. Tucker, 'The Child as Beginning and End: Fifteenth and Sixteenth Century English Childhood', in *The History of Childhood: The Untold Story of Child Abuse*, ed. Lloyd De Mause (New York, 1974), pp. 229–58 (p. 233); cf. *The Bestiary*, ed. T. H. White (New York, 1965), p. 104. It is interesting to note that childhood itself can be seen as a disability, in the context of the Ages of Man theme, whereby infancy, the first age, is 'without wit, strength or cunning and may do nothing that profits' (Pynson's *The Kalendar of Shepherdes* of 1506, quoted in Tucker, 'The Child as Beginning and End', p. 230); here one may also note the emphasis on profit and in the light of Gleeson's theories discussed in Irina Metzler, *Disability in Medieval Europe: Thinking about Physical Impairment during the High Middle Ages, c. 1100–1400* (London and New York, 2006), pp. 24–6, where one may observe how notions of the profitableness of something or someone begin to creep in towards the end of the Middle Ages.

[14] Cf. Lynn Thorndike, *A History of Magic and Experimental Science*, vol. I (New York and London, 1923), pp. 400–3.

[15] From writings known as the Pseudo-Clementines, translated by Rufinus, in *The Recognitions*, IX, 9, cited by Thorndike, *A History of Magic and Experimental Science*, vol. I, p. 414.

[16] I use 'defective' loosely here, implying both physically different and having character 'defects'.

the tenth century, mentions a woman who conceived by a priest and whose child was born without bones, which demonstrates, sneers the chronicler, that her repentance had not been stiffened with true contrition.[17] Gratian in the mid twelfth century cites a letter by Boniface suggesting that corrupt sexual unions would produce corrupt children.[18] And in an early fifteenth-century sermon Bernardino of Siena links neglect of filial duty with the punishment of begetting crippled, ugly, foolish and corrupt children.[19] However, a seemingly dissenting theory was proposed on the grounds of logical reasoning by Albertus Magnus, who turned the emergent notion of hereditary traits on its head. Possibly with a hint of irony Albertus claims that wise fathers beget foolish children, while foolish parents breed wise offspring: 'wise men mostly produce defective, foolish (fatui) children ... because he who is good at study is bad at sex (malus in venero acto)', since 'sex is the most foolish act a wise man commits in all his life', therefore the reverse must be true as well, and 'simple men' have wise offspring.[20] Nevertheless, medieval notions of heredity were far from comparable with the modern Mendelian, never mind genetic, concept of heredity, despite occasional random similarities. Although mid sixteenth century, Ambroise Paré's work on monsters is still pertinent for discussion of the Middle Ages, since he cites many medieval examples of monstrosities, but also in mindset he is not far from medieval understandings of the monstrous. In chapter 13 he cites examples of monsters that are created by hereditary diseases, where intellectual disability and epilepsy are mentioned in close conjunction: 'also if the father and the mother are fools usually the children are scarcely if ever intelligent (similarly epileptics give birth to children who are subject to epilepsy)'.[21]

By way of cultural comparison some evidence from the Islamic world may be useful, such as ideas from early twentieth-century Palestine cited by Dols:

17 Patricia Skinner, *Health and Medicine in Early Medieval Southern Italy* (Leiden, 1997), p. 49.

18 Gratian, *Decretum*, 1.56.10, referenced in Boswell, *Kindness of Strangers*, p. 338.

19 Bernardino of Siena, *Sermo de honore parentum*, in *Opera Omnia*, ed. P. P. Collegii Bonaventurae (Florence, 1956), vol. III, Sermo 17, pp. 311–18. See also S. Shahar, *Growing Old in the Middle Ages* (London and New York, 1997), p. 90. Children who neglect their aged parents would in due course be punished with a short life, poverty and the engendering themselves of sons who would be crippled, ugly, foolish and corrupt, and who would in turn treat their parents badly.

20 *Albert the Great: Questions concerning Aristotle's On Animals*, trans. Irven M. Resnick and Kenneth F. Kitchell Jr., Fathers of the Church: Medieval Continuation 9 (Washington, DC, 2008), Book 18, Question 4, pp. 537–8: 'Why wise men and philosophers very often generate foolish children'; Albertus Magnus, *Quaestiones super De Animalibus*, in *Opera Omnia*, ed. B. Geyer (Münster, 1955), vol. XII, p. 299; this English translation by Goodey, *A History of Intelligence and 'Intellectual Disability'*, p. 242.

21 Ambroise Paré, *On Monsters and Marvels*, trans. Janis L. Palliser (Chicago and London, 1983), p. 47, although a footnote draws attention to the fact that the line on epileptics is a posthumous addition to the original text.

'Insanity could also be inherited; some people believed that *coitus nudus*, intercourse in the open, or during menstruation affected the mental state of the child.'[22] And in the *hadith*, the pious traditions in Islam, in treatises on Prophetic medicine the aetiology of mental disorder is sometimes mentioned, for instance by Ibn Qayyim al-Jawziya (d. 1350), *The Medicine of the Prophet*, who says that 'a man who does not perform *ghusl*, or major ablutions, before sexual intercourse is responsible if his wife gives birth to a mentally retarded child'.[23]

Most discussions in medieval treatises centre on the method used in intercourse. Any deviation from the one prescribed method (the so-called missionary position) was seen either to avoid the main purpose of the act, namely procreation, or if a child was conceived by any other method then it would 'suffer deformities because of its parents' aberrant practices'.[24] A popular work falsely ascribed in the Middle Ages to Albertus Magnus, *De secretum mulierum* (On the Secrets of Women), mentions three main reasons why defective children are born: firstly, if the woman did not lie absolutely still but actually moved during intercourse, the male seed 'might be divided and a defective child conceived';[25] secondly, the woman should not let her thoughts wander during intercourse, but she should concentrate on what is going on, otherwise if at the critical moment she thought of something else, e.g. some animal like a cow, the child might turn out to resemble one;[26] and thirdly, any non-standard coital position might result in birth defects in those children who were the results of their parents' experiments in the conjugal bed.[27]

Here we have an example of the immensely influential concept of the maternal imagination. During intercourse and/or pregnancy, the mother can be imprinted by images that she sees, which will affect the shape and nature of the unborn or even unconceived child. This belief can be traced back to at least the Old Testament, where in Genesis 30:25–43 Jacob placed striped branches in front of the sheep of Laban, so that all the offspring of that flock

22 Michael W. Dols, *Majnûn: The Madman in Medieval Islamic Society*, ed. Diana E. Immisch (Oxford, 1992), p. 239. See also S. H. Stephan, 'Lunacy in Palestinian Folklore', *Journal of the Palestine Oriental Society* 5 (1925), 1–16 (pp. 4–7).

23 Dols, *Majnûn*, p. 245.

24 Helen Rodnite Lemay, 'Human Sexuality in Twelfth- through Fifteenth-Century Scientific Writings', in *Sexual Practices and the Medieval Church*, ed. Vern. L. Bullough and James Brundage (Buffalo, NY, 1982), pp. 187–205 (p. 201).

25 Lemay, 'Human Sexuality', p. 203. Cf. Commentary on *De secretis mulierum* (Venice, 1508), fol. E6v.

26 On this topic of the power of the maternal imagination to influence the physical appearance of the child, see Marie-Hélène Huet, *Monstrous Imagination* (Cambridge, MA and London, 1993), which deals mainly with Renaissance and Early Modern notions of imagination, but discusses some of the earlier ideas as well.

27 Cf. James A. Brundage, *Law, Sex and Christian Society in Medieval Europe* (Chicago, IL, 1987), pp. 451–2.

were born with striped fleeces, which Jacob claimed as his own. The topic is picked up in the early second century in a gynaecological text by Soranus, and again in Augustine's treatise *Against Julian*, both of which tell the story of a disfigured Cyprian tyrant who had beautiful works of art placed in the bedroom, so that his wife would look at those during sex rather than him, and thus he would not father a disfigured child.[28] Similarly, in the aforementioned thirteenth-century bestiary it is said that

> many people think that pregnant women should not look at ugly beasts such as apes and monkeys, in case they should bring children into the world who resemble these caricatures. For women's nature is such that they produce offspring according to the image they see or have in mind at the moment of ecstasy as they conceive.[29]

In the Renaissance, such classically-inspired ideas sustained and renewed their popularity; for example, in his astrological treatise *Liber de vita* of 1489, Marsilio Ficino mentions that 'people who are making babies often imprint on their faces not only their own actions but even what they are imagining',[30] thus extending the maternal to a paternal imagination as well. In wealthy Italian households it became important to surround potential parents with desirable images, located strategically so that they could be regarded at key moments. Leon Battista Alberti repeated this belief in *De re aedificatoria* (1452) with regard to painted portraits in the bedchamber: 'Wherever man and wife come together, it is advisable only to hang portraits of men of dignity and handsome appearance; for they say that this may have a great influence on the fertility of the mother and the appearance of future offspring.'[31]

Additionally, astrological explanations were offered. An example can be found in the twelfth-century text *Causae et curae* by Hildegard of Bingen: though men know the proper time for agricultural activities yet they beget their own offspring at any time without regard to the proper period in their lives or to the 'time of the moon', and defective children are the likely outcome of such heedlessness.[32] In the more scientific work, as opposed to spurious texts attributed to him, Albertus Magnus (c. 1206–80) argues that deformed births could be a result of particular causes, which would be related to the

28 Jacqueline Marie Musacchio, *The Art and Ritual of Childbirth in Renaissance Italy* (New Haven, CT and London, 1999), p. 128.

29 *Bestiary MS Bodley 764*, trans. Richard Barber (Woodbridge, 1999), p. 106.

30 Marsilio Ficino, *The Book of Life*, trans. Charles Boer (Irving, TX, 1980), p. 143.

31 Leon Battista Alberti, *On the Art of Building in Ten Books*, trans. Joseph Rykwert (Cambridge, MA and London, 1988), p. 299. See also Musacchio, *The Art and Ritual of Childbirth*, p. 130.

32 Hildegard of Bingen, *Causae et curae*, ed. P. Kaiser (Leipzig, 1903), pp. 17–18, 77–8. See also Mary M. McLaughlin, 'Survivors and Surrogates: Children and Parents form the Ninth to the Thirteenth Centuries', in *The History of Childhood*, ed. De Mause, pp. 101–81 (p. 147 n. 44).

paternal seed and the maternal reception thereof, while general causes could include the location and the relationship of the stars at the time of conception.[33] Albertus is not exactly certain which one of these causes is responsible, but he notes that some planetary conjunctions are recognised as particularly malicious, and points out that conception and birth should be avoided at such times. Specific problems might arise with regard to children born under a new moon, as they might be defective in sense and discretion.[34] Albertus claims to have seen himself the results of astrologically mistimed conceptions on two occasions, where human beings were born with truncated arms and legs who 'figuram corporis humani non habebit' (will not have the appearance of a human body).[35]

For a popular expression of similar ideas one can look even farther back, finding them in Old English texts, which seems to indicate the antiquity and the persistence of these notions, whereby the characters and the fates of children are influenced by the position of the moon on the day they are born.[36]

We find that the food consumed by the pregnant woman could have an influence on the shape of the child as well, according to the same Anglo-Saxon culture which produced such astrological treatises. In a collection of medical, astrological and magical texts we find the notions that 'if a woman is four or five months pregnant and she frequently eats nuts or acorns or any fresh fruit then it sometimes happens because of that that the child is stupid'; furthermore, if the expectant mother eats flesh of bull, ram, buck, boar or gander 'or that of any animal which can beget, then it sometimes happens

33 This is a summary of Albertus Magnus, *Physica*, Liber II, tract. 2, cap. 17, in *Alberti Magni Opera Omnia*, vol. IV, pars I, ed. Paul Hossfeld (Münster, 1987), pp. 123–5; the pertinent passage with regard to the origin of abnormal births (such as six-fingered children or conversely those lacking members or of conjoined twins) is at p. 125. See also B. B. Price, 'The Physical Astronomy and Astrology of Albertus Magnus', in *Albertus Magnus and the Sciences*, ed. J. A. Weisheipl (Toronto, 1980), pp. 180–1.

34 Albertus Magnus, *De natura boni*, tract. 2, pars 3, cap. 2, 2, 3, A, 1, 1, Prima interpretatio 'illuminatrix', in *Alberti Magni Opera Omnia*, vol. XXV, pars I, ed. E. Filthaut (Münster, 1974), p. 49 §125. Albertus is here following the ideas of Firmicus Maternus, *Matheseos*, IV, c1, n. 10; see Price, 'The Physical Astronomy', pp. 180–1.

35 Albertus Magnus, *Problemata determinata*, p. 35; an edition is given by James A. Weisheipl, 'The Problemata determinata XLIII, Ascribed to Albertus Magnus (1271)', *Mediaeval Studies* 22 (1960), 303–54 (pp. 349–50). The editor, Weisheipl, added a note that Albertus did not just transmit these stories, but had apparently observed such monstrous births himself (p. 349 n. 59). See Price, 'The Physical Astronomy', pp. 180–1.

36 Sentiments along those lines can be found in London, British Library, MS Cotton Tiberius A. iii. Cf. A. L. Meaney, 'Women, Witchcraft and Magic in Anglo-Saxon England', in *Superstition and Popular Medicine in Anglo-Saxon England*, ed. D. G. Scragg (Manchester, 1989), p. 19; on the antiquity of the idea cf. M. Förster, 'Vom Fortleben antiker Sammellunare in englischen und anderen Volkssprachen', *Anglia* 67-68 (1944), 1–171, especially pp. 94–5.

because of that that the child is humpbacked and deformed [?]'.[37] It is worth pointing out that all the meat the pregnant woman should avoid consuming is from male animals, and only the male of the species has the capability to beget, as we shall see.

Here we also touch on concern with the very modern topic of maternal nutrition. Soranus, practising medicine under emperors Trajan and Hadrian, had already said in his *Gynaecology* that pregnant women should be challenged in their desires 'for harmful things', by telling them that what is harmful to the stomach is also harmful to the foetus 'because the fetus obtains food which is neither clean nor suitable, but only such food as a body in bad condition can supply'.[38]

If a parent was particularly blamed for inappropriate behaviour that negatively influenced the development of the baby, it was the mother. A handful of examples from both the very early and very late Middle Ages may illustrate this point. In the fifth century Nemesius, compiler of an influential tractate on the soul, also looked at child development, and with regard to the causes of unfavourable bodily temperament stated: 'if the surroundings are dry, bodies become dry, if not all in the same way, and if a mother lives an unhealthy life and is luxurious her children will in consequence be born with a poor bodily temperament and wayward in their impulses.'[39] The effects of bodily temperament had been emphasised by Galen in his work *Quod animi mores*, but antecedents to this idea were already in Plato, *Timaeus* 86–87, a text in turn cited by Galen.[40] Bartholomäus Metlinger, author of the first paediatric handbook, *Ein regiment der jungen kinder* in the German vernacular, printed at Augsburg in 1473, had this to say on the causes of epilepsy:

> The first cause may be inordinate behaviour of the mother who carries the child, so there may be no hemming her desires, whether good or bad, or a defect (*blödigkeit*) in the being of the head of the fruit [i.e. the foetus], which sometimes comes through influence of the heavenly bodies [i.e. stars and planets]. But if epilepsy (*vergicht*) comes in children after birth, then the cause is the milk of the wetnurse, or that one suckles it inordinately, that is on the one hand too little, on the other hand too much, or that one always gives him more

37 The original text is in MS Cotton Tiberius A. iii, fols 40v–41r, 'Peri Didaxeion', and an edited version of the original Old English can be found in *Leechdoms, Wortcunning and Starcraft of Early England*, ed. T. O. Cockayne, 3 vols, Rolls Series 35, parts 1–3 (London, 1864–66), vol. 3, pp. 144–5. Modern English in M. L. Cameron, *Anglo-Saxon Medicine* (Cambridge, 1993), p. 183.

38 *Soranus' Gynecology*, trans. Owsei Temkin (Baltimore, MD, 1956), Book I, ch. 53, pp. 53–4.

39 *Nemesius: On the Nature of Man*, trans. (with introduction and notes) R. W. Sharples and P. J. van der Eijk, Translated Texts for Historians 49 (Liverpool, 2008), Section 40 [116.10], p. 199.

40 *That the Faculties of the Soul Follow the Mixtures of the Body*, 6, 49.12-51.11.

than he can bear or digest, also fright, fear and lack of care (*unbehütnuß*) of the children.[41]

Unsurprisingly, of the many substances ingested by both mother and father which can damage the sperm or the unborn child, excessive alcohol consumption is cautioned against. Soranus remarked on what we would now call foetal alcohol syndrome, stating that in the cases of nurses who abuse alcohol the bad effects are carried through into the milk, and thus babies may become 'sluggish and comatose and sometimes even afflicted with tremor, apoplexy, and convulsions just as suckling pigs become comatose and stupefied when the sow has eaten dregs'. The ideal 'wet nurse should be "self-controlled" so as to abstain from coitus, drinking, lewdness, and any other such pleasure and incontinence'; drinking harms the wet nurse's soul as well as her body, thus spoiling her milk, and heavy alcohol-induced sleep may cause her to neglect the newborn or even fall 'down upon it in a dangerous way'.[42] Furthermore, an Anglo-Saxon medical tract warned women against becoming drunk.[43] In his chronicle Thietmar of Merseburg (d. 1018) tells the story of Uffo, a citizen of Magdeburg, who while very drunk forced his wife Gelusa to have intercourse with him on the feast day of the Holy Innocents (28 December); Gelusa became pregnant and to her horror gave birth prematurely to a child with crippled toes, blaming herself and her husband; him for the improper request, herself for obeying him.[44] Writing around 1300, in chapter 25 of his *Lilium medicinae*, Bernard de Gordon repeats the advice of Soranus against alcohol consumption by the nurse: 'Since epilepsy comes rather often to children and infants through inebriation and wine-bibing and poor diet on the part of the nurse ... the routine of the nurse should be corrected.'[45] In the early fifteenth century Giovanni Morelli notes in the *Ricordi* that 'a man should not be drunk when his children were conceived or they would be weak, stunted, or (possibly even worse) female'.[46] And that same century Leon Battista Alberti writes in *I libri della famiglia*: 'The doctors say, and they

41 See *Quellen zur Geschichte der Epilepsie*, ed. Helmut Heintel, Hubers Klassiker der Medizin und der Naturwissenschaften Band XIV (Berne, Stuttgart and Vienna, 1975), pp. 34–5. My translation. The Augsburg edition of 1473, fols 13a–14b discuss epilepsy.

42 *Soranus' Gynecology*, Book II, ch. 19, pp. 92–3.

43 A. Hagen, *A Second Handbook of Anglo-Saxon Food and Drink: Production and Distribution* (Hockwold cum Wittom, Norfolk, 1995), p. 192.

44 Thietmar von Merseburg, *Chronik*, ed. Werner Trillmich, FSGA Band 9 (Darmstadt, 2002), p. 28: see also Kai P. Jankrift, *Mit Gott und schwarzer Magie. Medizin im Mittelalter* (Darmstadt, 2005), p. 53. According to Thietmar, the newborn baby boy died soon after his baptism, which at least cleansed him of the misdemeanour of his parents and assured him a place among the innocent infants in heaven.

45 See 'Bernard of Gordon on Epilepsy', trans. W. G. Lennox, *Annals of Medical History*, 3rd series, 3 (1941), 372–83 (p. 377).

46 A. Lynn Martin, *Alcohol, Sex, and Gender in Late Medieval and Early Modern Europe* (Basingstoke, 2001), p. 44.

give ample reasons, that if a mother or father are low and troubled because of drink ... it is reasonable to expect the children to manifest these troubles. Sometimes, in fact, they will be leprous, epileptic, deformed, or incomplete in their limbs and defective.'[47]

Popularly disseminated notions on improper sexual conduct can also be found in religious literature aimed at what might be termed a mass-market: penitentials, preaching and sermon tracts. Here the argument based on sex and sin is expanded upon, and damaging factors such as pregnancy, lactation or menstruation are considered. Robert of Flamborough, in the *Liber penitentialis* (1208–13), warned that children conceived during pregnancy (disregard the biological impossibility for the moment), during menstruation, or before a previous child was weaned, would be lame, leprous, given to seizures, deformed or shortlived.[48] Note that all three inopportune times Robert refers to are times that were believed to be infertile periods, in other words naturally contraceptive periods. With the absence of modern over-nutrition, in the past (as still in many traditional societies) the lack of nutrition influenced female fertility to the extent that the physical demands of breastfeeding on the body tended to prevent conception during that time. As we know from medieval childcare manuals, breastfeeding would ideally have continued until children were weaned at around two years of age.[49] Conception during these two years was then unlikely. Many modern hunter-gatherer societies equally do not wean children until two years old, and have lower levels of calorific intake than Western women, so among such peoples births tend to be spaced out at two-year intervals.[50] One could speculate that precisely because of the lack of conception during such times, which medieval people, especially women, may well have been aware of,[51] they were forbidden by moralists, as intercourse

47 Cited by Martin, *Alcohol, Sex, and Gender*, p. 45.

48 *Liber penitentialis*, Liber quartus, §288, ed. J.-J. Firth, Pontifical Institute for Mediaeval Studies, Studies and Texts 18 (Toronto, 1971), pp. 197–8. A little further on he wrote that at times the vices of semen are carried forward to the foetus, so that children are conceived with leprosy, elephantiasis, and are corrupted by too small or too large limbs (Liber quintus, §288, p. 238). See also Boswell, *Kindness of Strangers*, p. 338.

49 On breastfeeding see Shulamith Shahar, *Childhood in the Middle Ages* (London and New York, 1990), pp. 77–83. This practice is corroborated by Simon Mays, archaeologist, from evidence in dental remains of infants at Wharram Percy in a report by English Heritage, 'Human Osteology at Wharram Percy: Life and Death in a Medieval Village', http://www.english-heritage.org.uk/publications/conservation-bulletin-45/cb45p22-23.pdf (accessed 28 August 2014).

50 My family doctor informed me that because modern Western women are overfed, the old pattern of infertility during breastfeeding no longer applies, only in cases of nutritional deficiencies in the mother, but acknowledged that this would have been the prevailing pattern in the past.

51 On issues of contraception, see the seminal work by J. T. Noonan, *Contraception: A History of Its Treatment by the Catholic Theologians and Canonists* (Cambridge, MA, 1966); also J. M. Riddle, 'Oral Contraceptives and Early-Term Abortifacients during

then would have been for pleasure only and not for procreative purposes. In his *Sermons*, Berthold of Regensburg adds to such lists of physical deformities the dangers of deafness, mean spiritedness and demonic possession;[52] again, potential disability and moral defectiveness in children is ascribed to their conception at forbidden times, to which Berthold adds the six weeks immediately after childbirth (yet another infertile period), and furthermore notes that nobles and burghers are less prone to such sins than the peasantry. In his sermon on matrimony, he writes:

> All the children who are conceived at such times you rarely will gaze at with a loving look; for it is either possessed by the devil, leprous, epileptic, humpbacked, blind, crippled, dumb, foolish or has a head like a mallet. ... And this happens mainly to peasants and ignorant people. It does not happen to noble people and burghers in towns.[53]

A thirteenth-century French church synod proclaimed that the children conceived from illicit sex would be born humpbacked, crippled, or deformed in some way.[54] From a fourteenth-century manuscript we have the usual prohibition of sexual activity during menstruation, lactation and pregnancy, and the prediction that children born from such unions would be leprous, lunatic or possessed.[55] And an early fifteenth-century book of homilies, basing its knowledge on St Jerome, provides the full catalogue, stating that 'children conceived during maternal menstruation would be lepers, maimed, unshapely, witless, crooked, blind, lame, dumb deaf and of many othre mescheues'.[56]

Of the three inopportune, even proscribed, times of conception, menstruation was singled out as particularly important to avoid if parents wanted to

Classical Antiquity and the Middle Ages', *Past & Present* 132 (1991), 3–32; and P. A. Biller, 'Birth-Control in the West in the Thirteenth and Early Fourteenth Centuries', *Past & Present* 94 (1982), 3–26. That medieval people were probably well aware of the 'safe periods' is backed up by the fact that as early as the sixth century Aetio of Amida, a Byzantine court physician, recognised the existence of a less fertile or even infertile period at the beginning and at the end of the menstrual cycle; see Vern L. Bullough and James A. Brundage (eds), *Sexual Practices in the Medieval Church* (Buffalo, NY, 1982), p. 16.

52 Berthold von Regensburg, *Vollständige Ausgabe Seiner Predigten*, ed. F. Pfeiffer, 2 vols (Vienna, 1862), vol. 1, pp. 322–4, see also Boswell, *Kindness of Strangers*, p. 338.

53 Sermon XXI, 'Von der Ê', Berthold von Regensburg, *Vollständige Ausgabe*, vol. 1, p. 323, see also McLaughlin, 'Survivors and Surrogates', p. 147 n. 44.

54 Synodal de l'Ouest, 96, in *Les Statuts synodaux français du XIIIe siècle*, ed. and trans. Odette Pontal, 2 vols (Paris, 1971), Collection de documents inédits sur l'histoire de France, Section de Philologie et d'Histoire 9, 15. See also Boswell, *Kindness of Strangers*, pp. 338–9.

55 Cf. *inter alia* MS Bayerische Staatsbibliothek clm 18404 (s. XIV), fol. 128r, referenced in Boswell, *Kindness of Strangers*, p. 403.

56 London, British Library, MS Harley 45, fol. 119v, referenced in Carole Rawcliffe, *Leprosy in Medieval England* (Woodbridge, 2006), p. 82.

prevent the conception of impaired children. Menstruation was regarded as dangerous by scholastic authorities, using arguments in part derived from Aristotle. Aristotle had argued in *Generation of Animals*, IV, 3–5 that foetal aberrations should be blamed on a divergent movement of the female matter, and an imbalance of female matter with the formative sperm. While acknowledging that during the medieval period two competing and widely debated models of conception existed – the single-sex and the two-seed theories – it is, for the purposes of discussing medieval notions of birth defects, almost irrelevant to which theory a medieval authority subscribed. Misogyny was ingrained enough to find ample scope in both theoretical models for almost exclusive 'blame' on the woman. Broadly put, according to the single-sex model of natural science, the menses (or *menstruum*, female seed) accumulates gradually over each cycle as a kind of formless matter. Only the male seed has form itself and is pure maleness. The female simply receives the seed and nurtures it, but does not generate. By extension of this reasoning the female is of necessity defective; an idea that is theologically backed up by Genesis, where Eve's creation out of Adam's bent rib made Eve herself deviant from the male norm. The clearest expression of this kind of argument can be found in Albertus Magnus' *De animalibus*,[57] where, moving on from the premise of menses as formless matter, he reiterates the practical advice given by theologians and physicians alike that semen has the best chances of 'forming' the menses in the earlier part of the cycle. If conception takes place during a later stage of the cycle, however, there is a sliding scale of degradation and degeneration: having missed the ideal time for generating male offspring, the next best would be female children, hence only slightly deformed, followed by the severely defective (disabled) progeny, and lastly and worst no offspring at all[58] – the *horror vacui* of medieval philosophy. It is worth just repeating this descending scale from perfect male, to slightly imperfect female, to certainly imperfect deformity, to nothing.

Such notions are also apparent in medical texts, for instance the *Lilium medicinae* of Bernard de Gordon, where conception during menstruation is blamed for the birth of an epileptic child: 'When a person is begotten during

57 This is a summary of the explanation given by Albertus Magnus, *De animalibus*, Libri XXVI, Liber 15, tract. II, cap. 6, entitled 'De natura spermatis et menstrui tam feminae quam masculi quam habet secundum quod est principium generationis', §101–12, ed. Hermann Stadler, Beiträge zur Geschichte der Philosophie des Mittelalters, Texte und Untersuchungen 16 (Münster, 1920), pp. 1035–40; Sarah Alison Miller, *Medieval Monstrosity and the Female Body* (New York, 2010), has a chapter on gynaecology which looks at blood, seed and monstrous births through the lens of the Pseudo-Albertine *De secretis mulierum*, dated to the late thirteenth or early fourteenth century, providing a useful summary of Greek and Roman medico-philosophical discourse and its assimilation by medieval natural philosophers.

58 Charles T. Wood, 'The Doctor's Dilemma: Sin, Salvation, and the Menstrual Cycle in Medieval Thought', *Speculum* 56 (1981), 715–16.

the time of menstruation or from unclean seed, or if the parents are epileptic, and if after his birth he falls into epilepsy, such a person does not seem curable.'[59] Another famous physician and Bernard's contemporary, John of Gaddesden in his *Rosa anglica*, states similar things about the aetiology of congenital epilepsy.[60]

The effects of malconception could have a straightforward causal link, a rational explanation even. In discussing the origin of dwarfs, for example, Albertus Magnus describes a nine-year-old girl whom he had seen in Cologne who had not yet reached the height of a one-year-old boy. He followed the argument of Avicenna, which was perfectly scientific by the standards of the day, explaining that the lack of growth was due to the fact that at the moment of conception only a part of the paternal seed had reached the maternal uterus.[61] During the same century, writing c. 1276, Giles of Rome in his more general discussion of embryology *De formatione corporis humani in utero* holds a rather neutral opinion, stating blandly that although normally the male seed generates a male foetus from the menstruum, nothing in nature is so stable and fixed that things cannot go wrong sometimes, which is obvious from the fact that occasionally monsters are born with deformed members.[62] The medieval scientific approach was one that regarded all material creation as inherently imperfect, hence birth defects and congenital disability were not just individual markers on a sliding scale of imperfection, but also natural events to be expected.

We encounter the themes of religious analogy and potential disability, which run through so many of medieval moral texts, in a tract by John Gori of San Gemignano (c. 1260–c. 1323), a Dominican hagiographer and moral theologian, who compares the care that must be given to the newborn infant to the care that must be had for the soul of the *conversus*, the newly converted Christian; infants must be swaddled in order to straighten their limbs 'since

59 Owsei Temkin, *The Falling Sickness: A History of Epilepsy from the Greeks to the Beginnings of Modern Neurology*, 2nd edn (Baltimore, 1971), pp. 131–2, citing Bernard de Gordon, *Lilium medicinae* [*Omnium aegritudinum a vertice ad calcem, opus praeclariss. quod lilium medicinae appellatur*, Paris, 1542, fol. 119r].

60 Ioannes Anglicus, *Praxis medica, rosa anglica dicta*, recens edita opera ac studio clar. V. Doct. Philippi Schopffi, Medici Physici Durlacensis, 2 vols (Augsburg, 1595), p. 50. John of Gaddesden copied what Bernard de Gordon wrote on the subject virtually verbatim. See 'John of Gaddesden on Epilepsy', trans. W. G. Lennox, *Annals of Medical History*, 3rd series, 1 (1939), 283–307 (p. 294): 'When a child is conceived at the time of menstruation, or from unclean semen, or his parents are epileptics, then the child inherits epilepsy; this type does not seem to be curable, because after the child leaves the womb from such evil causes his complexion is fixed.'

61 *Kleine Menschen – Große Kunst. Kleinwuchs aus künstlerischer und medizinischer Sicht*, ed. A. Enderle, D. Meyerhöfer and G. Unverfehrt (Hamm, 1992), p. 34; see also H. Balss, *Albertus Magnus als Zoologe* (Munich, 1928), p. 15.

62 M. Anthony Hewson, *Giles of Rome and the Medieval Theory of Conception* (London, 1975), p. 187.

they are easily malformed'.[63] Swaddling done incorrectly could actually cause more damage than good, as Aldobrandino of Siena points out in 1256, in his treatise *Le régime du corps*, composed for Beatrix of Provence, mother-in-law of Louis IX of France:

> And when one wishes to swaddle [the baby], the members should be gently couched and arranged so as to give them a good shape … for just as wax when it is soft takes whatever form one wishes to give to it, so also the child takes the form which its nurse gives to it. And for this reason … beauty and ugliness are due in large measure to nurses.[64]

But other medical treatment could also be dangerous. The aetiology of mental retardation according to Avicenna (980–1037), in his *Canon of Medicine*, might be influenced by malpractice, in that with regard to medical treatments one should be cautious about applying cupping-glasses to the forehead for 'it impairs the activity of the intellect, making the offspring dull and forgetful, with poor reasoning powers and permanent infirmity'.[65]

Prevention of disability and disease could be attempted by all sorts of means, which in modern discourse might be described as ranging from the medical, via the religious, to the downright magical, although of course the medieval period would not have made such distinctions. For example, sacred texts and the books in which they were written assumed a status almost of bodily relics, since their possession was believed to promise protection. In one of the Old English *Lives of St Margaret*, chapter 19 states: 'And where the book of my martyrdom is [kept] may there not be born a child who is blind or lame or dumb or deaf or afflicted by an unclean spirit'.[66] Another version of the same chapter gives the variant that in such a house no 'unhal' child would be born, no cripple, dumb, deaf, blind or witless child[67] so here an allusion is made to the 'witless' child, the child with intellectual disabilities in modern

63 Goodich, *From Birth to Old Age*, p. 88. Disabilities arising out of malpractice would in today's medical parlance be termed perinatal of course, rather than classed as congenital disabilities, but for the purposes of the present discussion, they are included here as pertaining to the broader category of neonatal medical problems.

64 Aldobrandino of Siena, *Le régime du corps*, composed in 1256 for Beatrix of Provençe, mother-in-law of Louis IX of France, in *Medieval Medicine: A Reader*, ed. Faith Wallis (Toronto, 2010), p. 496.

65 Avicenna, *A Treatise on the Canon of Medicine of Avicenna: Incorporating a Translation of the First Book*, ed. and trans. Oskar Cameron Gruner (London, 1930), pp. 509–10: 'General Discourse upon the Treatment of Disease', Book I, Part IV, section 21, 1032, concerning application to the forehead, 'most people have a horror of applying cupping-glasses here, as they believe that the senses and intellect will suffer thereby'. See also R. C. Scheerenberger, *A History of Mental Retardation* (Baltimore, MD and London, 1983), p. 28.

66 *The Old English Lives of St Margaret*, ed. Mary Clayton and Hugh Magennis, Cambridge Studies in Anglo-Saxon England 9 (Cambridge, 1994), pp. 132–3.

67 *The Old English Lives of St Margaret*, p. 168.

parlance, as well as to the usual list of physical impairments. And in German literature, too, we encounter this concept. In 1172 Priester Wernher in his *Life of Mary* praises his text like a talisman: 'where these books are kept the Virgin will ensure that no child will be crooked [crippled] or blind'.[68]

Lastly, it is useful to look at some reactions to congenital disability, starting with a series of warnings against marriage and pregnancy. The so-called Acts of Thomas, dated to around AD 200, which in many ways deviate significantly from the established canonical Gospels of the New Testament, include a passage on the absolute value of sexual abstinence. To underpin these views, the writer points out that the majority of children conceived would in any case be oppressed by devils and turn out to be either lunatic (literally: drawn to the moon, that is perhaps epileptic), half withered, blind, deaf, dumb, paralytic or stupid (μωρος in the Greek); should they in fact be born healthy they would be doing useless acts and maladjusted in their behaviour, such as committing adultery, murder, theft or fornication.[69] The sentiment of such exhortations against sexual activity is picked up again and again throughout the Middle Ages. For example, from *Hali Meidenhad*, a thirteenth-century didactic treatise, stems this passage on the possibility or *chance* that the child may be disabled: 'For if it is [misborn], as often happens, and one of its limbs is missing or has some kind of defect, it is a grief to [its mother] and shame to all of its family, a reproach for malicious tongues, and the talk of everyone.'[70] In similar vein, Lotario de Segni (the future pope Innocent III) writes in his influential treatise *De miseria humanae conditionis*:

> For there are children who even at birth are so deformed and disfigured, that one should rather regard them as caricatures than as humans. It may have been better for them had they never seen the light of day, since they have nothing to expect other than being shown about like monsters and handed around like spectacular objects. Not a few of these are born with crippled limbs or dulled senses. At their aspect friends are miserable, the parents are embarrassed by such children, and relatives shun them.[71]

68 Priester Wernher, *Driu liet von der maget*, ed. Carl Wesle (Halle a. d. Saale, 1927), lines 3028ff, cited in Claudia Brinker-von der Heyde, *Die literarische Welt des Mittelalters* (Darmstadt, 2007), p. 117.

69 Edgar Kellenberger, *Der Schutz der Einfältigen. Menschen mit einer geistigen Behinderung in der Bibel und in weiteren Quellen* (Zurich, 2011), p. 103, referring to Acts of Thomas, ch. 12: for German translation, see *Neutestamentliche Apokryphen*, ed. W. Schneemelcher, Band 2, 6th edn (Tübingen, 1997), p. 308; *The Apocryphal New Testament*, trans. M. R. James (Oxford, 1924), available online at http://gnosis.org/library/actthom.htm (accessed 28 January 2013).

70 'Hali Meidenhad', in *Medieval English Prose for Women: Selections from the Katherine Group and Ancrene Wisse*, ed. and trans. Bella Millett and Jocelyn Wogan-Browne (Oxford, 1990), pp. 30–1.

71 *De miseria humanae conditionis* (bk 1, ch. 5), in Lotario de Segni (Papst Innozenz III),

More on the sins of the parents can be found in a Middle English version of *Dives et Pauper* looking at children afflicted by illness: 'Also God smytyght hem wyt sekenesse and myschef sumtyme for the fadrys synne and the modrys, for they lovyn hem to mechil and welyn goon to hell to makyn hem riche and grete in this world';[72] here it is not just the parents' (sexual) sin but the excessive love of their offspring that is punished by illness.

Interestingly, dissenting voices sometimes ran counter to the prevailing trend that parents were becoming ever more lax in their morals and committing ever greater sexual sins, which would have increased the number of deformed and disabled births. The Anglo-Norman text *The Mirror of Justices*, written about 1290, includes instructions for the coroner. It says that the ancient custom of having a coroner's viewing in cases of an 'infant monster who had nothing of humanity, or had more of the beast than man in them' was dying out, according to the writer, because of the general decrease in those consequences of sinfulness that had taken place in recent times.[73] Here the theme of monstrous births as a result of sexual sins is inverted from the majority view that medieval texts generally presented, and a progressive improvement of Christian morals is cited as reason for the concomitant decrease of birth defects.

With regard to the question of how medieval people *may* have reacted to the birth of children perceived as defective or impaired, Boswell has posited that children born visibly and recognisably impaired, and believed to have been born so due to sexual lapses of their parents, would either have been discreetly abandoned or, if the parents could afford it, placed in a monastery;[74] he

Vom Elend des menschlichen Daseins, trans. (with introduction) Carl-Friedrich Geyer, Philosophische Texte und Studien 24 (Hildesheim, 1990), p. 46.

72 *Dives and Pauper*, ed. P. Heath Barnum, 2 vols, EETS o.s. 275 (Oxford, 1976) and 280 (1980), vol. 1, p. 129. See also Carole Rawcliffe, *Medicine and Society in Later Medieval England* (Stroud, 1995), p. 8.

73 Faye Getz, *Medicine in the English Middle Ages* (Princeton, 1998), p. 73. See also *The Mirror of Justices*, ed. William Joseph Whittaker, Selden Society 7 (London, 1895), pp. 29–32.

74 Boswell, *Kindness of Strangers*, p. 339, cf. Caesarius von Heisterbach, *Dialogus miraculorum*, bk. 10 ch. 42, ed. J. Strange (Cologne, 1851); also *The Dialogue on Miracles*, trans. H. von E. Scott and C. C. Swinton Bland (with introduction by G. G. Coulton), 2 vols (London, 1929), recording the baptism of a deformed child who was obviously not abandoned; children may be abandoned later, though, when their deformities became more apparent or less likely to be cured, as Boswell (*Kindness of Strangers*, p. 339) assumed. He mentioned in this context one Margaret of Metola, born achondroplastic, blind, hunchbacked, and lame who was abandoned in the fourteenth century by her parents at the age of sixteen after she was not cured at the shrine of Città-di-Castello; cf. Michael Goodich, *Vita Perfecta: The Ideal of Sainthood in the Thirteenth Century*, Monogr. Geschichte des Mittelalters 25 (Stuttgart, 1982). On the abandonment of disabled children to monasteries see also the work on child oblation by Mayke de Jong, *In Samuel's Image: Child Oblation in the Early Medieval West* (Leiden, 1996), pp. 168–9, who argued that this was not just about 'dumping misfits', but that, in the case of a

assumes that such practice would have continued through to the later Middle Ages: 'Families were driven to abandon, as before [in the earlier Middle Ages], by poverty, by illegitimacy, by defect or ill health of children, and by the church's continued insistence that infant deformity resulted from parental incontinence.'[75] This is an interesting point. The idea is that the abandonment, and even infanticide, of impaired children may have increased with the promulgation of moral notions about the origins of defective children by the Church; if parents are constantly reminded of their sins – and they must have sinned, otherwise how could the deformed babies be explained? – then they may well have found it more difficult for emotional reasons, social pressure and peer behaviour to bring up and care for such infants.

It is also worth briefly considering medieval thoughts on what happened to disabled children who died, since medieval life expectancy at birth was generally very low (for even 'normal' and healthy neonates) so that severely disabled babies had a low chance of surviving beyond a short term. The brief answer can be summed up according to their baptismal status. If they had been baptised, they would go to heaven, as little innocents, since they died before being culpable. If they died pre-baptism, they went to limbo, a notion expressed by Dante in *Inferno*, IV. 31–42, probably following Thomas Aquinas on this, who argues with regard to unborn foetuses/unborn souls: 'Now those who die in their mothers' wombs can never be born again: therefore neither can they rise again.'[76]

While the question of the occurrence of infanticide in medieval culture is beyond the scope of this essay,[77] it is worth drawing attention at least to the *possibility* of infanticide as a parental reaction to the birth of a congenitally disabled child. For late Antiquity the question of infanticide receives a theoretical affirmative in the advice of Soranus in his *Gynaecology* on how to identify the infant that is 'not worth rearing' in contrast to the one that is:

> when put on the earth it immediately cries with proper vigour; for one that lives for some length of time without crying, or cries but weakly, is suspected of behaving so on account of some unfavorable condition. Also by the fact that

crippled son, for instance, the placement in a monastery would allow the child to 'develop his talents in directions not requiring physical prowess'.

75 Boswell, *Kindness of Strangers*, p. 403.

76 *Summa theologiae*, 75.2, obj.5. This incidentally is the foundation of the theological argument against abortion.

77 Among the growing literature on medieval infanticide two seminal studies stand out: the pioneering article by R. C. Trexler, 'Infanticide in Florence: New Sources and First Results', *History of Childhood Quarterly* 1 (1973), 98–116, and Boswell's *The Kindness of Strangers*; for an overview from a biomedical perspective see G. B. Ferngren, 'The Status of Defective Newborns from Late Antiquity to the Reformation', in *Euthanasia and the Newborn: Criteria for Infanticide in the Twentieth Century*, ed. R. McMillan, H. Engelhardt and S. F. Spicker (Dordrecht and Boston, 1986), pp. 47–64.

> it is perfect in all its parts, members and senses … that the natural functions of every <member> are neither sluggish nor weak; that the joints bend and stretch; that it has due size and shape and is properly sensitive in every respect. … And by conditions contrary to those mentioned, the infant not worth rearing is recognised.[78]

To conclude, according to medieval notions, congenital disability could be caused by seven factors impinging on the developing foetus or on the new-born child: the relationship of the microcosm to the macrocosm; the dangers of the 'wrong' sexual intercourse by the parents; the maternal imagination; astrological influences; the nutrition of the pregnant mother, and to a lesser degree that of the foetus, here especially concerns over alcohol; intercourse during inopportune conditions of the female body, such as pregnancy or lactation; and especially due to menstruation.

Medieval notions of congenital disability were thus extremely gendered, in that the prime cause for any disability present (or observable) at birth, or within the first few weeks in the life of an infant, tended to be blamed on some failing of the mother. One should remember, however, that this blame was not exclusively placed on the mother, even if in a majority of arguments the maternal physiology, maternal behaviour or moral laxitude were identified as factors. In that minority of causations where paternal blame was identified, it was alongside maternal error, for instance, when conception took place under astrologically disadvantageous stars, both parents could be blamed for not having heeded advice correctly; or where the husband forced his wife to have intercourse against her better judgement, as in the case of Uffo and Gelusa mentioned above, where Gelusa too is admonished for not having resisted her husband's ill-fated behaviour. Since in medieval medical discourse, taken on from classical traditions, the female tended to be viewed purely as a vessel receiving the procreative powers that resided exclusively in the male,[79] it was readily assumed that when things went wrong, this was the result of maternal malfunctioning, whether at a purely anatomical or at a moral level, which caused the pristine paternal seed deposited in the maternal body to be corrupted. In a sense all of humanity, since the Fall resulting from Original Sin, was corrupted. The sublunar, postlapsarian material world was inherently imperfect, a view of the world that to a degree equalised the gender differences again in the light of the overall misery of earthly, corporeal being, whether male or female. Trying to reconstruct medieval mentalities, congenital disability, or birth defects, can thus be viewed as just one element among many indicators

78 *Soranus' Gynecology*, Book II, ch. 10, p. 80.

79 This refers to the single-sex model of classical/medieval generation, but the alternative two-sex model, whereby both maternal and paternal seeds contribute to the growth of a foetus, still regards the female as the junior partner, of lesser importance than the male; see Joan Cadden, *Meanings of Sex Difference in the Middle Ages: Medicine, Science, and Culture* (Cambridge, 1993).

of the fragility of the physical cosmos. In a theology that postulated an overall imperfect world, the birth of an 'imperfect child' would be no more and no less than an expression of human fallacy as a whole, and by elevating such an event from a personal tragedy to a wider world-view, in contrast to the modern individualised and medicalised approach, the parental reaction to giving birth to a disabled child was potentially mitigated by regarding such an event as part of a wider, divinely ordained and purposeful cosmic order.

9

MARKING THE FACE, CURING THE SOUL? READING THE DISFIGUREMENT OF WOMEN IN THE LATER MIDDLE AGES*

Patricia Skinner

The facial disfigurement of women, whether through deliberate mutilation, accidental injury or the ravages of disease, was and still is a subject that evokes strong reactions, both positive (sympathy for the victim, attempts at rehabilitation and/or reconstruction of the damaged features, psychological counselling) and negative (shock or repulsion at the appearance of the victim, the passing of judgement or calculation of fault that led to the disfigurement, her rejection from the community).[1] Whilst men, too, might suffer traumatic facial damage, the gendered assumption that a woman valued and was valued for her beauty (regardless of the number of onlookers permitted to see her face) was and still is a strong element in the *habitus* of many communities. Our evolution as human beings has led us to scrutinise the face before all other features, to determine community membership (is s/he one of us?), recognition (who is s/he?), likely reception (is s/he friendly?) and subjective value (is s/he pleasing to the eye?).[2] Any disruption of the facial features confuses such signals, and may even send out misleading ones to the viewer (for example, if features are missing, or paralysis or disease limits facial expressions). The equation of beauty with good and ugliness with evil is a powerful idea.[3]

* I would like to thank Liz Herbert McAvoy for her invaluable advice during the preparation of this paper. This chapter forms part of a wider study of disfigurement in medieval Europe, funded by the Wellcome Trust (grant no 097469).

1 Some recent examples are discussed in Patricia Skinner, 'The Gendered Nose and its Lack: "Medieval" Nose-cutting and Its Modern Manifestations', *Journal of Women's History* 26, 1 (2014).

2 Vicki Bruce and Andy Young, *Face Perception* (London and New York, 2012). On identification see also Valentin Groebner, *Who are You? Identification, Deception and Surveillance in Early Modern Europe*, trans. Mark Kyburz and John Peck (New York, 2007).

3 Umberto Eco, *On Beauty: The History of a Western Idea* (London, 2004); Umberto Eco, *On Ugliness* (London, 2007).

Yet such categories are not set in stone. Dyan Elliot has pointed up the dangers of female beauty in the specific context of the medieval relationship between confessing women and their clerical confessors, and highlighted the increasing attention of commentators to preventing such relationships becoming carnal. Raymond of Peñafort, for example, recommended sitting opposite the penitent but not looking at her face during her confession. Moreover, the phenomenon of the frequently-confessing woman, she argues, came to be viewed not as a beneficial practice but a 'pathological' one.[4] Such terminology marks out one of the ways in which gender, religion and medicine – at least medical metaphors – could intersect, and has direct resonances with the case studies featured in this chapter.

This specific example, and a survey of later medieval texts, suggest that the period between 1150 and 1500 was one of increasing attention to the facial features of both men and women within and outside clerical circles, driven partly by increased exposure of western Europeans to peoples of different physical appearance, and partly by the rediscovery of the ancient pseudo-science of physiognomy, which claimed to read character traits from facial features. The link between the two trends is visible in high and late medieval depictions and perceptions of non-Christians, as Irven Resnick has demonstrated.[5] The latter field received a particular boost from Frederick II of Hohenstaufen's patronage of Michael Scottus (d. 1232), author of the *Liber Phisionomie*.[6] Scottus' work was copied, translated and excerpted in text compilations right up until the eighteenth century, and was in print by the 1470s. The textual popularity of the work, which had originally formed only part of Scottus's encyclopaedic cosmology, the *Liber Introductorius*, owed much to the fact that physiognomy was viewed essentially as a branch of medicine, and many of the versions of the *Phisionomie* circulated in compilations alongside medical texts, as facial complexion was thought to reflect the balance of humours within the body, and thus had medical implications.

A third, and for this chapter the most influential, element in the focus on the face as a site of contemplation was the rise of an affective piety which, whilst it identified with and celebrated Christ's wounds (often through intense physical mortification), nevertheless sought to escape from the boundaries of the flesh, inspired by the heroes of late Antiquity and the early Middle Ages.[7] Women

4 Dyan Elliott, 'Women and Confession: From Empowerment to Pathology', in *Gendering the Master Narrative: Women and Power in the Middle Ages*, ed. Mary C. Erler and Maryanne Kowaleski (Ithaca, NY and London, 2003), pp. 31–51 (p. 44) for Raymond and p. 47 for pathology.

5 Irven M. Resnick, *Marks of Distinction: Christian Perceptions of Jews in the High Middle Ages* (Washington, DC, 2012), pp. 13–52, especially pp. 34ff .

6 The following discussion of Michael Scottus is based on Martin Porter, '*Windows of the Soul': Physiognomy in European Culture, 1470–1780* (Oxford, 2005), p. 11.

7 E.g. ascetics, and self-mortification such as that of Radegund of France. See also Patricia

were particularly attracted by this form of spiritual life,[8] and the association between bodily pain and the health of the soul has been explored as a key strand in later medieval religious thought.[9] Jesus's perfection, however, made him a challenging figure to contemplate. Commentators agreed that Jesus had been born with a perfect balance of humours, with 'exemplary complexion and physiognomy':[10] only those who matched this could truly take their place by his side. Christ's face, depicted in agony in the later writings of Julian of Norwich,[11] for example, was presented by St Clare of Assisi in a letter to Agnes of Prague as a 'spotless mirror', to be gazed upon every day in the quest for a closer spiritual connection.[12] To that end, bodily mortification could serve as a means of expressing humility before God, a small step on the path to salvation. For example, St Margaret of Hungary (d.1270), according to her biographer Garinus, mortified her body in numerous ways, including wearing old and vermin-ridden clothing. When the sisters in her Dominican convent protested and refused to sit next to her, she pointed it that it was only her body, not theirs, being tormented by bites (a debateable point!), and that she wished to be so lacerated out of the love of Christ.[13]

Cox Miller, 'Visceral Seeing: the Holy Body in Late Ancient Christianity', *Journal of Early Christian Studies* 12 (2004), 391–411.

8 See Ulrike Wiethaus, 'Sexuality, Gender and the Body in Late Medieval Women's Spirituality: Cases from Germany and the Netherlands', *Journal of Feminist Studies in Religion* 7 (1991), 35–52; Elizabeth A. Robertson, 'The Corporeality of Sanctity in the Life of St Margaret', in *Images of Sainthood in Medieval Europe*, ed. Renate Blumenfeld-Kosinski and Timea Szell (Ithaca, NY, 1991), pp. 268–87; Elizabeth Petroff, *Body and Soul: Essays on Medieval Women and Mysticism* (Oxford, 1994); and see the essays collected in *Intersections of Sexuality and the Divine in Medieval Culture: The Word Made Flesh*, ed. Susannah M. Chewning (Aldershot, 2005).

9 E.g. Carla Casagrande, 'Il dolore virtuoso: per una storia medievale della pazienza' ['Virtuous grief: towards a medieval history of patience'], in *Piacere e Dolore: materiali per una storia delle passioni nel Medioevo*, ed. Carla Casagrande and Silvana Vecchio (Florence, 2009), pp. 31–47; Jeremy J. Citrome, 'Medicine as Metaphor in the Middle English Cleanness', *Chaucer Review 35* (2001), 260–80.

10 Resnick, *Marks of Distinction*, p. 32.

11 Julian of Norwich, 'A Revelation of Love', 10.1–8, in *The Writings of Julian of Norwich: A Vision Showed to a Devout Women and a Revelation of Love*, ed. Nicholas Watson and Jacqueline Jenkins (Turnhout, 2005), pp. 157–9: 'And after this, I saw with bodely sight in the face of the crucifixe that hung before me, in the which I beheld continually a parte of his passion: dispite, spitting, solewing, and buffeting, and many languring paines, mo than I can tell, and often changing of colour. And one time I saw how halfe the face, beginning at the ere, overyede with drye bloud till it beclosed into the mid face. And after that the other halfe beclosed on the same wise, and therewhiles it vanished in this party, even as it cam. / This saw I bodely, swemly, and darkely.' I thank Liz Herbert McAvoy for pointing me towards this text.

12 Joan Mueller, *Clare of Assisi: The Letters to Agnes* (Collegeville, MN, 2003), fourth letter, p. 87.

13 *AA.SS. vol. III, 28 January*, De B. Margaritae Hungariae Virginis, p. 517: 'permittatis corpus meum amore Jesu Christi Domini Nostri ab istis vermibus lacerari'.

This chapter, however, explores a series of contradictions inherent in high- and late-medieval responses to women's facial disfigurement, as presented in three works of hagiography. Deriving almost entirely from texts recording the male gaze, it considers the troubled relationship between women's beauty and their spiritual health. Religious texts, in particular, present the abnegation and destruction of a beautiful face, through often drastic, physical injury, as one option available to women in search of salvation, although such mutilation in secular life had quite different meaning, as we shall see. Throughout, therefore, the chapter will move between the fleshly reality of the wounded or damaged face, and the possibilities that existed, within medical and surgical fields, for its care; and the concerns of the victims and observers for their spiritual health, and how this might be assisted, or not, by bearing their physical deformities or even self-inflicting them. Whilst a damaged face might represent the threat of social disability – the removal of beauty tantamount to destroying a woman's chances of marriage (a theme implicit in the responses of the saint's family members), the texts themselves do not explore the potential for permanent, physical impairment. The tense relationship between religion and medicine is revealed in hagiographic texts, whilst gender clearly played a part in the ways hagiographers constructed their stories of the mutilations themselves.

Central to the chapter will be a consideration of three holy women, Oda of Brabant (d. 1158), St Margaret of Hungary (d. 1270) and St Margaret of Cortona (d. 1297),[14] each of whose lives feature an episode of actual or near mutilation of the face. They have featured in passing in studies of female sainthood, but have not been considered as a group nor set into their historical environment. They differ considerably in how the hagiographer presents facial mutilation, both in terms of why the saints should consider self-mutilating, and the responses they received to their desire to do so. Were such differences conditioned by geography, or by changes over a century and a half in attitudes towards facial disfigurement? What purpose was such mutilation held to serve? And how did it fit into the wider, secular world of corporal punishment and ideas of healing the body and soul?

To place these lives into their chronological context, the central and later Middle Ages has traditionally been represented as a period of European history that saw a sharp increase of threatened and actual violence towards the body. Johan Huizinga long ago characterised these centuries as 'the special period of judicial cruelty' and during which, according to Sean McGlynn, judicial punishment 'exceeded Old Testament notions of an eye for an eye',[15] and mutilation as a tool of justice reached its peak. This, too,

14 *AA.SS. vol. XI, 20 April*, Vita Ven. Oda Praemonstratensis; *AA.SS. vol. III, 28 January*, De B. Margaritae Hungariae Virginis; *AA.SS. vol. VI 22 February*, De B. Margarita Poenit. Tertii Ord. S. Francisci Cortonae in Etruria, respectively.

15 Johan Huizinga, *The Waning of the Middle Ages*, trans. F. Hoffman (London, 1955), especially his much-cited Chapter 1, 'The Violent Tenor of Life'. A useful critique of

attracts Valentin Groebner's attention: his essays argue for a period during which violence to the body (and face) reached a particular peak of terror and intensity and, when used in a judicial setting, was intended to render its victims 'formless [Ungestalt]' in society.[16] The greater emphasis on the death penalty in later medieval England, it is also suggested, led to the development in that region of more forms of mutilation offered to the offender as 'clemency'.[17] From being a merciful punishment for crimes meriting the death penalty, mutilation took on a life of its own as a marker not only of criminality but also of immorality, blurring the boundaries between crime and sin and inflicting a permanent record of a temporary aberration on the body of the perpetrator. In her recent consideration of such penalties, Irina Metzler aptly draws attention to the distinction between mutilation of the limbs, which left the victim with an 'orthopaedic impairment', and mutilation of the face (including blinding), which could lead to sensory deprivation.[18] Saintly self-mutilation, therefore, carried with it a risk – intended as a means to humble the pride of a woman in her own facial beauty, it might lead to complications of bleeding, infection, permanent loss of senses or even death. (Loss of sensory perception, of course, might be a welcome side effect, if denying oneself the ability to taste and smell – a possibility if the nose was damaged or removed – represented a further denial of worldly pleasures.) Facial mutilation was commonly threatened in legal codes for sexual misdemeanours such as adultery or pimping, and women emerge here far more frequently than men as the intended targets. In Groebner's words, 'Defacement … meant inscribing a complex story

Huizinga's influence is Malcolm Vale, 'Aristocratic Violence: Trial by Battle in the Later Middle Ages', in *Violence in Medieval Society*, ed. Richard W. Kaeuper (Woodbridge, 2000), pp. 159–81, which comments: 'Huizinga clearly went too far and overstated his case' (p. 161). Sean McGlynn, *By Sword and Fire: Cruelty and Atrocity in Medieval Warfare* (London, 2008), p. 10.

16 Valentin Groebner, *Defaced: the Visual Culture of Violence in the Later Middle Ages*, trans. Pamela Selwyn (New York, 2004). He is careful to point out, however, that the records of punishments that modern historians use to reconstruct medieval violence 'arose as political texts' and were intended, primarily, to express the effectiveness of state control: *Defaced*, p. 43.

17 McGlynn, *By Sword and Fire*, p. 13. This shift is made explicit in the so-called laws of William the Conqueror, although the precise origin of the statement attributed to him, that 'no one should be killed or hanged for any crime (culpa), but let their eyes be taken out and their testicles cut off' ['Interdico etiam ne quis occidatur aut suspendatur pro aliqua culpa, sed eruantur oculi et testiculi abscidantur'], quoted in *Gesetze der Angelsachsen*, ed. F. Lieberman, 3 vols (Halle, 1903–16), vol. 1, p. 488, is a matter of controversy: see Patrick Wormald, *The Making of English Law: King Alfred to the Twelfth Century*, I (Oxford, 1999), p. 404. The clause relating to testicles, of course, also demonstrates that the perpetrator was assumed to have been male.

18 Irina Metzler, *A Social History of Disability in the Middle Ages: Cultural Considerations of Physical Impairment* (London and New York, 2013), p. 13.

of sin and sanction onto the body of someone defenceless'.[19] For a female penitent such as the three women under discussion here, therefore, it may have seemed a logical culmination of their endeavours to remove themselves from secular concerns.

This period also saw a resurgence in the transmission of medical knowledge and texts, and these often included recipes to heal facial blemishes or disguise them with cosmetics.[20] It was a short step from here to the non-therapeutic use of make-up. The enhancement of facial beauty in this way in its turn caused greater ambivalence – for whom was such enhancement intended and what purpose did it serve?[21] There was a difference between a flawless face and a decorated one, and Christian moralists since Tertullian had been quick to condemn the use of cosmetics.[22] By 1500, too, surgical intervention on damaged faces was beginning to be considered in texts: significantly, one of the earliest examples of such cosmetic surgery texts, the *Manual of Wound Care* of Heinrich von Pfolspeundt, comes from Germany, where actual instances of facial mutilation, rather than just threats, were recorded.[23]

The faces of our three saints, then, were potentially sites of gendered discussion surrounding beauty, religious devotion, sickness and cure. But they were also mirrors of wider prevailing attitudes towards female agency, appearance and sexuality.

19 Groebner, *Defaced*, p. 87.

20 Carmen Caballero Navas, 'The Care of Women's Health and Beauty: an Experience Shared by Medieval Jewish and Christian Women', *Journal of Medieval History* 34 (2008), 146–63; Geneviève Dumas, 'Le soin des cheveux et des poils: quelques pratiques cosmétiques (XIII-XVI siècles)', in *La chevelure dans la littérature et l'art du moyen age*, ed. Chantal Connochie-Bourgne (Aix-en-Provence, 2004), pp. 129–41; Laurence Moulinier-Brogi, 'Esthétique et soins du corps dans les traités médicaux latins à la fin du moyen age', *Médiévales* 46 (2004), 55–71. It is significant that the treatise 'On women's cosmetics', circulating under the name of the female medical practitioner Trota of Salerno, has been shown to be male-authored: see Monica Green, *The Trotula: A Medieval Compendium of Women's Medicine* (Philadelphia, 2001).

21 Christine Martineau-Genieys, 'Modèles, maquillage et misogynie, à travers les textes littéraires français du moyen age', in *Les soins de beauté, moyen age-début des temps modernes*, ed. Denis Menjot (Nice, 2004), pp. 31–50; Susan Udry, 'Robert de Blois and Geoffroy de la Tour Landry on Feminine Beauty: Two Late-Medieval French Conduct Books', *Essays in Medieval Studies* 19 (2002), 70–89.

22 Marie-Geneviève Grossel, 'Entre médecine et magie: les gestes de beauté (l'Ornatus Mulierum)', in *Le geste et les gestes au moyen age: colloque* (Aix-en-Provence, 1998), pp. 255–72, traces the subsequent history of misogynist attitudes towards cosmetic enhancements.

23 Heinrich von Pfolspeundt, *Buch der Bündt-Ertznei (1460)*, ed. H. Haeser and A. Middeldorpf (Berlin, 1868), especially surgical rebuilding of the nose, pp. 29–31; Groebner, *Defaced*, pp. 68–70.

BEAUTY AND THE BEAST

It is taken as read that the sight of a mutilated female face could engender horror and shock in the medieval viewer, and that this generated (and possibly exaggerated) the reports we now have of its occurrence. It was precisely this response that the Franciscan missionary William of Rubruck intended to elicit when he reported his encounter with the wife of the Mongol leader 'Scacatai' in 1253. William commented that:

> De qua credebam in veritate, quod amputasset sibi nasum inter oculos ut simior esset: nihil enim habebat ibi de naso, et unxerat locum ilium quodam unguento nigro, et etiam supercilia: quod erat turpissimum in oculis nostris.
>
> [I was really under the impression that she had amputated the bridge of her nose so as to be more snub-nosed, for she had no trace of a nose here, and she had smeared that spot and her eyebrows as well with some black ointment, which to us looked thoroughly dreadful.]

Elsewhere he deduced from this that such flatness was a marker of beauty within Mongol culture, and that 'Quæ minus habet de naso pulchrior reputatur. Deturpant etiam turpiter pinguedine facies suas' [the less nose one has, the more beautiful she is considered, and they disfigure themselves horribly, moreover, by painting their faces].[24] William's comments are of course designed to convey to the western European readers of his report – most notably King Louis IX of France to whom he addressed it – the strangeness of his hosts. Part of the process of 'othering' the Mongols was to draw contrasts between their behaviours and those of Westerners, and the appearance and practices of the women, although not strictly a matter with which a Franciscan friar should have been concerned, was just one noticeable difference among many.[25] There is, however, another dimension to William's sketch of the Mongol women: although he highlights the flatness of their noses as 'hideous' and attributes at least one case to deliberate surgery,[26] he does

24 *The principal navigations, voyages, traffiques, and discoveries of the English nation*, collected by Richard Hakluyt, ed. Edmund Goldsmid (Edinburgh, 1885–90), vol. 8, cc. 12 and 8 respectively, digitised at http://ebooks.adelaide.edu.au/h/hakluyt/voyages/rubruquis/ accessed 5 September 2013. English translations: *The Mission of Friar William of Rubruck*, trans. Peter Jackson with notes by Peter Jackson and David Morgan, Hakluyt Society 2nd series 173 (London, 1990), c.X.2 (p. 100) and c.VI.5 (p. 89).

25 Contrast William of Malmesbury's depiction of the Turks during the First Crusade, where gender seems to be paramount in both his framing of the enemy and criticism of females among the crusaders: Kirsten A. Fenton, 'Gendering the First Crusade in William of Malmesbury's *Gesta Regum Anglorum*', in *Intersections of Gender, Religion and Ethnicity in the Middle Ages*, ed. Cordelia Beattie and Kirsten Fenton (London, 2011), pp. 125–39.

26 On the relationship of the Church with surgery, and the increasing anxiety expressed from the twelfth century onward, see Marie-Christine Pouchelle, *The Body and Surgery in the Middle Ages*, trans. R. Morris (Oxford, 1990), pp. 20-1.

not draw any comparisons about the meaning of this facial feature in his own world. Yet the bridgeless or flattened nose was commonly thought in the later medieval West to be a sign of leprosy, which itself was associated with dubious morality,[27] whilst a deliberately cut or maimed nose came increasingly to signify a punishment for sexual misdemeanour on the woman's part.[28] He left it to his readers to make such connections.

The *Vita* of St Margaret of Hungary (d. 1270), however, provides a striking counterpart to William's text. For, against the same background of Mongol aggression, this Hungarian princess, given to the Dominican order in childhood, stated that, should the 'Tartars' invade Hungary, she would cut off her lips to ensure they found her so repulsive as to leave her unviolated.[29] Yet her hagiographer relates that when repelling (Western) suitors for her hand in marriage, she declared that she would rather cut off her nose and lips, *and* gouge out her eyes, than marry any of the three royal suitors proposed.[30] Herein lies the paradox of facial damage for women. The account of Margaret's threat of self-mutilation to preserve her virginity against both pagan aggressors and Christian suitors belonged to a long tradition of 'the heroics of virginity': St Brigit of Ireland was said to have gouged out her own eye to avoid marriage, whilst one of the most celebrated cases of collective self-mutilation was that of Abbess Ebba and the nuns at Coldingham in England, faced with the prospect of Viking invaders.[31] Nevertheless the action that Margaret was proposing – which in the context of the approaching pagan

27 Carole Rawcliffe sounds a note of caution, however, against assuming that lepers were so regarded across Europe: see *Leprosy in Medieval England* (Woodbridge, 2006), pp. 131–3. See Antje M. Schelberg, 'The Beauty and the Beast? Medieval Ideas on Physical Appearance and Their Psychological Meaning with Regard to Leprosy Sufferers', in *The Myths of Medieval Leprosy: A Collection of Essays*, ed. Antje M. Schelberg (Göttingen, 2006), pp. 35–50.

28 Skinner, 'The Gendered Nose and its Lack'. It is worth noting, however, that as early as the eighth century Byzantine law had associated nose-slitting with a string of irregular sexual relations with nuns, virgins, god-daughters, close female relatives and prepubescent girls. In these cases it was the male perpetrator who was targeted, with the woman only punished if she had consented. In cases of adultery, both the male perpetrator and the adulterous wife had their noses slit: *A Manual of Roman Law: The Ecloga of Leo III and Constantine V of Isauria at Constantinople, AD 726*, ed. E. H. Freshfield (Cambridge, 1926), ch. XVII, clauses 23–7, 30–4.

29 *AA.SS. vol. III, 28 January*, De B. Margaritae Hungariae Virginis, p. 518: 'Ait Margarita, "Ego scio, quid faciam: labia mea detruncabo, et cum inde viderint me deturpatam, dimittent intactam".'

30 *AA.SS. vol. III, 28 January*, De B. Margaritae Hungariae Virginis, p. 518: 'respondit, quod prius praecideret sibi nasum ac labia, et oculos erueret, quam cujuscumque matrimonio consentiret'.

31 Lisa Bitel, *Land of Women: Tales of Sex and Gender from Early Ireland* (Ithaca, NY, 1996), p. 35 for Brigit; Shari Horner, *The Discourse of Enclosure: Representing Women in Old English Literature* (New York, 2001), p. 120 for Ebba. Jane Tibbetts Schulenberg discusses the early medieval precursors to Margaret: 'The Heroics of Virginity: Brides of

Mongols had strong parallels with Ebba's –would not only leave her open to wound-related infection or even death, but also render her face similar to mutilated criminals, adulterers, pimps and fornicators. A generation earlier than William's expedition and Margaret's *vita*, legal texts were being promulgated in southern Europe which threatened the slitting of women's noses (and thus flattening them in grotesque form) for instances of sexual misdemeanours. For example, the laws of Frederick II for Sicily (based on earlier provisions of King Roger II) imposed nose-slitting on adulteresses and mothers who pimped their daughters.[32] The chronology matters: such a measure had been unknown in western Europe before the eleventh century (although, as we have seen, it was mentioned in earlier Byzantine law). Thus earlier examples of threatened or actual self-mutilation differed starkly from Margaret's message to her parents: if they forced her to break her monastic vow, they gave her no choice but to carry out an action that would reduce her –irremediably – to the status of marked whore.

JUDGEMENTS

The fear of sexual violation, then, drove Margaret's intention to maim herself, mirroring contemporary legal punishments for sexual and other transgressions. Like most of the cases considered in this chapter, however, it was merely the *threat* of self-mutilation, rather than its actual practice, that was an effective deterrent. This is a point somewhat overlooked by those convinced that the high and late Middle Ages were a theatre of cruelty. Moreover, we need to ask how Margaret's religious commitment, and its subsequent reporting in hagiography, may or may not reflect the secular world. The records we have of actual judicial processes often stop at a court's verdict – the sentence of mutilation, rather than its actual execution – and women form a very small minority of those so sentenced. In fact, cases of women actually being judicially mutilated are quite rare, and not all examples were for cases of immorality. Helen Carrel has argued that 'The threat of harsh punishment, which was then ultimately remitted, was a set piece of medieval legal practice', and suggests that, although mutilation was prescribed for many offences, it was rarely put into practice after the late thirteenth century.[33] Margaret's

Christ and Sacrificial Mutilation', in *Women in the Middle Ages and Renaissance: Literary and Historical Perspectives*, ed. Mary Beth Rose (Syracuse, NY, 1986), pp. 29–72.

32 *Die Konstitutionen Friedrichs II für das Königsreich Sizilien*, ed. Wolfgang Stürner, *MGH*, Constitutiones et Acta Publica Imperatorum et Regum II, Supplement (Hanover, 1996), Book III.74 (p. 439: husband has right to remove adulterous wife's nose); 79 (p. 442: pimps suffer same penalty as adulterers); 80 (p. 442: mothers who pimp their daughters to have noses cut off). These laws were, however, attributed to King Roger II (r. 1130–54), and were repeated in the constitutions under Frederick's name: ibid., III.84-5 (pp. 446–7), but mitigated for those in poverty.

33 Helen Carrel, 'The Ideology of Punishment in Late Medieval English Towns', *Social*

threat, therefore, might be understood as just that – its extremity designed to convey her deep-seated religious commitment through the idea of radical, physical self-harm, invoking an image in the reader's mind but not carried out in practice.

Elsewhere in the secular world, the late fifteenth- and early sixteenth-century German and Swiss urban records studied by Groebner reveal definitive evidence of actual facial mutilation taking place, but the targeting of the face of suspected or actual adulterers outlasted formal, juridical 'mirror punishments' by the authorities by the fifteenth century, and seems to have been an extreme, and unsanctioned, act of anger carried out on the face of a spouse suspected of adultery, or her/his lover, or even on the innocent partner of the lover. Such 'private' attacks, Groebner suggests, were still driven by the association of adultery with facial punishment, but these incidents make it into the records so that the *attackers* might be censured (somewhat lightly, given the injuries they inflicted).[34]

This unofficial understanding of violent, facial punishment against women for their perceived lapses may already have been an accepted social norm in other regions by the thirteenth century. Again, evidence comes from the records of proceedings against the perpetrator of the violence. A hearing before the *podestà*'s court in Venice in May 1291 centred on the assault of Bertholota Paduano of Torcello by a priest from the island of Burano. Bertholota testified that when she defended her friend Maria against the priest's slanderous words:

> et percussit dictam Bertholotam sub oculo sinistro cum digito, et postea cum pugno bis per caput, scilicet semel per vultum iuxta nasum, talieter quod sanguis exivit ei per buccam et per nasum et alia vice iuxta aurem, et postea iniuravit ei dicens, 'Turpis vilis meretrix, nunc aliquantulum feci vincdictam [*sic*] de te, vade acceptum bastardos quos fecisti de Valentio, quia sum dolens et tristis quod non proieci ipsam in aquam'.
>
> [The above parish priest raised his hand and hit the above Bertholota with his hand below her left eye, and then twice with his fist on her head: that is, on her face by her nose, so that blood began to flow from her mouth and nose, and

History 34 (2009), 301–20 (pp. 307–8). The process of mitigation, if not total mercy, is illustrated in the Shropshire eyre court record of 1203. A certain Alice, who with others was implicated in the murder of an unnamed woman in Lilleshall, had fled to Staffordshire, where she was apprehended with some of the chattels of the slain woman. Taken back to Shropshire for questioning, she first denied being involved, then claimed before the county court that she had been forced by the malefactors to conceal them, for which she had been given the goods. At the eyre court, however, she withdrew this story. 'Therefore', continues the record, 'she has deserved death, but by way of dispensation let her eyes be torn out [*eruantur ei occuli*]': see *Select Pleas of the Crown, voume I: AD 1200–1225*, ed. F. W. Maitland (London, 1888), no. 77, p. 34.

34 Valentin Groebner, 'Losing Face, Saving Face: Noses and Honour in the Later Medieval Town', *History Workshop Journal* 40 (1995), 1–15; Groebner, *Defaced*, p. 76.

> another way by her ear, and afterwards he injured her, saying: 'You shameful and vile whore, *now I have given you a little punishment* [my emphasis], go, and take the bastards you had by Valentio with you, for I am grieving and sad that I did not throw her [Maria] in the water.']

Further witnesses added that they heard the priest say,

> 'Illa turpis meretrix; modo feci quod cupivi et, nisi fuisset pro presbitero qui eam defensavit, male apparassem eam.'
>
> ['She is a filthy whore; now I have done what I wanted to do, and had it not been for the priest who defended her, it would have gone badly for her.'][35]

We do not know how this case ended – presumably the clerical perpetrator of the assault would have objected to being hauled up before the secular *podestà's* court and the case may well have been referred to his clerical superiors, which would explain the lack of sentencing as it survives in the *podestà's* records. What the hearing did to Bertholota's reputation is also unknown, but the record is revealing in how it presents the case, and what it chooses to include. Arguably, the victim's physical appearance after the attack (temporarily bloodied face and black eyes, and more permanently a probable broken nose) would have raised questions about her status as a respectable woman, but it is striking that she is named in the record whilst her assailant is not, and that her reputation as a whore was rehearsed in court (twice) and then written down.[36] The case itself may therefore have been more punitive on *her* than on him, and this may have been the latter's intention.[37] He was, after all, a priest, and may well have considered himself within his rights to challenge Bertholota's (and Maria's, for that matter) way of conducting their lives, particularly if Bertholota's children had been born out of wedlock as the record suggests. But it is clear that there was a distinction to be drawn between legally-sanctioned punishment, controlled by the Venetian state, and the violence occasioned by this individual's sense of outrage against the women.[38] Religion is present here

35 *Podestà di Torcello, Domenico Viglari (1290–1291)*, ed. Paolo Zolli (Venice, 1966), pp. 14–16. The full transcript of the hearing is translated into English in *Medieval Writings on Secular Women*, ed. Patricia Skinner and Elisabeth van Houts (London, 2011), pp. 156–8.

36 On the power of rumour and slander, see the essays in *Fama: The Politics of Talk and Reputation in Medieval Europe*, ed. Thelma Fenster and Daniel Lord Smail (Ithaca, 2003) and Jesús Ángel Solórzana Telechea, 'Fama Publica, Infamy and Defamation: Judicial Violence and Social Control of Crimes against Sexual Morals in Medieval Castile', *Journal of Medieval History* 33 (2007), 398–413.

37 Medieval court cases often revolved around much wider issues of community adhesion than the specific matter at hand, as illustrated by Chris Wickham, 'Gossip and Resistance among the Medieval Peasantry', *Past & Present* 160 (1998), 3–20.

38 In fact Venetian law does not appear to have prescribed corporal punishment for sexual offences: an adulterous wife simply lost her dowry: Linda Guzzetti, 'Separations and Separated Couples in Fourteenth-Century Venice', in *Marriage in Italy, 1300–1650*, ed.

of course – the assailant was a priest – but his actions were hardly designed to bring Bertholota to repentance.

The theme of the punished fornicator brings us to our second holy woman, in the form of St Margaret of Cortona. Her lengthy *vita*, consisting almost entirely of Margaret's dialogues with Christ (and thus effectively positioning her in a face-to-face relationship with him), centres on Margaret's remorse at her previous life of sexual freedom that had resulted in her bearing an illegitimate child. Margaret was apparently strikingly beautiful, and the motif of denying this beauty recurs throughout the life, as she struggles ever closer to her true love, Christ himself. Early in the life Christ says:

> 'Recordare, quod tui aspectus decorem, quem hactenus in mei magnam injuriam conservare conata es, imo et augere, adeo abhorrere et odire coepisti, ut nunc abstinentia, nunc lapidis allisione, nunc pulveris ollarum appositione, nunc diminutione frequenti sanguinis, delere desiderasti.'
>
> ['Remember how you previously endeavoured to maintain and even increase your beautiful appearance, much to my injury, and now you have begun to abhor and hate it, so that now you desire to rub it out with fasting, by dashing your skin with stones, by covering it with dust, and by frequent bleeding.'][39]

But such trials are not yet enough – when Margaret asks Christ to call her 'daughter', he replies rather tersely, 'Non adhuc vocaberis filia, quia filia peccati es; cum vero a tuis vitiis integraliter per generalem confessionem iterum purgata fueris, te inter filias numerabo' ['You won't be called daughter yet, for you are the daughter of sin. Only when you are completely purged of your vices by constant confession, then I will count you among my daughters.'].[40] This handily reminds us that Margaret had to overcome not only her past life, but her very status as woman, as a daughter of Eve, whose original sin marked her with a sexuality that fasting, scarification and the denial of bodily comforts could only control, not destroy. Margaret's request to become a recluse is also refused, by God, who has other plans for her.[41] The *vita* was written by Margaret's confessor, and he has a major role to play as she becomes increas-

Trevor Dean and K. J. P. Lowe (Cambridge, 1998), pp. 249–74 (p. 254). Having children out of wedlock seems only to have become a live issue if it threatened the stability of the Venetian nobility, leading to the bastard-exclusion law of 1376: Stanley Chojnacki, 'Nobility, Women and the State: Marriage Regulation in Venice, 1420–1530', in ibid., pp. 128–51 (p. 136).

39 *AA.SS. vol. VI 22 February*, De B. Margarita Poenit. Tertii Ord. S. Francisci Cortonae in Etruria, *Vita*, c.I.6, p. 305.

40 *AA.SS. vol. VI 22 February*, De B. Margarita Poenit. Tertii Ord. S. Francisci Cortonae in Etruria, *Vita*, c.II.22, p. 308.

41 *AA.SS. vol. VI 22* February, De B. Margarita Poenit. Tertii Ord. S. Francisci Cortonae in Etruria, *Vita*, c.II.27, p. 309: 'Cur postulas, ut te in cella recludam? … Vade, et non te recludas, quo usque te abscondere volam'. This frees the way for Margaret to become a Tertiary.

ingly frustrated by her failure to achieve her goal.[42] Seeing that her abstinence is not destroying the beauty of her face fast enough, she secretly hides a razor and asks her confessor's permission to use it to cut off her nose and top lip, for 'Et merito, inquit, hoc vigilanter desidero, quia vultus mea decor multorum animas vulneravit' ['I deserve it and strongly wish it, since the beauty of my face has injured the souls of many'].[43] But he refuses permission, and threatens not to hear her confession again if she carries out her intent. Margaret's later request to Christ, to afflict her with leprosy, meets a similar refusal. If she wanted to reach Christ, the message appears to be that she had to do it the hard way, not by quick solutions such as enclosure, self-harm or disease.

INVERTING SICKNESS AND HEALTH

There is a strong thread of medical allusion running through the *vita* of Margaret of Cortona, centred on Margaret's desire to rid herself of her facial beauty. Many of her actions seem to be rather ill-conceived – regular bleeding, after all, was meant to be a therapeutic act,[44] rather than a deleterious one, and raises the question of whether we should read her slow journey towards Christ as effecting some kind of 'cure' for an affliction incurred by her previously sinful life. She is not permitted to mutilate herself, her confessor explains, because she would lose too much blood, or the wound would change into another type of evil.[45] Although it is not stated explicitly, the inference is that the only wound capable of resisting such 'infection' is Christ's own wound. Her desire to draw her own blood, therefore, might be worse than the 'ill' – her beauty – she is trying to cure. Similarly, in seeking to be afflicted with leprosy, she is taking too easy a path. The disease might well disfigure her and prevent her beauty from causing further offence to Christ ('ne de cetero te offendam'), but in fact the disease is presented almost as a comfort: Christ comments that 'quod ei [Christ] sufficerent poenae suae, quia cum lepra secura esset, sed cum tentationibus et infirmitate corporea ipsam conservabat in timore

42 Beverly Kienzle, 'Margherita of Cortona: Women, Preaching and the Writing of Hagiography', *Medieval Sermon Studies* 54 (2010), 38–50: she explores this relationship between life and text.

43 *AA.SS. vol. VI 22 February*, De B. Margarita Poenit. Tertii Ord. S. Francisci Cortonae in Etruria, *Vita*, c.II.40, p. 311.

44 Pedro Gil-Sotres, 'Derivation and Revulsion: the Theory and Practice of Medieval Phlebotomy', in *Practical Medicine from Salerno to the Black Death*, ed. Luis García-Ballester, Roger French, Jon Arrizabalaga and Andrew Cunningham (Cambridge, 1994), pp. 110–55.

45 *AA.SS. vol. VI 22 February*, De B. Margarita Poenit. Tertii Ord. S. Francisci Cortonae in Etruria, *Vita*, c.II.40, p. 311: 'ex nimia sanguinis emanatione de vulnere posses deficere, vel vulnus in alterius speciem mali poterit transmutari'. The use of the verb *deficere* here offers two readings – either she will physically fail, i.e. run out of blood, or she will have failed in her mission through taking the quick option.

et gratia' ['with leprosy she would feel untroubled, but with temptations and corporeal weakness he was keeping her in fear and grace'].[46] By the thirteenth century, after all, lepers were increasingly being viewed as a means for the healthy to gain spiritual rewards through gifts to hospitals and the prayers of the afflicted, and thus being valorised rather than rejected for their condition. The message in the *vita* was that Margaret was not worthy even to join this special group. The message of patient submission having got through to her, she likens taking communion to a sick person coming to the doctor and getting medicine, and says she is still unworthy of this care.[47] By this time, she herself has become the reluctant object of veneration by the sick seeking cures through touching her.[48]

Margaret's *vita*, then, offers an interesting series of inversions regarding religion and medicine: she uses bleeding – a therapeutic act – to harm herself physically, seeks sickness to cure her bodily temptation, and wishes fervently to cut her face in order to destroy what she clearly sees as the root of her troubles, the beauty which she had previously deployed in her sinful life. The horror with which her confessor greets her proposal suggests that he sees her act as one of vanity (the 'alterius speciem mali'?), regardless of its intentions. Although in some respects the polar opposite to William of Rubruck's report of the Mongol women, whose nose-cutting is interpreted as a means to *acquire* beauty, the *vita* still seems to share that author's mistrust of women's agency. Self-mutilation of the face seems to have been gendered a specifically feminine practice. Despite medical metaphors of cutting away evil flesh circulating in the Church since its inception, the actual putting into practice of this on real bodies was always viewed with ambivalence.

This problem dogs the last, but earliest, tale of saintly self-mutilation under consideration here. Blessed Oda of Brabant (d. 1158) actually went ahead and cut off her own nose when threatened with marriage by her parents. Her *vita*, written by Philip of Harvengt, recounts:

> domumque veniens, in matris thalamam secessit. Firmatoque ostio super se, Deum in adjutorium suum orat intendere; et arrepto gladio, quem ad caput lectuli videt dependere, nasum suum festinat praecidere. Sed manus tremula nec docto in gladio percutere, dum nervorum superiorem duritiem ictu feminino non praevalet excutere; indignata sibi ait, "O ensis quam retusae es aciei, qui mordaci acumine nequis destruere meae decorem faciei!" Haec

[46] Ibid., c.V.118, p. 328.

[47] This is a motif found in other hagiographic texts, as is illustrated by Naoë Kukita Yoshikawa, 'Mysticism and Medicine: Holy Communion in the Vita of Marie d'Oignies and *The Book of Margery Kempe*', *Poetica* 72, Special Issue, Convergence/Divergence: The Politics and Late Medieval English Devotional and Medical Discourses, ed. Denis Renevey and Naoë Kukita Yoshikawa (Tokyo, 2009), 109–22.

[48] *AA.SS. vol. VI 22 February*, De B. Margarita Poenit. Tertii Ord. S. Francisci Cortonae in Etruria, *Vita*, c.V.131, p. 330 (communion) and c.IV.55, p. 314 (resisting the sick).

dicens, erexit se contra se, ferrumque pressit durius, et obliquo vulnere nares sibi detruncavit, pretiosumque rosei sanguineis rivulum in pelvim distillavit; sicque vultus sui genuinum splendorem admodum deturpavit.

[Coming home, she shut herself in her mother's bedroom. Having closed the door she began to pray to God for help; she seized the sword, which she saw hanging at the head of the bed, and hurried to cut off her nose. But her hand was shaking and she had not been trained to strike with a sword, and her feminine blow was not enough to cut through the greater hardness of the nerves. Indignantly she said, 'Oh sword that is considered sharp, how is it that your biting sharpness does not wish to destroy the beauty of my face?!' Saying this, she lifted it up to herself again, and pressing the blade harder, cut off her nose with a sideways stroke and caught the precious river of rosy blood in a basin; and thus she fully destroyed the beauty of her cheeks and face.][49]

The *vita* continues:

Ut non esset idonea huic nequam seculo conformari, elegit naso vivere pravo; et seductibilis formae speciem deformari, quam adulterino fuco falsa pulchritudine depingi, et lascivos oculos in se procaciter impingi;'cute sordida et humili cultu'; 'ornatu superfluo in modum vulpium caudis pulverem tergere, corpusque meretriciis fovere unguentis, quibus solet adulterorum nausea provocari.'

[So that she might not be shaped by the worthless ideals of secular life, she chose to live without a nose; and to deform the type of seductive cheeks that are painted with false beauty in adulterine red, and to dash the impudence of lascivious eyes.

She preferred to live in the house of Christ 'with a dirty face, cultivating humility', rather than 'polish herself up with overdone embellishments like a fox's tail, and pamper her body with whorish lotions, with which it is usual to provoke the vice of adultery'.][50]

For all the hagiographer's rhetoric, however, Oda was never formally canonised. Why? I should like to suggest that the face-cutting episode was in fact damaging to her reputation. Firstly, it is essentially an act of disobedience, carried out in secret in a bedroom, done without warning to her parents or confessor (unlike the two Margarets) and apparently premeditated (she catches the blood in a bowl – but is the hagiographer trying too hard here to insert a Eucharistic motif as well?) Moreover, unlike Margaret of Cortona, whose concealment of a razor suggested planning and a certain surgical precision, Oda's clumsy use of a sword renders the scene of her mutilation almost farcical in tone, although the detail that she cut her face sideways does perhaps suggest that the sword was inverted and that she was kneeling or leaning against it. Secondly, whilst Oda had been aided by prayer to God, her self-inflicted disfigurement was simply the means to an end – the

49 *AA.SS. vol. XI, 20 April*, Vita Ven. Oda Praemonstratensis, c.III.14, p. 774.

50 Ibid. Note here the attack on cosmetics.

preservation of her virginity. Even their horror at seeing their daughter did not immediately persuade her parents, however. As other, contemporary and later, lives of female saints demonstrate, going to such drastic lengths was extremely unusual. Christina of Markyate (d. 1155–66), for example, had eventually prevailed and seen her (unconsummated) marriage dissolved without such a demonstration, and by the thirteenth century merely the threat of self-mutilation was sufficient to indicate the firmness of purpose of both Margarets.[51] Oda's capitulation to the urge towards physical self-harm essentially marked her as less strong in purpose: Larissa Tracy, citing the work of Ruth Mazo Karras, has remarked that for male religious, autocastration was 'an easy way out because spiritual salvation came from overcoming sexual temptation through sheer force of will'.[52] In the same way, actual destruction of facial beauty, for women, deprived them of the opportunity to show that they could be more than simple temptresses, that they had overcome the internalised rhetoric of blame equating them with Eve and were capable of strength in the face of carnal challenges.

It is helpful at this point to consider other contemporary hagiography that dealt with the thorny question of mutilation in a judicial context. In theory, the Church was broadly in favour of judicial mutilation as an alternative to seeing someone put to death, since it offered the possibility of repentance, but the punishment of the body in this way did not on its own have any effect on the health of the criminal's soul,[53] even if it 'mirrored' the offence in the location of the mutilation (for example, cutting of the tongue was a prescribed punishment in late medieval secular law codes in France for blasphemy).[54] This disjuncture was as relevant to cases of self-mutilation as judicial punishments – bodily mortifications have even been described as 'penitential pantomimes' by Mitchell Merback, who emphasises the spectacle: 'For medieval people,

51 *The Life of Christina of Markyate*, ed. Samuel Fanous and Henrietta Leyser (Oxford, 2008).

52 Larissa Tracy, 'Introduction', in *Castration and Culture in the Middle Ages*, ed. Larissa Tracy (Cambridge, 2013), p. 11: Ruth Mazo Karras, *Sexuality in Medieval Europe: Doing Unto Others* (New York and London, 2005), p. 39.

53 G. R. Evans, *Law and Theology in the Middle Ages* (London and New York, 2002), pp. 8–19, outlines how medieval writers addressed the difference between sin (dangerous to the soul) and crime (leading to punishment of the body).

54 Nathalie Gonthier, *Le châtiment du crime au Moyen Âge (XIIe-XVIe siècles)* (Rennes, 1998), pp. 141–2. Escalating punishment of blasphemers in the Provençal code of 1472: from splitting of the upper lip for a second offence, to splitting the lower lip for the third and finally the cutting-out of the tongue: McGlynn, *By Sword and Fire*, p. 23. Only blinding seems to have been understood as 'a "deprivation of moral sight" by enacting it upon the bodies of criminals as the deprivation of sensory sight': Edward Wheatley, *Stumbling Blocks before the Blind: Medieval Constructions of a Disability* (Ann Arbor, MI, 2010), p. 22. Wheatley, ibid., pp. 36–7, highlights Alice's case, discussed above in note 33, but suggests that as the thirteenth century progressed the blinding of criminals, which had always been exceptional, became less frequent.

the experience of *seeing and imagining* a body that was ravaged and bleeding from tortures inflicted upon it lay at the centre of a constellation of religious doctrines, beliefs and devotional practices.'[55] But a wrongly-mutilated body could be problematical.[56] The anxieties surrounding corporal punishment are most clearly expressed in miracle stories, as saints strove to put right the physical defects of unjustly inflicted punishments. Thus a layman falsely accused of arson in c. 1177 was deprived of his eyes and testicles by his successful accuser – but as reported in the miracles of St William of York, this injustice was corrected by the saint, who caused both pairs to grow back.[57] In hagiographic tales such as this, mutilation was presented as the negative outcome of a miscarriage of secular justice. Moreover, the clergy were to be protected at all costs from the risk of this type of punishment: an English case of a cleric who had committed manslaughter c. 1163, for example, was dealt with by the episcopal court, and his punishment would be achieved 'through a decree of the archbishop [Thomas Becket], that was sanctioned by old and authentic canons, by a spiritual and not a corporal punishment (absque omni mutilatione vel deformatione membrorum)'.[58] The deceased Becket himself also assisted a certain Eilward of Westoning, restoring the man's eyesight and testicles after he had been unjustly blinded and castrated.[59]

Indeed, exploring clerical accounts of extreme violence done to the face in twelfth- and thirteenth-century Europe reveals that a substantial number of the reports are designed, just as in the hagiography, to evoke pity for the victim and condemn the tyranny of the perpetrator/s. Mutilation of the face was an extreme, an atrocity. I suggest therefore that it caused the writer of Oda's *vita* some difficulty in positioning it as a positive act. Rather, Oda's dramatic shedding of her own blood may have been spiritually meaningless and was also potentially life-threatening, if the effusion of blood described is

55 Mitchell T. Merback, *The Thief, the Cross and the Wheel: Pain and the Spectacle of Punishment in Medieval and Renaissance Europe* (London, 1999), pp. 19–20.

56 It might be satirised, as in Adam of Bremen's eleventh-century portrayal of the archbishop of Hamburg-Bremen, Adalbert, throwing people into prison and 'joking that bodily affliction was good for the soul (asserens cum risu afflictionem corporis animae utilem)': Adam von Bremen, Hamburgische Kirchengeschichte, ed. Bernard Schmeidler, *MGH SRG* in usum scholarum II (Hanover, 1917), Book III, 56 (57), p. 202. Or, as in later texts directed at holy women, excessive self-harm might be actively discouraged: see below, note 61.

57 *English Lawsuits from William I to Richard I*, vol. 2, ed. Raoul C. Van Caenegem, Selden Society Publications 107 (London, 1991), case 504. John Hudson, 'Violence, Theft and the Making of the English Common Law', in *Crime and Punishment in the Middle Ages*, ed. T. H. Haskett (Victoria, BC, 1998), pp. 19–35 (p. 31), highlights the element of vengeance visible in this case, in that the accuser, rather than the court, carried out the 'punishment'.

58 *English Lawsuits*, vol. 2, case 416.

59 The *Miracula* of Benedict of Peterborough, reproduced in *English Lawsuits*, vol. 2, case 471B.

anything to go by. Her hagiographer seems to have been aware of this for, after persuading her parents that she should now become a nun, Oda experienced another physical trial, this time through God's intervention, rather than her own:

> Illa namque viridis ac robusta membrorum compactio, indigesta ciborum cruditate, soluta est; et corruptis humoribus, nitidae cutis superficies maculosis tumoribus infecta est. Attendentes igitur, Sorores virginae speciem faciei in pallorem gelidum tam celeriter immutatam; et cutem, quae fuerat vitro clarior, quibusdam in locis inflatione vitiosa jam rugatam; suspicatae sunt eam leprae contagio praegravari.
>
> [She, unable to digest the rough food, was weakened by the joining-together of her youthful and strong limbs; and with the corrupt humours, the shining surface of her skin was infected with mottled tumours. The sisters, seeing the virgin's face so quickly transformed into a frosty pallor, and her skin, which had been clearer than glass, corrupted in reddened and swollen places, suspected that she was infected with leprosy.][60]

She was rapidly confined and isolated, suffering the social death of the leper within the community, but in fact this was a test of her humility and patience – she was not leprous at all, recovered and was made prioress. Again a sickness is seen as a redemptive strategy in the hagiography: only when Oda submitted patiently to an illness sent by God was she able fully to embrace her religious life. (And as we have already seen, 'leprosy' only worked as a redeeming condition if the person suffering it did not expect or request it.) This message of submission – and of moderation – is of course conveyed strongly by the guide for anchoresses, the *Ancrene Wisse*, composed in England in the early thirteenth century. Whilst its author was openly contemptuous of those who sought to preserve their bodily health whilst neglecting their spiritual strength, the guide also sought to control the urge to mortify the flesh, stating that such self-inflicted torments as beating, drawing blood or wearing garments designed to abrade the skin were only to be done with the confessor's permission.[61]

Almost all of the facial mutilations discussed so far, whether carried out or not, would have involved heavy bleeding and the risk of infection (and we have already seen this acknowledged in metaphorical terms in Margaret of Cortona's *vita*). We do not know whether a medieval surgeon was regularly on hand to attend the aftermath of judicial punishments: the report dated 1172 of the restoration of Eilward's lost eyes and testicles, this time by Thomas

60 *AA.SS. vol. XI, 20 April*, Vita Ven. Oda Praemonstratensis c.V.20, p. 776

61 *Ancrene Wisse: A Corrected Edition of the Text in Cambridge, Corpus Christi College MS 402 with variants from other manuscripts*, ed. Bella Millett EETS o.s. 325 (Oxford, 2005), Parts 6.11, p. 139 (care of health) and 8.16, p. 158 (mortification). Modern English translation in *Ancrene Wisse: Guide for Anchoresses*, trans. Bella Millett (Exeter, 2009), with same pagination as edition.

Becket himself, indicates that some care was available. Thus as the miracle of restoration of his sight occurred, 'malagma cereum, quod sive ad extrahendas orbium vacuorum purulentias seu ad ipsa cilia claudenda fuerat appositum' ['he scratched and removed with his fingernail the wax and the emollient which had been applied to eliminate the pus'].[62] But the fact that Oda's face was permanently disfigured, to the horror of her parents (and, it seems, to the discomfort of some of her fellow nuns), meant that had she remained in the secular world, she would have been stigmatised for life by the confusing message of her damaged face. From English examples of the following century, we know that men who had accidentally become disfigured often approached the court to have it put in writing that their injuries were not a result of criminal penalties: this seems to confirm how such deformities would be scrutinised within the community.[63] For all that later medieval Europe saw a flourishing in both medical and surgical knowledge, wounds to the face were (and remain) the hardest to conceal.

MARKING, STIGMA, CURE

It is this sense of disproportionate damage, I argue, that made facial disfigurement such a powerful motif for hagiographers. As Erving Goffman points out, the ancient Greek term 'stigma', in the sense of a bodily sign exposing something unusual or bad about the moral status of the bearer, retained its meaning until relatively recently, when the behaviour or characteristic itself, rather than the physical sign, became known by that term.[64] Shlomo Shoham points to the shaved head and segregation of the medieval penitent as an example of stigmatising the wrongdoer visibly in order to act as a deterrent to those viewing the offender.[65] As is well known, however, the term *stigma* took on an entirely different significance in the later Middle Ages. Rather than isolating the bearer, the term was used to describe bodily signs of holy grace, as manifested, for example, on the bodies of St Francis (1181/2–1226) and of St Catherine of Siena (1347–80).[66] The key difference, however, is

62 The *Miracula* of Benedict of Peterborough, reproduced in *English Lawsuits*, vol. 2, ed. Van Caenegem, case 471B.

63 Patent Roll records cited by Andrew G. Miller, '"Tails" of Masculinity: Knights, Clerics and the Mutilation of Horses in Medieval England', *Speculum* 88 (2013), 958–95 (p. 977).

64 Erving Goffman, *Stigma: Notes on the Management of Spoiled Identity* (Englewood Cliffs, NJ, 1963, repr. London, 1990), p. 11.

65 S. Giora Shoham, *The Mark of Cain: the Stigma Theory of Crime and Social Deviation* (Jerusalem, 1970), p. 7.

66 St Francis: *The Stigmata of Francis of Assisi: New Studies, New Perspectives*, ed. Jacques Delarun et al. (New York, 2006). St Catherine: *A Companion to St Catherine of Siena*, ed. Carolyn Muessig, George Ferzoco and Beverley Kienzle (Leiden, 2011). On stigmata see Carolyn Muessig, 'The Stigmata Debate in Theology and Art in the Late Middle Ages', in

that the marks (invisible in Catherine's case) were placed on their bodies by God, not self-inflicted. Nevertheless, it is striking that the *vitae* of three women, all following different orders for their religious vocation (Oda was a Praemonstratensian, Margaret of Hungary a Dominican and Margaret of Cortona a Franciscan Tertiary), should explore the issue of bodily marking as a sign of spiritual devotion. Nor were Francis and Catherine alone in their acquisition of holy markings: John Coakley highlights the case of Christina of Stommeln, whose visions included bloody violence and who also received *stigmata* to her body.[67] But it is significant, it seems to me, that a century later Catherine's *vita* reports her request to God to keep her *stigmata* invisible: Raymond rather presents it as an example of her humility, but was this to set her apart from the growing number of stigmatics?

The major difference between these examples and our cases is, of course, that *stigmata* were a spontaneous phenomenon, rather than a calculated act, and herein lies the tension between the desire to mortify the flesh and the prevalent attitudes in twelfth- and thirteenth-century secular Europe to the facially-mutilated. The *vitae* of the three holy women discussed in this essay all explored facial mutilation as a possible way of expressing their commitment to a chaste or virginal life. But the dangers of following this path were all too apparent against a secular world in which facial mutilation was a sign of wrongdoing.

To some extent, the geographical separation of the three women's *vitae*, situated as they were in Flanders, Italy and Hungary, is mitigated by the obvious similarities in their message about submission to God (and their confessors). Yet they each convey something of their specific location: it may be no coincidence that the only *actual* mutilation recorded is from northern Europe, where judicial penalties targeted on the face are, if not commonplace, at least well known and better documented in the sources. Margaret of Hungary's *vita*, on the other hand, was able to draw upon the potential for physical martyrdom in the face of a pagan hoard, perhaps inspired by earlier models of sainthood. Margaret of Cortona's life, however, needed a different reason to justify her desire for penitential mutilation, and so focuses far more on her previous, secular life in the cosmopolitan, urban world of late medieval Italy.

There are strong parallels in the tales of mutilation, however, with contemporary hagiography about male saints. Larissa Tracy, exploring images in the *South English Legendary*, comments that 'Castration may have been taboo in hagiography as a genre because the authors did not want to align their saints with the criminals against which the sentence was historically

The Authority of the Word: Reflecting on Image and Text in Northern Europe, 1400–1700, ed. Celeste Brusati, Karl Enenkel and Walter Melion (Leiden, 2011), pp. 481–504.

67 John W. Coakley, *Women, Men and Spiritual Power: Female Saints and their Male Collaborators* (New York, 2006), pp. 89–110.

applied'.[68] Whilst the *vitae* discussed here did not entirely elide the subject of a similarly-charged form of mutilation – they demonstrated that women's sexuality and allure to men was thought to reside in facial beauty – they presented the problem as to some extent 'contained' by the fact that female religious needed the authority of their male confessors before putting their impulses to self-harm into practice. Oda's case was meant to be shocking on several levels, but it most effectively showed up her weakness: women's ultimate vanity, as highlighted by these texts, lay in imagining that a physical change could rid any of them of their main 'affliction', which was simply being female. Of all three saintly careers, Margaret of Cortona's is most concerned with this theme, since she had led the most 'sinful' life of the three, and it is also the most valuable for exploring intersections of medicine, religion and gender. She, after all, had the lengthiest consultation with 'Christus Medicus': the motif of Christ as doctor was well established, even if it does not explicitly appear in the *vita*. But no amount of bodily isolation, mutilation or self-denial, to the point of weakness and illness, could substitute for inner qualities such as patience, humility and submission. Only then would these women truly *see* the 'doctor', and achieve a 'cure'.

[68] Larissa Tracy, '"Al defouleden is holie bodi": Castration, the Sexualization of Torture and Anxieties of Identity in the *South English Legendary*', in *Castration and Culture*, ed. Tracy, pp. 87–107 (p. 96).

10

DID DRUNKENNESS DIM THE SIGHT? MEDIEVAL UNDERSTANDINGS AND RESPONSES TO BLINDNESS IN MEDICAL AND RELIGIOUS DISCOURSE*

Joy Hawkins

> Hechinge and smertinge of yȝen comen somtyme of outward þings, as of ... poudir þat hurtiþ the yȝen and þe tendir substaunce þerof, and of smoke þat dymmeþ iȝen and makeþ hem smerte, and of colde wynde smytinge þe spirit of siȝte; also of hot aier ... grete briȝtnes of þe sonne ... of vnordinate diete and of contynuel dronkenes þat dymmeþ the siȝt; of fleischlich liking and ofte seruyse of Venus þat corrumpiþ and dissolueþ þe spiritis ... somtyme of inward matere and causis, as of humours hote or colde, drye oþer moiste.[1]

The thirteenth-century encyclopaedist, Bartholomaeus Anglicus, whose work was later translated into the vernacular by John Trevisa, included excessive alcohol consumption in his list of the possible causes of blindness; individuals who constantly deluged their body with unhealthy liquids would inevitably damage their eyesight. Bartholomaeus' statement underscores the medieval theological and medical belief that most sufferers were responsible, at least in part, for their misfortunes. Classical Greek authorities had stressed that it was essential to keep the four humours – blood, phlegm, black and yellow bile – in balance by carefully following a regulated lifestyle appropriate to one's age, gender and environment. These ideas were readily adopted and fostered by the medieval Church as they accorded perfectly with the Christian belief that individuals should be personally responsible for following a regimen that was geared to restraint and moderation. For example, the Apocryphal Book

* This chapter has been developed from sections in my doctoral thesis: Joy Hawkins, 'The Blind in Later Medieval England: Medical, Social and Religious Responses', unpublished Ph.D. thesis, University of East Anglia, 2011. My thanks go to Professor Carole Rawcliffe for her advice and encouragement throughout the supervision of my research.

1 Bartholomaeus Anglicus, *On the Properties of Things: John Trevisa's Translation of Bartholomaeus Anglicus' De Proprietatibus Rerum*, ed. M. C. Seymour et al., 3 vols (Oxford, 1975–88), vol. 1, pp. 359–60.

of Sirach warned that too much wine would make even the wisest of men go astray.[2] However, as Bartholomaeus' entry shows, there were many different causes of eye complaints; in addition to failing to maintain one's humoral balance, an act as simple as staring at the sun or lengthy exposure to a cold wind could upset the eye's delicate equilibrium.

Because theologians often (but not always) equated disability with sin, some surveys of the disabled in the period before industrialisation take it as read that those with sensory impairments, such as blindness, must have been pushed to the margins of society or even completely excluded, and were forced to beg or join troops of wandering minstrels in order to earn a living.[3] Family members suffering from physical and sensory disabilities have been described as burdens, reliant upon their kin to support them and unable to contribute to the household economy in return.[4] Studies based on this assumption fail to acknowledge that, in practice, each person suffering from a physical impairment would have been treated according to his or her particular needs. This chapter will demonstrate that responses to blindness varied according to the circumstance, cause and severity of the individual's impairment, and that not all didactic literature treated the blind with uniform negativity. A degree of overlap can be seen in the advice offered in medical and theological discourse; indeed, each often informed the other, with both offering reassurance as well as a course of action to aid the physically impaired.

The medieval Church taught that disease, suffering and blindness were only unleashed on mankind after Adam and Eve committed Original Sin. In the Garden of Eden, Adam and Eve's humours had been perfectly balanced with neither black nor yellow bile, the two most likely to cause bodily ailments, predominating. According to Hildegard of Bingen (1098–1179), the twelfth-century nun and polymath, when Adam and Eve were expelled from Paradise, 'black bile coagulated in [their] blood', which resulted in the loss of man's innate humoral balance, leading to the corruption of body and soul.[5] The image of Eve succumbing to the serpent's enticement was commonplace

2 Sirach 19:2. Biblical quotations are taken from *The Holy Bible containing the Old and New Testaments in the Earliest English Versions made from the Latin Vulgate by John Wycliffe and his Followers*, ed. J. Forshall and F. Madden, 4 vols (Oxford, 1850).

3 Brendan Gleeson, *Geographies of Disability* (New York, 1999), p. 63; M. A. Winzer, 'Disability and Society before the Eighteenth Century: Dread and Despair', in *The Disability Studies Reader*, ed. L. J. Davis (New York, 1997), pp. 75–109 (p. 80); David T. Mitchell, 'Foreword', in Henri-Jacques Stiker, *A History of Disability*, trans. William Sayer (Ann Arbor, MI, 1999), pp. ix–xi.

4 C. Safilios-Rothschild, *The Sociology and Social Psychology of Disability and Rehabilitation* (New York, 1970), p. 12: 'The disabled have always been "problematic" for *all* societies throughout history, since they could not usually perform their social responsibilities satisfactorily.' Also see Winzer, 'Disability and Society', pp. 76, 91–2.

5 Hildegard of Bingen, *On Natural Philosophy and Medicine: Selections from Cause et cure*, trans. Margaret Berger (Cambridge, 1999), p. 43.

throughout medieval Europe, adorning the walls of churches and decorating manuscripts, as a constant reminder to the viewer of what had been lost.

In his influential work, *The City of God*, St Augustine of Hippo (d. 430) explained that every person carried with him or her the legacy of Original Sin, but any further, personal sin would make matters infinitely worse.[6] It was important, therefore, to keep the humours in balance to maintain the health of the whole body. This was not always an easy task, however, as some organs in the body were much more prone to ailments and disease. The French surgeon Henri de Mondeville (d. c. 1320) was quick to point out that the eyes were a particularly fragile organ whose delicate nature could easily be damaged by even a slight degree of instability.[7] Medical authorities understood that most eye complaints were caused by an excess or deficit of one of the four humours, usually exacerbated by a poor regimen, but theologians went one step further, making the connection between a person's misconduct and his or her poor health. They taught that any of the seven deadly sins, but especially gluttony and lust, could have a direct and detrimental effect on the eyesight by destabilising the complex network of humours and spirits that made vision possible.

Excessive alcohol consumption was particularly frowned upon by theologians and medical authorities alike. Drunkenness was regarded as a type of gluttony, and was, therefore, a mortal sin against God.[8] The *Fasciculus morum*, a fourteenth-century handbook offering advice to preachers, explained that gluttons risked damaging their health because those who ate or drank excessively could 'literally lose their eyesight'.[9] Furthermore, gluttons and drunkards spent most of their time in the tavern, which was known to be a favourite haunt of the devil. In his analysis of *The Book of Vices and Virtues* (c. 1340), Morton Bloomfield points out that the tavern was regarded as 'the chapel of Satan' because, whilst 'God does His miracles in His church; the devil does his, which are the opposite, in the tavern. Instead of making the blind see, the devil makes blind those who can see.'[10] The *Fasciculus morum* uses similarly comparative religious language, emphasising that those who 'make their pilgrimage to the tavern' would 'lose their sight' as well as 'their ability to walk'.[11] Such evidence clearly reflects the medieval belief that sin

6 St Augustine, *Concerning the City of God Against the Pagans*, trans. Henry Bettenson (London, 1972; repr. 2003), p. 1067.

7 Marie-Christine Pouchelle, *The Body and Surgery in the Middle Ages*, trans. Rosemary Morris (New Brunswick, NJ, 1990), p. 119.

8 *Fasciculus Morum: A Fourteenth-Century Preacher's Handbook*, ed. and trans. Siegfried Wenzel (University Park, PA, 1989), p. 633; *Middle English Sermons*, ed. W. O. Ross, EETS o.s. 209 (Oxford, 1940; repr. 1960), p. 56.

9 *Fasciculus Morum*, p. 635.

10 Morton W. Bloomfield, *The Seven Deadly Sins* (East Lansing, MI, 1952; repr. 1967), p. 183; *The Book of Vices and Virtues*, ed. W. Nelson Francis, EETS o.s. 217 (Oxford, 1942), pp. 53–4.

11 *Fasciculus Morum*, pp. 433, 637.

and blindness, both physical and spiritual, were closely interrelated, and that anyone of loose moral behaviour would be more likely to suffer from associated eye complaints.

Since man had lost his perfect humoral balance in the Garden of Eden, it followed that the detrimental effect gluttony and drunkenness had on the body system was explained in terms of humoral theory. When any food or drink was consumed, it passed straight from the mouth to the stomach, where it was cooked as if in an oven.[12] The degree of heat in the stomach was fundamental to the health of the entire body. Too much alcohol would overheat the body, deluging it with unhealthy liquid. Medical authorities frequently classified wine as a hot and dry substance and, therefore, if an excess was introduced into the body system this would cause the stomach to over-heat, burning the food, destroying its nutrients and producing dangerous choleric toxins.[13]

Once foodstuffs had been converted into a mixture known as 'chyle' in the stomach, it was transported along the portal vein to the liver where it was transformed through a secondary cooking process into black and yellow bile, phlegm and, crucially, blood.[14] Blood was the most important substance in the body, as it conveyed the rest of the humoral matter through the veins and arteries. The vital and animal spirits were created directly from this venous blood, and thus an immoderate diet would make them weak and sick, which helps to explain how 'contynuel dronkenes' would dull the animal and vital spirits, which in turn would 'dym the sight'.[15] The idea of living a *via media* was readily fostered by the medieval Church as it accorded perfectly with the Christian belief that individuals should be personally responsible for following a regimen that was geared towards restraint and moderation. Those who failed to follow this advice risked their physical and spiritual health. Preachers who readily warned their congregations of the consequences of gluttony enlisted the support of medical authorities to lend force to their argument, combining medical theory with biblical teachings to emphasise their point. Indeed, the author of the *Fasciculus morum* uses the following tale as one such example to make congregations clearly understand why gluttony was to be scorned. A blind man complained of hunger to his guide, and asked if they might stop to eat. Failing to listen to the boy who was leading him, who advised that it was not a good place to rest, the impetuous man attempted to make his own way,

12 *Secretum secretorum: Nine English Versions*, ed. M. A. Manzalaoui, EETS e.s. 276 (Oxford, 1977), p. 51.

13 Ken Albala, 'To Your Health: Wine as Food and Medicine in Mid-Sixteenth-Century Italy', in *Alcohol: A Social and Cultural History*, ed. Mack P. Holt (Oxford, 2006), pp. 11–24 (p. 14). Also see E. Ruth Harvey, *The Inward Wits: Psychological Theory in the Middle Ages and Renaissance* (London, 1975), p. 26.

14 Nancy Siraisi, *Medieval and Early Renaissance Medicine: An Introduction to Knowledge and Practice* (Chicago, 1990), p. 106.

15 Bartholomaeus Anglicus, *On the Properties of Things*, vol. 1, p. 360.

'stumbled and nearly broke his neck'. Without any further mishap, they made their way to:

> an eating place where they were given delicious but raw and unhealthy food; so the boy warned the blind man not to eat any of it. But he said: 'I have a first-class stomach' and ate greedily and so made himself sick.[16]

In this exemplum the preacher is making an obvious connection between physical and spiritual blindness to his audience.

It was not, however, solely gluttony that was thought to cause blindness; lust was also believed to have a detrimental effect on both a person's moral and physiological well-being. Excessive quantities of semen were thought to corrupt the blood, causing illness and potentially damaging the sight. One cautionary tale, attributed to the influential Dominican friar, Albert the Great (d. 1280), reinforces this idea. It describes a monk who went blind from having 'desired a beautiful lady seventy times before matins was rung'. After his death, an autopsy revealed that his brain was reduced to the 'size of a pomegranate', whilst his eyes had been 'destroyed'. Albert interpreted this as a 'sign that coitus drains ... the brain'. Both the brain and the eyes were phlegmatic in nature and therefore especially vulnerable to the physiological upheavals in the body caused by sexual excess.[17] As happened when one ate too much hot or spicy food, the generation of too much innate heat during sexual intercourse, or from having too many libidinous thoughts, would cause the stomach to overheat and produce burnt humours which, in turn, corrupted the entire venous system.

It was not just the physical act of sexual intercourse that could have a negative impact on the body system. Medical authorities and theologians both warned of the dangers of a lustful gaze. Indeed, a man who looked at a woman lecherously was often believed to be as culpable as if he had performed the deed. According to *Handlyng Synne*, a vernacular guide to spiritual health, adapted from the Anglo-Norman *Mannuel de pechiez* (c. 1260) by the Gilbertine monk, Robert Mannyng (d. c. 1338), man can 'synne yn lechery, yn þe lokyng of þyn yghe'. He warns his readers not to look at 'wymmen ouer mochyl' as 'syghte makeþ mennys þoghtes fykyl'.[18] It is of little surprise, therefore, that in the medieval period, the moment of the Fall was associated with sight more than any other sense, including touch. Gerald of Wales in his guide to the clergy explained that 'Eve would not have touched the tree unless she had first gazed upon it heedlessly'.[19] Suzannah Biernoff observes that

16 *Fasciculus Morum*, p. 637.

17 Albert the Great, *Questions on Animals*, quoted in D. Jacquard and C. Thomasset, *Sexuality and Medicine in the Middle Ages*, trans. M. Adamson (Oxford, 1998), pp. 55–6.

18 *Robert of Brunne's 'Handlyng Synne'*, ed. F. J. Furnivall, 2 parts in 1 vol., EETS o.s. 119, 123 (London, 1901), pp. 242, 258, 280.

19 Gerald of Wales, *The Jewel of the Church: A Translation of Gemma Ecclesiastica by*

Eve was 'seduced by the pleasant looking fruit, and tempted by the serpent's promise of omniscience … A desiring gaze foreshadows the original sin.'[20] The conviction that sin could enter the body through the eye was a common trope in medieval homiletic literature and sermons, reinforced by medical texts which taught that the eye could absorb a copy of the object which was gazed upon which would, in turn, have a direct impact on the body system.[21] Thus it followed that one reason why the eyes were 'very quick to harm [the] soul' was because of their porous nature.[22] Whether the Aristotelian theory of the eye's passive intromission or the Galenic concept of extramission of vision was accepted, in both cases, the eye needed to be permeable to allow the copy of the image being viewed into the body.[23] Women's damp and fleshy bodies were similar in humoral composition to the phlegmatic eyes; it is little coincidence, therefore, that temptation and sin were frequently associated with sight. The eyes' desire to sin was regarded as being so great that even holy women could be prone to temptation; hence, anchoresses were encouraged to cover their windows with a thick black curtain because 'sin entered [Eve] first of all through her sight'.[24] Not only would the dark, dense cloth preclude any intrusion of, or interaction with, the outside world, but in addition the colour black would protect the delicate eyes as it was believed to 'hurt the eyes less' than other brighter colours which were regarded as damaging to the eyesight.[25]

The link between eyesight and sin was further reinforced by biblical examples of wrongdoers being deprived of their sight by a vengeful God. Exempla from the Bible alongside hagiographic texts describing God and his saints punishing sinners with blindness as a form of chastisement or in order to teach a lesson to the impious are hard to ignore.[26] Hagiographers clearly enjoyed recounting stories of saints who blinded their detractors. For instance, according to one twelfth-century miracle collection, St James deprived Gilbert, a keeper of hounds, of his sight as a penance for hunting on his feast day.[27] A saint revealing his power through such an act was a common

Giraldus Cambrensis, trans. J. Hagen (Leiden, 1979), p. 182.

20 Suzannah Biernoff, *Sight and Embodiment in the Middle Ages* (Basingstoke, 2002), p. 42.

21 Joy Hawkins, 'Sights for Sore Eyes: Vision and Health in Medieval England', in *On Light: Aspects and Responses*, ed. K. P. Clarke and Sarah Baccianti (Oxford, 2013), pp. 137–56 (pp. 139–40).

22 *Fasciculus Morum*, p. 651.

23 For a full explanation of the difference between these two opposing ideas and how they came to be reconciled during the Middle Ages, see Hawkins, 'Sights for Sore Eyes', pp. 139–40.

24 *Ancrene Wisse: Guide* for *Anchoresses*, trans. Bella Millett (Exeter, 2009), Part 2, p. 20.

25 *Ancrene Wisse*, Part 2, p. 21.

26 See for example, Deuteronomy 28:28–9: 'the Lord shall smyte thee with … blyndnesse'.

27 'The Miracles of the Hand of St James', ed. Brian Kemp, *Berkshire Archaeological Journal* 65 (1970), 1–19 (p. 13).

theme in miracle accounts: one of the most famous examples of divine retribution, retold throughout the medieval period, was that of Leofstan, a tenth-century abbot of Bury St Edmunds. On inspecting the open tomb of the abbey's patron saint, he wanted to verify whether the decapitated head of King Edmund had miraculously rejoined his body, as legend claimed. He therefore pulled the saint's head whilst a monk held onto the feet. They soon discovered that the two parts were firmly attached, but as a punishment for his sacrilege, Leofstan's hands were paralysed and he was struck blind and dumb.[28]

From such evidence, it is tempting to accept unquestioningly that there was an overriding belief throughout the Middle Ages that physical impairment, including a loss of sight, was an unavoidable consequence of sin, especially as the Bible taught that a bodily deformity could be a reflection of the person's diseased soul.[29] However, such assumptions are too simplistic and arise when studying the blind outside of their historical and cultural context. Indeed, more often than not, historians have demonstrated, such as Edward Wheatley in the case of France, that men and women who lost their sight 'through no blameworthy cause', as, for example, in an industrial accident, or through old age, usually received sympathy from their peers and society did its best to provide adequate care and shelter.[30] Medieval men and women were perfectly aware that their less than perfect humoral balance would further deteriorate with the passage of time. As the body aged, it cooled and dried out as it lost its vital internal moisture.[31] The eyes would become cold, dry and sore, which in turn caused irritation and poor sight. Far from being an inevitable consequence of sin, blindness was seen as a natural part of the human life-cycle; according to the thirteenth-century friar, Roger Bacon (d. 1292), it was as inescapable as white hair and wrinkles.[32] It should be of little surprise, therefore, that medieval communities cared for, rather than condemned, those who had gone blind through no fault of their own, and in particular the elderly.

The statutes of English craft guilds reveal empathy and a need to care for one's own in times of hardship.[33] Fourteenth-century fraternities showed a

28 Samsonis abbatis, 'Opus de miraculis Sancti Ædmundi', in *Memorials of St Edmund's Abbey*, ed. T. Arnold, Rolls Series 96 (London, 1890), pp. 133–4.

29 Luke 11:34–6.

30 See Edward Wheatley, *Stumbling Blocks before the Blind: Medieval Constructions of Disability* (Ann Arbor, MI, 2010) and Mark P. O'Tool, 'Disability and the Suppression of Historical Identity: Rediscovering the Professional Backgrounds of the Blind Residents of the Hôpital des Quinze-Vingts', in *Disability in the Middle Ages: Reconsiderations and Reverberations*, ed. Joshua R. Eyler (Farnham, 2010), pp. 11–24.

31 Galen's work, *On the Powers of Foods*, states that even if a person was fortunate enough to possess a balanced temperament, he or she 'cannot preserve it unchanged throughout the stages of life': Mark Grant, *Galen on Food and Diet* (London, 2000), p. 74.

32 Roger Bacon, *Opus majus*, trans. Robert B. Burke, 2 vols (New York, 1928; repr. 1962), vol. 2, p. 619.

33 Gervase Rosser, 'Communities of Parish and Guild in the Late Middle Ages', in *Parish,*

keen awareness of the occupational hazards and the economic implications of a long-term disability. The fear of losing one's livelihood through an industrial accident or old age, as well as the sympathy engendered if one of their own had suffered such a fate, led to several guilds offering a type of financial assistance against periods of penury or ill health, albeit rather limited by later standards. Such help would have gone some way to alleviate the poverty from which a whole family could suffer when its main breadwinner was incapacitated. Modest hand-outs were available for deserving cases throughout the Middle Ages; for example the Ludlow Palmer's guild, founded in 1284 by a group of burgesses, extended 'particular care' to members who were blind or mutilated.[34] One hundred years later, the Holy Trinity guild in Wisbech, Cambridgeshire, whose statutes date from 1379, offered (but did not necessarily always pay) 10d a week to members of their fraternity who 'by act of God be paralysed, dumb or blind', in the hope it would prevent them from having to resort to begging.[35]

A few respected members of guilds who lost their sight during their working lives may have received enough help to survive a potentially debilitating change of circumstance. Between 1373 and 1484, the Trinity Guild in Lynn, Norfolk, provided assistance to an average of twenty-five members each year, including men suffering from crippling injuries, disease and old age.[36] Although it has been argued that in practice guilds provided less than their statutes suggested, and that those promising assistance were often the wealthier fraternities whose members were less likely to require help,[37] the examples above demonstrate that the desire to help was certainly present among guild members, even if in reality it was not always followed through to the same extent. To ensure that funds were not squandered, guilds usually limited the financial help on offer, allocating moneys 'according to the merit and quality of the person concerned';[38] or only for those who found themselves in 'extreme' circumstances. The mid fourteenth-century statutes of the Corpus Christi Guild in Stretham, Cambridgeshire, included the loss of an eye as one such 'extreme' situation.[39] Losing one's sight, especially through an industrial accident or because of close work, would evoke compassion among other guild members.

Church and People: Local Studies in Lay Religion, 1350–1750, ed. S. J. Wright (London, 1988), pp. 29–55 (p. 37).

34 *Victoria County History of the County of Shropshire*, 11 vols, ed. W. Page (London, 1973), vol. 2, p. 134.

35 H. F. Westlake, *The Parish Gilds of Mediaeval England* (London, 1919), p. 148 and Ben McRee, 'Charity and Gild Solidarity in Late Medieval England', *Journal of British Studies* 32 (1993), 195–225 (p. 204).

36 McRee, 'Charity and Guild Solidarity', pp. 215–16.

37 McRee, 'Charity and Guild Solidarity', pp. 197–8, 200.

38 *Victoria County History of Shropshire*, vol. 2, p. 134.

39 V. R. Bainbridge, *Gilds in the Medieval Countryside: Social and Religious Change in Cambridgeshire, c.1350–1558* (Woodbridge, 1996), p. 114; Westlake, *Parish Gilds*, p. 145.

It is clear that fraternities felt a need to offer financial support when at all possible, as they would have been painfully aware of their own vulnerability.

The variety of guild statutes offering help to their members shows that there were many different industries that could prove potentially detrimental to workers' eyesight. Metalworkers, lime-burners, smiths and glass blowers all used furnaces to generate intense heat, prolonged exposure to which would seriously damage the eyes.[40] Not only the extreme heat, but the intensity of light, as well as stray sparks, could trigger short-term conditions such as excessive lacrimation and blurred eye-sight as well as longer-term problems including damage to the retina, which, if severe, might eventually result in blindness. Nor would metal and glass workers have suffered from the heat alone, since each of the processes they carried out while crushing, smelting and tempering produced noxious by-products.[41] Many trades and crafts used what today would be regarded as toxic substances, including lead and mercury. Bartholomaeus Anglicus, citing his fellow Franciscan, the philosopher Richard Rufus of Cornwall (d. c. 1260), emphasises the importance of brimstone and mercury (quicksilver), explaining that they 'ben þe element and matiere of þe which alle meltynge metalle is ymade'.[42] Bartholomaeus warned of the risks of heating and mixing quicksilver with other substances, as 'þe smoke þerof is most greuous to men'.[43] Not only were craftsmen at risk from exposure to these injurious substances, their eyes could also be strained by performing close work over long periods. This would be true of any craftsman, such as glovers and tailors, who produced intricate work in poor light. As these artisans grew older, their problems could become increasingly troublesome, and sufferers had to rely on the generosity of their peers. The 1354 statutes of the Little Company of Glovers of London ordained that a generous 10½d should be given each week to members of the fraternity who were impoverished because of blindness;[44] and in the fifteenth century, the Tailors' Guild built almshouses to provide subsidised accommodation for their elderly or disabled brethren.[45] Individuals who lost their sight through hard work, either through the demands of undertaking intricate work over

40 R. J. Charleston, 'Vessel Glass', in *English Medieval Industries: Craftsmen, Techniques, Products*, ed. J. Blair and N. Ramsay (London, 1991), pp. 237–64 (p. 240). Charlotte Roberts and Margaret Cox, *Health and Disease in Britain: From Prehistory to the Present Day* (Stroud, 2003), p. 235.

41 Ronald F. Homer, 'Tin, Lead and Pewter', in *A History of Technology*, ed. Charles Singer et al., 5 vols (Oxford, 1954–59), vol. 3, pp. 57–80 (pp. 59–60, 63); Roberts and Cox, *Health and Disease*, p. 237.

42 Bartholomaeus Anglicus, *On the Properties of Things*, vol. 2, p. 831.

43 Bartholomaeus Anglicus, *On the Properties of Things*, vol. 2, p. 832.

44 Westlake, *Parish Gilds*, p. 188.

45 Matthew Davies, 'The Tailors of London: Corporate Charity in the Late Medieval Town', in *Crown, Government and People in the Fifteenth Century*, ed. R. Archer (Stroud, 1995), pp. 161–90 (pp. 182–4); Rosser, 'Communities of Parish and Guild', pp. 37–8.

a long period of time or through a work-related accident, were often prioritised in the guilds' statutes. It is also possible that fraternities offered smaller amounts of informal help directly to such deserving cases without the details ever being recorded formally in the guild accounts.[46]

During the second half of the fifteenth century, the Glovers of Chester performed the play of the 'Healing of the Blind Man' as their contribution to the city's annual Mystery Cycle. In it, the blind man is singled out by Christ as a 'worthy object of … healing'.[47] Paraphrasing the Gospel of St John, the text explains that the man is not to blame for his disability and the actors performing the play urged the spectators to recognise the importance of offering support to those who were suffering from such ailments through no fault of their own. To reinforce this point, the boy who guided the blind man around the stage also acted as the audience's conscience. He implored them to 'remember … the poore and the blynd' and to give 'charitable almes' because each deserving pauper was their 'owne neighbour' and their 'own kynd'.[48] It is interesting to note that at the end of the play, the same boy walked among the crowd asking for alms; quite possibly this was one way in which the guild raised money to help the blind and infirm.[49] Documentary evidence reveals how such resources were distributed: on its guild day in 1492, for example, the Norwich guild of St George gave 4d in alms to 'Sir Stephyn the blynd prest'.[50]

A further indication of the extent to which guild members wanted to help their more unfortunate brethren is when affluent craftsmen left monetary bequests in their wills for this purpose. Three London goldsmiths each set aside legacies in the early fifteenth century for their blind brothers.[51] The eyes of goldsmiths were particularly exposed to risks from the fumes created when metals and other substances were heated. This was recognised by the guild when in 1341 the company in London gained a royal charter granting it the right to acquire land and use the ensuing rents for the 'sustenance of those of their mystery who have been blinded by fire and smoke of the glowing silver'.[52]

46 Caroline M. Barron, 'The Parish Fraternities of Medieval London', in *The Church in Pre-Reformation Society*, ed. Caroline M. Barron and Christopher Harper-Bill (Woodbridge, 1985), pp. 13–37 (p. 27).

47 P. J. P. Goldberg, 'Performing the Word of God: Corpus Christi Drama in the Northern Province', in *Life and Thought in the Northern Church, c.1100–1700*, ed. Diana Wood, Studies in Church History, Subsidia 12 (Woodbridge, 1999), pp. 145–70 (p. 165).

48 *The Chester Mystery Cycle*, ed. R. M. Lumiansky and D. Mills, EETS n.s. 3 (Oxford, 1974), p. 231.

49 *The Chester Mystery Cycle*, ed. David Mills (East Lansing, MI, 1992), p. 220.

50 Norfolk Record Office, NCR, 8/F, St George's Guild Account of Receipts and Expenses, 1491–92, no foliation.

51 The three goldsmiths were John Godman, Thomas Atte Haye and Richard Wethyhale: *Calendar of Wills Proved and Enrolled in the Court of Hustings, London A.D. 1258–A.D. 1688*, ed. R. Sharpe, 2 vols (London, 1890), vol. 2, pp. 364, 377, 446.

52 *Calendar of Patent Rolls, 1216–1509*, 54 vols (London, 1893-1916), *1340–43*, p. 221.

Testamentary provision was an important way for individuals to use their goods and money to pay for post-mortem intercession. The idea that the soul's journey could be expedited through the commendatory prayers of the living was an integral and reassuring part of the doctrine of Purgatory. The speed of the soul's transit depended in part on the quality as well as the number of the prayers offered after death, and the intercessions of blind men and women were considered especially powerful. It was not just those in guilds, therefore, who remembered the blind in their wills. Thomas de Bekyngton, bishop of Bath and Wells, who died in 1464, left 100s to be distributed among the poor parishioners of his first benefice, giving priority to those who were blind.[53] In several cases, testators reveal touching ties of kinship and community in their bequests: in 1515, Margery Dogett of Norwich gave her second best gown to 'blynde Margaret',[54] whilst in 1466, Katherine Pacok of York left her black gown lined with fur to a blind widow who had fallen on hard times, presumably because of her infirmity, and thus had been reduced to living in the cemetery of her parish church.[55]

In addition to wishing to care for those within their own communities, with whom they had a connection and familiarity, the Gospel stories preached from the pulpit urged congregations to care for the poor and needy. The duties all Christians were expected to perform were laid out in the Gospel of St Matthew. These charitable acts, including the provision of food, water, shelter and clothing, had to be discharged by anyone who hoped to enter the Kingdom of Heaven.[56] The wealthier members of society were especially bound to fulfil these obligations because it was believed that they would have a harder time getting to Paradise than the poor. Preachers followed the Gospel's lead and warned their congregations of the importance of almsgiving, as those weighed down by material goods would spend longer in Purgatory, always assuming they were fortunate enough to escape the fires of Hell altogether. Vivid accounts of the horrors of Purgatory were broadcast from the pulpit to persuade congregations of the need to shorten their ordeal by making provision for their souls in advance, through pious gift-giving. Mindful of their own spiritual needs, donors expected recipients to offer heartfelt and regular prayers on their behalf. Through their suffering the blind had gained an especial connection to God, and, in addition, they were subject to fewer

Further licences were granted in 1393 and 1402, showing that this was an ongoing problem: *1391–96*, pp. 219, 262 and *1401–05*, p. 58.

53 *Somerset Medieval Wills, 1383–1500*, ed. F. W. Weaver (London, 1901), p. 205.

54 Norman P. Tanner, *The Church in Medieval Norwich* (Toronto, 1984), p. 321.

55 York, York Minster Library, York, D/C Reg. 1, fol. 318v.

56 Matthew 25:35–6. The six acts of charity were: feeding the hungry, providing drink for the thirsty, giving shelter to the homeless, clothing the naked and visiting the sick and prisoners. A seventh act, burying the dead, was taken from Tobit 1:16–17, and the list of seven became the accepted number by the end of the Middle Ages.

distractions and thus were considered to be better able to concentrate on their intercessory prayers.[57] The blind, therefore, were regarded as being especially worthy recipients. From the fifteenth century there is evidence that a significant number of the wealthier guilds were founding or acquiring almshouses in order to accommodate their decrepit brethren and sisters.[58] Running an institute for their old and blind colleagues would help them to fulfil many of the works of charity listed above. In return they would enjoy the collective benefits of prayers and supplications whilst being reassured that they, too, might find accommodation if they became too old and disabled to work.

Almsgiving was an important and intrinsic aspect of Christian piety. The authors of religious texts, such as *The Book of Vices and Virtues* mentioned above, emphasised the spiritual and physical benefits of giving alms. It was even argued that unless one performed charitable acts the health of one's body and soul would decline.[59] *Regimina* instructed medieval men and women that it was essential to eat the correct foods and to follow a moderate lifestyle. Similarly, good deeds were a necessary part of a spiritual 'dyete' to maintain health.[60] Giving alms to the needy was compared to draining the body of an excess of bodily fluids through purging.[61] Freeing oneself from excessive wealth, which would weigh the soul down on the day of judgement, was an essential part of a spiritual regime, as important to the health of the soul as confession and penance. Moreover, Virginia Bainbridge observes that a common phrase used in the statutes of medieval fraternities was 'just as water extinguishes fire, so alms extinguishes sin'.[62] The act of almsgiving 'quenched' the effects of a transgression, 'making it less', which, in turn, diluted any residual 'wykkednes'.[63] Alms, therefore, could be given in atonement for specific sins that had already been committed, such as gluttony or lust, both of which could be injurious to the eyes. This approach to gift-giving meant that affluent men and women commonly regarded good works as a means of shortening their post-mortem ordeal. *The Book of Vices and Virtues* provided further advice, recommending that assistance should be directed towards specific groups or types of people who were considered to be 'worthy'.[64] The latter included the poor and blind, who reputedly embodied Christ-like

57 J. Agrimi and C. Crisciani, 'Charity and Aid in Medieval Christian Civilization', in *Western Medical Thought from Antiquity to the Middle Ages*, ed. M. D. Grmek (Cambridge, MA, 1998), pp. 170–96 (p. 174).

58 Patricia H. Cullum, 'Hospitals and Charitable Provision in Medieval Yorkshire', unpublished Ph.D. thesis, University of York, 1989, pp. 366–9.

59 *The Book of Vices and Virtues*, pp. ix, 199.

60 *Lydgate and Burgh's 'Secrees of Old Philisoffers': A Version of the Secreta Secretorum*, ed. Robert Steele, EETS e.s. 66 (London, 1894), p. 41.

61 *Fasciculus Morum*, p. 257.

62 Bainbridge, *Gilds in the Medieval Countryside*, pp. 101–2.

63 *Robert of Brunne's, 'Handlyng Synne'*, p. 227.

64 *The Book of Vices and Virtues*, p. 213.

qualities, and had been the focus of charity and healing in the Bible.[65] The blind were seen as being particularly deserving recipients of charity, who were put on earth by God to remind others of their Christian obligation to care for their less fortunate neighbours.

The positive response to the visually impaired from their Christian neighbours demonstrates that blindness could be equally considered a gift as a sign of sin. Indeed, in some homiletic texts, blindness is viewed as a divine gift to be utilised by the saints to strengthen their belief and bring them closer to God.[66] Good Christians who accepted their fate with humility hoped to be spared a far worse ordeal in Purgatory. When the prospect of intense and protracted agony in the next world was compared to the transitory nature of suffering on earth, blindness seemed almost a privilege, a mark of divine favour bestowed by a clement father. For this reason a saint or holy person could be blind or visually impaired without incurring any suspicion of sin. Those who bore their disabilities with meekness and resignation appeared particularly fortunate, because they were spared earthly distractions and could focus more clearly upon the light of heaven. A visual impairment could represent a sign of divine election, and it is for this reason that blindness increasingly became associated with piety and wisdom. Significantly, from the fourteenth century onwards, artists depicted the fathers of the Church wearing spectacles to indicate their inner piety and wisdom, as well as their learning. Matthew the Evangelist is sometimes depicted as needing eye-glasses in order to be able to consult his Gospel.[67] Such recurrent imagery would have offered a degree of reassurance to the hypermetropic members of the congregation that declining vision did not preclude them from cultivating inner sight. The saints certainly provided ample reassurance that blindness or impaired vision were not necessarily a punishment for sin, and that, if pain and disability could be borne with sufficient grace, then their fortitude would be rewarded in the afterlife. Problems of this kind actually allowed the sufferer to experience his or her purgatory on earth, shortening the soul's journey to heaven after death.

One sermon in the *Fasciculus morum* employs a commercial metaphor of profit and loss, making the concept of Purgatory relevant and comprehensible to merchants and tradesmen in the congregation. It explains in simple language that the 'body and soul are partners in delights and sins'; and that, like a party to fraud, the 'flesh, if it could, would like to steal away without punishment and leave all his debt with the soul'. However, Christ, here

65 Matthew 11:5.

66 Joy Hawkins, 'Seeing the Light? Blindness and Sanctity in Later Medieval England', in *Saints and Sanctity*, ed. Peter Clarke and Tony Claydon, Studies in Church History 47 (Woodbridge, 2011), pp. 148–58.

67 David Farmer, *The Oxford Dictionary of Saints*, 4th edn (Oxford, 1997), p. 340. St Matthew is illustrated wearing a pair of spectacles and consulting his Bible on the roodscreen of the parish church of St Agnes, Cawston, Norfolk.

compared to a mayor of a large city, 'out of his love for our soul, takes the body and restrains it and sends it infirmities, and thus he forces it to pay the part of the debt which belongs to it'.[68] Such teachings reiterated the belief that those experiencing disabling and painful illnesses were the fortunate ones who were being purged of their sins on earth, ready for a smooth passage to heaven. They were urged to welcome, and even embrace, pain and suffering, because God used disease as a test and a means for improving individuals who would eventually be destined for heaven. The Scriptures maintained that disability and disease were conferred by a benevolent God, because 'whom the Lord loveth he chasteneth'.[69]

Unlike Hell which was everlasting, Purgatory was a finite, intermediary world in which the soul was subjected to a trial rather than unremitting torture; however, it was still a place where one wished to spend as little time as possible. Consequently, medieval men and women wanted a quantifiable time frame whereby their earthly illnesses could be converted into an appropriate reduction in the sentence that awaited them after death; for each day of pain and discomfort, the sufferer hoped to be spared a specific amount of time in Purgatory. Preachers reassured their congregations that one day of earthly suffering, borne meekly, was of greater value than twenty in Purgatory.[70] This may have brought an element of comfort and hope to individuals for whom earthly medicine had not produced a cure. The fifteenth-century chantry priest, John Audelay, wrote a number of devotional poems in which he refers to himself as 'blynd Audlay'.[71] He believed that God was punishing him for his previous sinful behaviour but, faced with failing sight and hearing, he sought reassurance that his ordeal was not in vain. He believed he would be spared in the afterlife, as a merciful God would not punish any penitent twice:

> To haue thi payne, thi purgatorye,
> Out of this world or that thou dye,
> Fore God ponysche [punish] not twyse truly.[72]

Sinners could turn to the saints 'as powerful helpers and healers in time of need, whether bodily need or in the last spiritual extremity of death and the pains of Purgatory'.[73] One such 'powerful helper' was St Lutgarde (1182–1246),

68 *Fasciculus Morum*, p. 139.

69 Hebrews 12:6.

70 *Middle English Sermons*, p. 42.

71 John Audelay, *The Poems of John Audelay*, ed. E. K. Whiting, EETS o.s. 184 (Oxford, 1931), pp. xiv–xvi, 101. For further detail on John Audelay and his understanding of his bodily infirmities, see Takami Matsuda, 'Purgatory and Spiritual Healing in John Audelay's Poems', in this volume.

72 Audelay, *Poems*, p. 85.

73 Eamon Duffy, *The Stripping of the Altars: Traditional Religion in England c.1400–1580*, 2nd edn (New Haven, CT, 2005), p. 178.

a Cistercian nun who spent most of her adult life at the convent of Aywières in modern day Belgium and endured complete blindness for the last eleven years of her life. During her time as a nun she had been renowned for the efficacy of her prayers; allegedly there was no one whose intercession was 'more powerful in liberating souls from purgatory'.[74] After her death, a strong devotion to her cult developed and she became known as the patron saint of souls in Purgatory. The visually impaired would have identified particularly with a saint who had herself endured a similar trial, especially as in a posthumous miracle Lutgarde reputedly healed a nun whose eye had been torn out of its socket when impaled on a spike during prayer.[75] A sense of empathy and intimacy could certainly develop between the saint and supplicant when there was a shared experience; the blind could more confidently invoke Lutgarde's help to endure their pain patiently in order to achieve a swifter transit through Purgatory.[76]

It was not enough merely to suffer the ordeal of being blind; the *manner* in which the individual endured his or her disability was of equal, if not greater, importance. Those who resisted pain, or proved resentful or impatient, would fail their trial and either forfeit, or have to wait much longer for, the rewards of heavenly bliss. Since sickness was considered to be God's will, the sick and disabled were instructed to bear their afflictions calmly, not least because, according to the contemporary medical theory, 'perturbations of mind were dangerous', disrupting the vital and animal spirits further, and, in turn, damaging the immortal soul.[77] In order to reap the spiritual rewards from any physical ordeal it was essential to bear one's burden without complaint. William Langland (c. 1331–87) observed that:

> Blynde and bedreden and broken hire membres,
> That taken this mischief mekeliche, as mesels [lepers] and othere,
> Han as pleyn pardon as the Plowman hymselve.
> For love of hir lowe hertes Oure Lord hath hem graunted
> Hir penaunce and hir Purgatorie upon this erthe.[78]

The blind were constantly encouraged to welcome their suffering as a 'means of spiritual and physical purification' which would save them from protracted suffering after death.[79] If they failed to follow such advice and 'grumble[d]

74 Thomas Merton, *What Are These Wounds? The Life of a Cistercian Mystic: Saint Lutgarde of Aywières* (Dublin, 1980), pp. 49, 52, 113–14, 122, 139.

75 Merton, *What Are These Wounds?*, p. 156.

76 Duffy, *Stripping of the Altars*, p. 180.

77 Paul Slack, 'Mirrors of Health and Treasures of Poor Men: The Uses of the Vernacular Medical Literature of Tudor England', in *Health, Medicine and Mortality in the Sixteenth Century*, ed. Charles Webster (Cambridge, 1979), pp. 237–73 (p. 270).

78 William Langland, *The Vision of Piers Plowman: A Critical Edition of the B-Text*, ed. A. V. C. Schmidt (London, 1978), p. 82.

79 Slack, 'Mirrors of Health and Treasures of Poor Men', p. 270.

against Christ on account of [their] infirmities' their souls would be 'damned in eternity'.[80] It was the way in which an individual dealt with his or her illness that was important. The *Ancren Wisse* emphasises that the anchoress must 'accept her illness not just patiently, but very gladly'; only those who did so would be rewarded in the afterlife.[81]

It was, moreover, not only the sufferer who could benefit from affliction. Illness also provided an ideal opportunity for carers to exercise the virtues of patience and humility. For example, Francis Patrizzi of Sienna (d. 1328) 'was kept from becoming a hermit by the necessity of attending to his blind mother'. When he finally achieved his goal, he seemed to be more holy because of the enforced delay, and, presumably, because he had been caring for a relative who was blind.[82] Loss of sight, could, therefore, be seen as a form of spiritual medication not simply for the individual who was experiencing his or her Purgatory on earth, but also for those in good health who provided either physical support or material assistance. Such help could ease the difficult circumstances of the blind, and perhaps even, on occasion, help them to recover; additionally, good works were believed to strengthen the spiritual and physical well-being of the person who performed them.

As shown above, until recently, scholars have believed that the blind were somehow marginalised or excluded from society because their impairment acted as a form of stigma – an indication of sin. This chapter has demonstrated that this was rarely the case; in reality, medieval communities were far more pragmatic in their response to their blind members, recognising that many aspects of life could cause blindness, from a dietary imbalance to old age. Following the advice provided by medical authorities in *regimina*, it was recognised that moderation was vital 'in al thynge' to 'kepyth helthe', including 'in trauaill [and] in reste',[83] and thus it was important that the blind had the opportunity to perform small tasks and walk outside in the open air. Creative solutions were often sought in order to allow the blind and visually impaired to live fulfilling lives. Although slightly later than the main period covered by this survey, the Norwich Census of the Poor of 1570 shows that children were hired out to blind individuals to act as guides and helpers. From the age of about seven or eight, a child could be both a useful assistant and a companion to a sightless man or woman. An orphan or the youngest child of a poor family would be given board and lodging in return for acting

80 *Fasciculus Morum*, pp. 139–41.

81 *Ancrene Wisse*, Part 1, p. 19.

82 Richard Kieckhefer, *Unquiet Souls: Fourteenth-Century Saints and Their Religious Milieu* (Chicago, IL, 1984), p. 58. The nun who attended to St Lutgarde in her last years became well known for the patient care of her charge despite her initial 'repugnance' and 'impatience': Merton, *What Are These Wounds?*, pp. 122–3.

83 *Three Prose Versions of the Secreta secretorum*, Vol. 1, ed. Robert Steele, EETS e.s. 74 (London, 1898), p. 237.

as a guide. For instance, the household of Richard Sandlying, a fifty-four year old blind man, included a fatherless child of twelve who 'led Sandlyng about'.[84] Such a practice, however, already had a long tradition by the sixteenth century. As noted above, Christ's healing of the blind man annually recreated by the Glovers of Chester included a role for a boy to guide his steps, and Bartholomaeus Anglicus in his encyclopaedia mentions that a blind man might need a child to lead him about, as well as describing the drawbacks if the blind man does not treat his guide well.[85] Because of this reliance on others and the immense level of trust that had to be placed in another person, Bartholomaeus Anglicus, clearly influenced by the translations of Arabic medical writings produced by Constantine the African (d. c. 1099), proclaimed blindness to be the 'most wrecchid' of all physical impairments, and he even went as far as comparing it to a 'prison', confining the sufferer to a private world of darkness.[86] Added to this were the examples of God and his saints punishing sinners with blindness preached from the pulpit, which must have encouraged connections to be made between bodily deformity and sin, especially for women, for it was Eve who 'looked at the forbidden apple, and saw that it was beautiful and began to delight in gazing at it'. Her visual 'desire … overcame her' which led to her picking the apple from the tree.[87] Consequently, disease and disability were acknowledged to be an inescapable consequence of human life, as a result of this Original Sin in the Garden of Eden.

Although every man and woman carried the weight of Eve's burden, rarely were individuals expected to shoulder the blame completely, unless of course the person was believed to have brought the suffering upon him or herself by failing to adhere to a moderate and balanced regimen, for example by succumbing to gluttony. Medical and didactic texts equally underscored the eyes' fragility; the eyes were considered to be the weakest of the senses, 'ruined by the least bit of dust and wind', or, as Bartholomaeus underscored, too much wine.[88] Medieval men and women were expected to take special care of this most precious of their senses, but if disaster was to strike, then their ailment or injury, if endured with sufficient humility and patience, was thought to relieve

84 *The Norwich Census of the Poor 1570,* ed. J. F. Pound, Norfolk Record Society 40 (London, 1971), p. 66.

85 Bartholomaeus Anglicus, *On the Properties of Things,* vol. 1, p. 365.

86 Bartholomaeus Anglicus, *On the Properties of Things*, vol. 1, pp. 364–5. See also Monica H. Green, 'Constantine the African', in *Medical Science, Technology, and Medicine: An Encyclopedia*, ed. Thomas Glick, Steven J. Livesey and Faith Wallis (New York and Abingdon, 2005), pp. 145–7.

87 *Ancrene Wisse*, Part 2, p. 21.

88 *Fasciculus Morum*, p. 653; this is very similar to Henri de Mondeville's belief that 'a single grain of corrosive matter is more harmful to [the eye] than a hundred would be to feet or jaws': Pouchelle, *Body and Surgery*, p. 119.

the soul from some of its purgatorial toils.[89] Indeed, as has been shown above, the blind often held a privileged position as they were considered to be among God's elect as not only were they an earthly reminder of Christ's suffering, but their disability also protected them from the distractions and potential threats associated with a wanton gaze. In turn, those caring for the blind would also reap rewards in the afterlife, and consequently communities cared tenderly and sympathetically for those who had lost their eyesight through hard work, old age or an industrial accident.[90] If physical and sensory impairments were placed in order of the benefit to the soul, blindness certainly would have been ranked highly. Such examples reveal the variation in the understandings of and responses to blindness during this period. By studying a physical impairment such as blindness, therefore, we are offered a fascinating insight into the medieval mindset. Blindness is in some way an exceptional case, yet it is indicative of the complexity of responses to disease, a tangled web of explanations and understandings, that we simplify at our peril.

89 Carole Rawcliffe, *Medicine for the Soul: The Life, Death and Resurrection of an English Medieval Hospital, St Giles's, Norwich, c. 1249–1550* (Stroud, 1999), p. 7.

90 Carole Hill includes an interesting discussion of 'the expected reciprocity of powerful intercessory prayer': see *Women and Religion in Late Medieval Norwich* (Woodbridge, 2010), pp. 114–16.

11

BETWEEN PALLIATIVE CARE AND CURING THE SOUL: MEDICAL AND RELIGIOUS RESPONSES TO LEPROSY IN FRANCE AND ENGLAND, C. 1100–C. 1500

Elma Brenner

Although leprosy affected only a small minority of people in the Middle Ages, its presence is very much felt in the sermons, literature and material culture of the period. In the past twenty-five years, historians have paid increasing attention to the social and religious dimensions of responses to leprosy, and have underlined the extent to which Christian society took responsibility for the needs of lepers, albeit placing them at a physical distance in *leprosaria*.[1] Indeed, the leprous were a major focus of charity, particularly in the twelfth and thirteenth centuries.[2] It was widely recognised by contemporaries that leprosy could not be cured through medical intervention: thus, the care of the leprous focused on the alleviation of their physical suffering and the attainment of salvation for their souls. Since leprosy was a chronic illness that often afflicted individuals for a number of years, the care of sufferers needed to take into account their long-term needs and gradual physical deterioration.

This chapter explores the intersection between bodily care and spiritual care within and outside *leprosaria* in northern France and England between 1100 and 1500, particularly in the region of Normandy. *Leprosaria*, often monastic institutions equipped with a chapel and religious personnel, provided spiritual facilities for their leprous residents, including the performance of Mass, confession, funerary rites, burial and commemoration. However, *leprosarium* statutes reveal that these communities also tended the bodies of the sick,

1 See, in particular, François-Olivier Touati, *Maladie et société au Moyen Âge: la lèpre, les lépreux et les léproseries dans la province ecclésiastique de Sens jusqu'au milieu du XIVe siècle*, Bibliothèque du Moyen Âge 11 (Brussels, 1998); Carole Rawcliffe, *Leprosy in Medieval England* (Woodbridge, 2006). For a historiographical overview, see Elma Brenner, 'Recent Perspectives on Leprosy in Medieval Western Europe', *History Compass* 8 (2010), 388–406.

2 See Carole Rawcliffe, 'Learning to Love the Leper: Aspects of Institutional Charity in Anglo-Norman England', *Anglo-Norman Studies* 23 (2000), 231–50; Elma Brenner, *Leprosy and Charity in Medieval Rouen* (Woodbridge, forthcoming 2015/2016).

through dietary regulation, bathing, exercise, the supply of clothing and shelter, bloodletting, the dressing of sores and other measures. In theory at least, therefore, the overall environment of the *leprosarium* was highly beneficial to both soul and body.

Much as was the case for members of healthy society, the experience of leprous individuals was shaped by their gender, social status and degree of access to medical care. Within *leprosaria*, particular emphasis was placed on the chastity of leprous women, whose pursuit of a religious vocation needed to be protected, and who were associated in medical texts with the sexual transmission of the disease. Some high status, wealthy lepers apparently did not enter *leprosaria*, receiving private care from medical practitioners. The Montpellier physician Bernard de Gordon (fl. 1283–1308), for example, treated a leprous countess.[3] By the later Middle Ages, medical practitioners and lay officials examined suspected cases of the disease and issued formal diagnoses, often at a financial cost to examinees. The chapter will discuss both accounts of such examinations and other documents that shed light on the broader social context and consequences of (mis)diagnosis.[4]

At the lowest end of the social spectrum, many poor lepers had a wandering, itinerant existence, sometimes staying temporarily at *leprosaria* or entering cities to solicit alms. Those lepers who lived predominantly outside *leprosaria* did not follow the religious life observed by their counterparts within these institutions, nor did they receive diagnostic attention or benefit from the finely tuned bodily regimen that leper houses could offer.[5] Although the treatments provided by elite practitioners confirm that secular medicine did address the problem of leprosy in this period, the majority of contemporary responses to the disease were shaped by a combination of religious and medical concepts, and by the belief that the ultimate salvation of the leper's soul was of primary importance.

LEPROSY IN RELIGIOUS DISCOURSE

At the Third Lateran Council in 1179, a canon was issued (Canon 23) instructing that groups of 'leprosis qui cum sanis habitare non possunt et ad ecclesiam cum aliis convenire' ['lepers, who cannot dwell with the healthy

3 London, Wellcome Library, MS 130 (Bernard de Gordon, *Practica medicinalis (Lilium medicinae)*, fourteenth century), fol. 18r; Bernard de Gordon, *Practica seu Lilium medicinae* (Naples, 1480), fols 26v–27r; Luke Demaitre, *Leprosy in Premodern Medicine: A Malady of the Whole Body* (Baltimore, MD, 2007), pp. 21, 172–3.

4 For the consequences of (mis)diagnosis, see London, Wellcome Library, MS 5133/1 (agreement for a leprous man to be admitted to the *leprosarium* of Saint-Ladre, Pontoise, 17 May 1412) and MS 5133/3 (letter from the duke of Lorraine, c. 1487, protecting the interests of a man wrongly accused of having leprosy).

5 The terms '*leprosarium*' and 'leper house' are used interchangeably in this chapter.

nor come to church with others'] should have their own church, cemetery and priest.[6] This decree suggests a widespread acceptance that lepers should be segregated from mainstream society, perhaps because of concern about contagion, but also perhaps as a result of the view that they required special bodily and spiritual care. At the same time, however, it makes it clear that lepers were still understood to be members of the Christian community, and that it was considered important for them to have the essential facilities they needed as Christians. In the thirteenth century, sermons addressed specifically to lepers confirm that they were still perceived to be very much part of the Church.[7] At this time, as the concept of Purgatory (formalised at the second Council of Lyons in 1274–5) became increasingly well established, causing heightened concern about the future fate of souls, leprosy featured in discourse concerning sin and penitence. Nicole Bériou argues that the disease could be seen 'comme un signe par lequel Dieu incitait l'homme à la pénitence, qui serait guérison et résurrection de son âme mortellement atteinte par la lèpre du péché' ['as a sign by which God incited man to penitence, for the cure and resurrection of his soul mortally afflicted by the leprosy of sin'].[8]

The understanding of leprosy as a physical manifestation of sin was linked to ideas about its causation: like some other diseases, it was associated with excessive (and by implication immoral) sexual activity, resulting from the lasciviousness of sufferers. Here, sex was understood within the broader framework of the 'non-naturals', physical factors and psychological states that brought about health or illness. Sex was relevant to two of the non-naturals: the purgation of bodily fluids and exercise (other non-naturals were air and the broader environment, sleep, food and drink, and emotional well-being). It was believed that excessive sex adversely affected the body's humoral balance, by causing the blood to become too hot and by draining too many fluids from the body. Medical works of the thirteenth and fourteenth centuries clearly evidence the belief that leprosy could be caused by sex, although sexual intercourse was often secondary within the overall consideration of the disease's aetiology. In his discussion of the causes of leprosy in his *Lilium medicinae* (completed 1305), Bernard de Gordon adds the anecdote that a leprous countess in his care became pregnant by a bachelor of medicine who treated her, who then contracted the disease from her. There is a strong moral tone to Bernard's advice that 'caveat igitur quilibet coire cum muliere leprosa' ['one

6 *Decrees of the Ecumenical Councils*, ed. and trans. Norman P. Tanner, 2 vols (London and Washington, DC, 1990), vol. 1, pp. 222–3.

7 Nicole Bériou, 'Les Lépreux sous le regard des prédicateurs d'après les collections de sermons *ad status* du XIIIème siècle', in Nicole Bériou and François-Olivier Touati, *Voluntate dei leprosus: les Lépreux entre conversion et exclusion aux XIIème et XIIIème siècles* (Spoleto, 1991), pp. 33–80 (pp. 37–8).

8 Bériou, 'Les Lépreux sous le regard des prédicateurs', pp. 36–7.

should beware of having intercourse with a leprous woman'].[9] Indeed, women were primarily attributed with sexual transmission: it was held that leprous females infected male partners but not *vice versa*, and that a woman who had intercourse with a leprous man would transmit the disease to a subsequent partner (particularly her next partner) while not contracting leprosy herself. This latter notion was linked to the understanding that the uterus was hard and cold, meaning that it retained infected semen but did not itself absorb it.[10] These ideas attributed prostitutes, who had multiple partners within a short space of time, with a key role in transmitting leprosy, thus increasing the immoral associations of the disease.[11] Such notions also indicate that misogyny and anxieties about sex helped to shape ideas about how leprosy was caused and transferred from one person to another.[12]

Yet although leprosy was associated with sin, there is also much evidence to suggest that lepers were viewed as a quasi-religious group, chosen by God to suffer on earth and be saved. Although there is an apparent tension here between the notions of sinfulness and divine favour, this may be reconciled by viewing lepers as sinners specially selected for redemption. The language of late twelfth- and early thirteenth-century documents suggests that the idea that God intervened to inflict leprosy on an individual was particularly strong at this time. An entry of 1188 in the cartulary of the *leprosarium* of Grand-Beaulieu at Chartres, for example, refers to Nivelon, son of Geoffrey du Grandpont, 'Dei voluntate lepra sigillatus' ['marked with leprosy by the will of God'], who gave himself and various revenues and possessions to the leper house.[13] Lepers were also associated with the physical suffering of Christ on the cross, a theme (*Christus quasi leprosus*) that drew upon the description of Christ as a leper in the Latin Vulgate Bible.[14] In his division of society into thirty *status* (religious and lay categories), the French preacher Jacques de Vitry (c. 1165–1240) placed lepers in the highest category of the laity, alongside other sick and poor people, pilgrims, mourners and crusaders. These lay people were being tested by God, and were thus closer to the religious (clerics, followed by monks, followed by members of fraternities)

9 Wellcome Library, MS 130, fol. 18r; de Gordon, *Practica seu Lilium medicinae*, fols 26v–27r (transcription is from this 1480 edition); Demaitre, *Leprosy*, pp. 21, 172–3.

10 Demaitre, *Leprosy*, pp. 171–4; Danielle Jacquart and Claude Thomasset, *Sexuality and Medicine in the Middle Ages*, trans. Matthew Adamson (Cambridge, 1988), pp. 185–90.

11 Jacquart and Thomasset, *Sexuality and Medicine*, p. 190.

12 Demaitre, *Leprosy*, p. 174.

13 *Cartulaire de la léproserie du Grand-Beaulieu et du prieuré de Notre-Dame de la Bourdinière*, ed. René Merlet and Maurice Jusselin (Chartres, 1909), p. 54 (no. 132); François-Olivier Touati, 'Les Léproseries aux XIIème et XIIIème siècles, lieux de conversion?', in Bériou and Touati, *Voluntate dei leprosus*, pp. 1–32 (pp. 14–15); Touati, *Maladie*, pp. 190, 196–7.

14 Rawcliffe, *Leprosy*, pp. 60–3.

than the rest of the laity.[15] Entry to a *leprosarium*, where lepers would pursue a religious life, often living in common according to a rule, was in many instances viewed as a process of conversion.[16]

Lepers' special relationship with God made them powerful intercessors, and the generosity of charitable benefactors to the leprous, reflected above all in the foundation of numerous *leprosaria* in France and England between the twelfth and fourteenth centuries, partly reflects donors' perception that their own souls would benefit from lepers' reciprocal prayers. Assistance to lepers also enabled benefactors to engage in most of the six biblical works of mercy (feeding the hungry, giving drink to the thirsty, granting hospitality to strangers, clothing the naked and visiting the sick and prisoners; another work, burying the dead, was added in the Middle Ages). These pious works were essential to attaining salvation, since at the Last Judgement Christ only admits those who have fulfilled these works to heaven (Matthew 25.31–46). In addition, lepers were a focus of practices of piety, as evidenced by the recurrent theme of the kissing of lepers and the washing of their feet in hagiographical writings such as the life of Hugh, bishop of Lincoln (1186–1200).[17] The charity and piety for lepers underlines the religious dimensions of responses to leprosy and the care of its sufferers.

LEPROSY AND GENDER

The majority of *leprosaria* were mixed communities – yet within these institutions, men and women were strictly segregated. Many of the larger *leprosaria*, such as Mont-aux-Malades at Rouen, followed the Augustinian rule, and the separation of men and women reflects the concern one would expect for chastity within a monastic community. It also enabled sick men and women to be cared for in a discreet manner, without the intrusion of the opposite sex, and ensured that the leprous and the non-leprous (religious and lay staff) of either sex occupied distinct living quarters. In the 1260s, Mont-aux-Malades was understood to have five separate communities, of Augustinian canons, lay brothers, lay sisters, male lepers and female lepers.[18] Statutes for the leper house at Sherburn, county Durham, confirmed in the early fourteenth century, reveal that the leprous sisters were accommodated in a separate house

15 Bériou, 'Les Lépreux', pp. 39–40.

16 See Touati, 'Les Léproseries', pp. 11–19.

17 Catherine Peyroux, 'The Leper's Kiss', in *Monks and Nuns, Saints and Outcasts: Religion in Medieval Society, Essays in Honor of Lester K. Little*, ed. Sharon Farmer and Barbara H. Rosenwein (Ithaca, NY, 2000), pp. 172–88; Rawcliffe, *Leprosy*, pp. 144–7.

18 *Regestrum visitationum archiepiscopi Rothomagensis: Journal des visites pastorales d'Eude Rigaud, archevêque de Rouen. MCCXLVIII–MCCLXIX*, ed. Théodose Bonnin (Rouen, 1852), p. 513; *The Register of Eudes of Rouen*, ed. Jeremiah F. O'Sullivan and trans. Sidney M. Brown (New York, 1964), p. 585 (1 April 1264 [= 1265]).

above the chapel; furthermore, the leprous brothers and sisters attended two separate daily Masses, although they did unite in the chapel for the great Mass on Sundays and feast days.[19]

Rules laid down by Peter de Collemezzo, archbishop of Rouen (1236–44) in May 1237 to correct discipline at Mont-aux-Malades indicate that there was especial concern to protect the seclusion of leprous women: 'Item, ad duo ostia claustri sororum clauda fieri volumus quod duabus sororibus non supportis, quarum una sana sit et alia leprosa eorum custodia commitatur' ['we wish for the two doors to the cloister of the sisters to be closed, and for their guard to be entrusted to two sisters *non supportis*, one healthy and one leprous'].[20] Similarly, at Sherburn following the great Mass, 'the sisters will return to their own house and their door will be shut'.[21] The statutes of the *leprosarium* of Amiens in northern France, confirmed on 21 July 1305, prohibited brothers and sisters from entering each other's accommodation; if exceptionally women entered the men's houses to attend a man's burial, they were to do so in groups of two or three, 'teles dont on ne puist avoir nulle malvaise souppechon' ['so that there should be no bad suspicion'].[22]

A handful of *leprosaria* in England (at Westminster, Maiden Bradley, Woodstock and Thanington outside Canterbury), and at least one such institution in Normandy (Salle-aux-Puelles outside Rouen), offered provision only to women, thus further ensuring that the chastity and religious vocation of female lepers were protected. However, the statutes of a mixed *leprosarium* in Normandy, Saint-Ladre at Les Andelys (south of Rouen), compiled before 1380, testify to the awareness that the sexual activity of men as well as women within leper communities needed to be curbed. Any married male member of the community who had intercourse with his wife would be expelled for a year and a day; the same penalty applied if a man slept with one of the sisters of the house. If a sister became pregnant as a result of such an encounter, or if she had intercourse with an 'homme sain' ['healthy man'], she would be expelled. If she was pregnant when she first entered the *leprosarium*, she would have to leave until she had given birth; if she became pregnant again subsequently, she would be permanently expelled.[23]

19 'Constitutiones Hospitalis domus leprosorum de Shirburne', translated in Peter Richards, *The Medieval Leper and his Northern Heirs* (Cambridge, 1977; repr. Woodbridge, 2000), pp. 125–8 (p. 125).

20 Paris, Archives nationales, S4889B, dossier 13, doc. (xxi), fols 1r–2r (fol. 2r). I have not ascertained the exact meaning of 'non supportis': perhaps these were sisters who did not have private financial support, and thus had to fulfil certain duties in the *leprosarium* to 'earn their keep'.

21 'Constitutiones Hospitalis domus leprosorum de Shirburne', p. 125.

22 'Statuts de la léproserie d'Amiens', in *Statuts d'Hôtels-Dieu et de léproseries: recueil de textes du XIIe au XIVe siècle*, ed. Léon Le Grand (Paris, 1901), pp. 224–30 (p. 225).

23 'Statuts de la léproserie des Andelys', in *Statuts d'Hôtels-Dieu et de léproseries*, ed. Le Grand, pp. 246–52 (pp. 247–8). On Saint-Ladre of Les Andelys, see Jean Fournée, 'Les

It is not clear whether the Les Andelys statutes refer to the leprous or non-leprous members of the community: they could well refer to both, since, like a sick individual, a healthy lay person who served the sick at a *leprosarium* could be married when he or she entered the house. Nonetheless, the reference to the possibility of a sister engaging in carnal activity with a healthy man suggests that the brothers and sisters here are primarily considered to be leprous. Entry to the leper house of Les Andelys was restricted to members of the burgess class, and was refused to those of illegitimate birth.[24] As well as ensuring chastity, therefore, the statutes' provisions against sexual activity and pregnancy relate to the expectation of good moral and social standards within and outside the community. Such concern is also evident in statutes for the *leprosarium* of St Julian near St Albans, revised in 1344, which instructed that, if a married man entered, not only he but also his wife who remained outside must take a vow of chastity.[25] The Les Andelys provisions could also reflect ideas about the transmission of leprosy from mother to child, as well as between sexual partners. Leprosy was understood to be hereditary in key medieval medical writings such as the *Canon* of Avicenna (lived c. 980–1037) and the works of Constantine the African (d. between 1085 and 1098), and this notion was increasingly widely held by medical authors from the fourteenth century onwards.[26] However, it does not necessarily follow that the staff and patrons of *leprosaria* were aware of these learned ideas, nor that, in drawing up rules for leper communities, they were preoccupied with preventing the spread of the disease. Given the monastic character of such communities, a concern about chastity and morality, that encompassed the behaviour of both women and men, appears the more likely explanation for these tenets in the Les Andelys statutes and similar prescriptions in other ordinances for *leprosaria*.

EXAMINATION AND DIAGNOSIS

Formal examinations of individuals suspected of having leprosy took place in western Europe from at least the thirteenth century, and continued until the early eighteenth century. Examinations reflect the need to identify cases of the disease and, in the Middle Ages, to arrange for confirmed lepers to live apart from mainstream society. From the fourteenth century, particularly following the Black Death, the separation of lepers was motivated by notions of contagion via corrupt air (miasma). Earlier on, segregation

Maladreries et les vocables de leurs chapelles', *Lèpre et lépreux en Normandie, Cahiers Léopold Delisle* 46 (1997), 49–142 (pp. 90–1).

24 'Statuts de la léproserie des Andelys', p. 247.

25 'Statuta Hospitalis de Sancto Juliano', translated in Richards, *Medieval Leper*, pp. 129–36 (pp. 130–1).

26 Demaitre, *Leprosy*, pp. 155–6.

reflected other social and religious concerns, including the belief that lepers themselves would benefit from the bodily and spiritual care offered by *leprosaria*. The *iudicium leprosorum* was a legal procedure particularly prevalent in northern Europe, involving an examination followed by a judgement that determined the fate of the individual concerned. The certificates issued to individuals enabled them either to gain entry to a *leprosarium* or to prove that they were free from leprosy.[27] Although priests were involved in earlier examinations, from the mid-thirteenth century, these procedures were increasingly secular in nature, overseen by physicians, surgeons and municipal officers. The earliest evidence that the historian Luke Demaitre has found for the involvement of physicians comes from Siena (Italy) in 1250, where a certain Pierzivallus was judged to be leprous by four physicians. The growing role of physicians and surgeons in the examination of suspected leprosy sufferers marks what Demaitre terms 'the medicalization of the diagnosis of leprosy'.[28] These practitioners followed a formal procedure involving the verbal questioning of the individual being examined, a physical examination of the exterior and interior of the body (including the inspection of blood and urine), and deliberation among the practitioners. They searched for unequivocal signs of the presence of leprosy, and referred to medical theory in identifying and interpreting these signs.[29] Despite the dominance of physicians, surgeons and barbers, the juries involved in these examinations could also include the residents and administrators of *leprosaria*. There was great variety in the composition of juries across Europe and over time.[30]

As was the case elsewhere, leprosy examinations took place in France from the thirteenth century onwards. An important source of information about leprosy and leper houses in the region of Upper Normandy is the *Register* of Eudes Rigaud, archbishop of Rouen (1248–76), a set of visitation records compiled between 1248 and 1269. On 6 September 1268, when visiting the abbey of Le Tréport, in the far north of Normandy on the coast, Eudes Rigaud found that: 'Frater Ricardus, quondam prior, suspectus habebatur de morbo lepre, et tunc precepimus ei quod coram aliquibus monachis cum eo missis examinationem subiret' ['Brother Richard, formerly a prior (of a priory dependent on the abbey), was held suspected of the disease of leprosy: thus, we ordered that he should undergo an examination in the presence of some monks sent with him'].[31] The monk may have relinquished his office as prior as a result of his illness. The archbishop's instruction indicates that

27 Demaitre, *Leprosy*, Chapter 2 and pp. 197–8.

28 Demaitre, *Leprosy*, pp. 35–9.

29 Demaitre, *Leprosy*, pp. 197–201.

30 Demaitre, *Leprosy*, pp. 35–7.

31 *Regestrum*, p. 609; *Register*, p. 701. Although I am citing the published English translation of Eudes Rigaud's *Register*, the translations given are my own.

the examination was performed outside the abbey itself; yet monks were to accompany Richard, perhaps to verify the outcome on behalf of the community. Plausibly, this examination could have been performed by one or more physicians or surgeons. However, it had a strong ecclesiastical flavour, being ordered by the archbishop and witnessed by monks.

During his visitations, Archbishop Eudes Rigaud was not consistent in instructing that the *iudicium* should be performed on individuals suspected of having leprosy, suggesting that this was certainly not a firmly established practice in Upper Normandy at this time. At the abbey of Bec-Hellouin (south-west of Rouen) a few months earlier, on 3 April 1268, he had encountered another suspected leper, Brother Nicholas of Lendy. However, in this instance he merely advised the abbot 'quod dictum fratrem N. abinde amoveret' ['that he should remove the said brother N. (Nicholas) from there'], and was informed that the abbot would send him to Saint-Lambert, a dependent priory where there was only one other monk.[32] Thus, there was no mention of an examination, or indeed of a leper house – though Saint-Lambert was considered an ideal place, 'ubi non est frequentia hominum, ubique beneficium aeris et multa infirmitatis sue levimenta habere posset' ['where there is not the crowding of people, and where he can have the benefit of the air and much mitigation of his infirmity'].[33] The reference here to crowding may suggest that the archbishop was concerned about leprosy and contagion. However, overall he appears to have had Nicholas of Lendy's needs in mind, believing that good air (one of the non-naturals), and presumably a peaceful, quiet environment, would alleviate his physical suffering. The impression is that it was already accepted that Nicholas indeed had leprosy.

Another example of the examination of a suspected leper concerns one of Eudes Rigaud's predecessors as archbishop of Rouen. When Theobald of Amiens (1222–29) was elected as archbishop on 5 March 1222, his election was opposed by the party of another candidate, William de *Canapello*, which introduced a rumour that Theobald was leprous. Canon law prohibited the promotion of a leper to high ecclesiastical office, yet it is likely that the opposing party was also appealing to certain fears and prejudices about leprosy. Pope Honorius III (1216–27) sent three judges delegate, the bishop of Sées, the dean of Amiens, and the archdeacon of Rheims, to examine whether Theobald was leprous; they were to be assisted by doctors. This suggests that, already by the first quarter of the thirteenth century, physicians were involved in leprosy examinations in northern France. Nonetheless, in the examination of a prospective archbishop, they had a secondary role, assisting three high-status ecclesiastics. It was found that Theobald of Amiens was free

[32] *Regestrum*, p. 623; *Register*, p. 717.

[33] *Regestrum*, p. 623; *Register*, p. 717.

from leprosy, and he was formally consecrated as archbishop on 4 September 1222.[34]

While there was evidently great concern regarding whether a prospective archbishop had leprosy, a case from the fifteenth century reveals the taking of precautions regarding a lower-status ecclesiastic, a parish priest, suspected of having the disease. A register of the deliberations of the cathedral chapter of Rouen records, under Tuesday, 20 February 1452 (= 1453), 'iudicationem seu visitationem' ['the judgement or visitation'] of Jean Gaultier, parish priest of Saint-Michel, Rouen, by three physicians and two surgeons.[35] It was established that, while he was not to be segregated, 'se abstinendum a magnis hominibus communicacionibus [et] ab administratione' ['he should abstain from extensive communication with men, (and) from administration (of the sacraments)'].[36] These instructions testify to the fact that diagnoses could fall into a grey area: it would appear that the practitioners who examined Jean Gaultier detected some signs of leprosy but did not consider the disease to be sufficiently advanced for him to have to enter a *leprosarium*. Nonetheless, they were concerned that he might transmit the disease to others and, apparently, required him to relinquish his duties as a parish priest.

A positive leprosy diagnosis had a major impact on a person's social identity, circumstances and future. In the late fifteenth or early sixteenth century (between 1487 and 1507), Duke René II (1451–1508) of Lorraine, a duchy in the north-east of modern-day France, issued a letter confirming that Jehan Jacquemin, a burgess residing in the suburbs of the town of Saint-Dié, was not leprous. Jehan had been maliciously accused of being infected, and had appealed for the duke's assistance. Duke René's physicians found that he was 'non infecte de ladite lepre … quil nous a fait exposciste a ester a tort condempne' ['not infected with the said leprosy … he has shown us that he was wrongly condemned'].[37] Provision was made for Jehan to be compensated financially, and it was established that he could freely move about as he had done prior to the accusation, and could come into contact with other people.[38]

The fact that Jehan Jacquemin had actively solicited this certificate from the duke suggests that it was deeply important to individuals' social standing and situation to rectify matters when they were (as they claimed and others corroborated) misdiagnosed with leprosy. The document also indicates the

34 Vincent Tabbagh, *Fasti ecclesiae gallicanae: Répertoire prosopographique des évêques, dignitaires et chanoines de France de 1200 à 1500. Tome II: diocèse de Rouen* (Turnhout, 1998), pp. 80–1; Jörg Peltzer, *Canon Law, Careers and Conquest: Episcopal Elections in Normandy and Greater Anjou, c. 1140–c. 1230* (Cambridge, 2008), pp. 84–6.

35 Rouen, Archives départementales de Seine-Maritime, G2134, fol. 225r.

36 Ibid.

37 Wellcome Library, MS 5133/3, fol. 1r.

38 Ibid.

practical implications of a positive diagnosis at this time: while it is not clear whether Jehan had entered a *leprosarium*, his freedom of movement in mainstream society had evidently been inhibited, perhaps simply as a result of stigma. He had also incurred financial costs, possibly through having been required to pay for his original examination and through being prevented from pursuing his usual livelihood. As well as providing evidence of these practical issues, the document evokes an atmosphere of accusation, rumour and the stigmatisation of lepers and leprosy. It refers to a certain 'menasseur' who had threatened Jehan, and concludes with the duke's expression of concern that his subjects should not be troubled and molested.[39] This suggests that an accusation of leprosy could be used as a means to attack a person; the power of such aggression derived from fear of the disease and suspicion of leprosy sufferers by the end of the Middle Ages.

THE BODILY CARE OF LEPERS

Although responses to leprosy and its sufferers could reflect fear and negativity, particularly from the fourteenth century onwards, it is also evident that a great deal of care was provided to some leprous individuals. Within the *leprosarium*, the sick were assured of the fundamental necessities for survival: sustenance, warmth and shelter. A document marking the entry of Jehan Duquesnoy called 'le Bourguignon' to the *leprosarium* of Saint-Lazare at Aumône near Pontoise (north-west of Paris), issued on Tuesday 17 May 1412, makes this explicit: the master would provide him with 'boire mengier feu lit hostel et toutes ses autres neccessitez' ['drink, food, fire, bed, accommodation and all his other necessities'].[40] Like the leper house at Les Andelys, the Pontoise *leprosarium* only admitted those of burgess status; Jehan Duquesnoy was apparently to live very comfortably there, in a private room with his bed, linen sheets, table cloths and other possessions.[41] While all these facilities would undoubtedly have supported his physical well-being, they suggest that this *leprosarium*'s purpose was understood in terms of the provision more of hospitality – a fundamental monastic duty and the origin of the model of the hospital – than of medical care.

Nonetheless, in many *leprosaria* bodily care was available that accorded with the key medical concepts of the bodily humours and the non-naturals. In the Galenic understanding of medicine that prevailed in the Middle Ages, health was understood to derive from a balance of the four humours (blood, yellow bile, black bile and phlegm), and to be affected by the behavioural, environmental and emotional factors that were known as non-naturals.

39 Ibid., fols 1r, 1v.

40 Wellcome Library, MS 5133/1.

41 Ibid.

Bloodletting was a key means of restoring and maintaining the humoral balance, by removing excessive and corrupt matter from the body. As well as being a fundamental tool of medical practice, performed by surgeons and barber-surgeons, bleeding was an important moment in the calendar within monastic communities.[42] Given that *leprosaria* were monastic institutions that sheltered the sick, one might expect that phlebotomy was among the facilities available to their residents. Indeed, the statutes of the *leprosarium* of Les Andelys provide for each resident to have 'pour sa saingnée, chascun mois, deux pos de vin' ['for his or her bleeding, every month, two pots of wine'].[43] Statutes for the female house of Salle-aux-Puelles outside Rouen, drawn up in August 1249, refer to the fact that residents could voluntarily undergo bloodletting by a female phlebotomist, and indicate that bleeding could take place outside the *leprosarium*.[44] The wine at Les Andelys presumably served to restore fluids and strength to those who had been bled, while the fact that residents could choose whether or not to undergo bleeding at Salle-aux-Puelles indicates that customs could be more flexible in a *leprosarium* than in a 'standard' monastery, taking into account the physical condition and preferences of individuals. In medical theory, it was held that bleeding was only truly effective in the very early stages of leprosy, since in the advanced stages the whole body was filled with contaminated humoral matter, making bleeding from any one point insufficient. Phlebotomy was advocated in certain instances: Avicenna and Albucassis (d. 1013) both recommended bleeding from the veins in the neck to lessen the breathing difficulties of advanced cases of the disease, and it was believed that bleeding leprous women who were unable to menstruate would remove the corrupt matter that they were retaining. Both cupping, a gentler treatment that stimulated blood flow to the surface of the body, and cautery, a much more dramatic form of intervention, were also included among treatments for leprosy.[45] Nonetheless, it is clear that bleeding was deployed cautiously on lepers, and contemporaries must have frequently observed, as the Les Andelys statutes indicate, that sufferers were considerably weakened as a result.[46]

Much of the provision offered to lepers also accorded with the non-naturals. Although leprosy is a debilitating and disabling disease, physical exercise would have been possible for those in the relatively early stages of sickness. At the *leprosarium* of Saint-Lazare in Falaise (Lower Normandy), the chapel roof had to be repaired twice in the later fifteenth century because of damage

42 See Mary K. K. H. Yearl, 'Medieval Monastic Customaries on *Minuti* and *Infirmi*', in *The Medieval Hospital and Medical Practice*, ed. Barbara S. Bowers, AVISTA Studies in the History of Medieval Technology, Science and Art 3 (Aldershot, 2007), pp. 175–94.

43 'Statuts de la léproserie des Andelys', p. 250.

44 *Regestrum*, pp. 101–2; *Register*, pp. 116–17.

45 Rawcliffe, *Leprosy*, pp. 232–8.

46 See Rawcliffe, *Leprosy*, pp. 233, 238.

caused by residents playing *jeu de paume*, a ball game.[47] Good air and a clean environment were considered very important to health, particularly following the Black Death, when the spread of disease was increasingly associated with corrupt air and stench.[48] The positioning of *leprosaria* outside towns and cities in semi-rural locations ensured that their residents breathed clean air and were protected from the pollution (caused by human and animal waste, and industrial processes such as tanning and the dyeing of cloth) of urban environments. A number of *leprosaria* in northern France and England, such as Mont-aux-Malades at Rouen, St Nicholas at Harbledown outside Canterbury, and Bartlemas outside Oxford, were situated on hills, where the air was considered to be very pure.

Leprosarium statutes frequently detail the food and drink to be given to the sick, also among the non-naturals. While in practical terms this was an essential aspect of community life that needed to be set down in such documents, it also shows an awareness that providing adequate sustenance and, sometimes, regulating the diet, was an important component of the bodily care of lepers. In general, in order to improve the humoral balance within the body, medical theory advised that the leprous should consume moist, mild food and drink, such as poultry, eggs, fresh fish, fresh bread, good quality pork and light wine.[49] The dietary instructions in the August 1249 ordinance for Salle-aux-Puelles outside Rouen very much fit with these recommendations: the leprous sisters were to have beer, wine and bread daily, fresh meat in the proper season, fish once a week at other times, and five eggs or three herrings on days when they did not eat other fish or meat. However, the statutes also prescribe that the non-leprous members of the community should share the same diet, drawing into question whether this regimen was in fact specifically tailored towards the physical needs of lepers.[50]

The Salle-aux-Puelles statutes and other ordinances also show awareness of the different degrees of severity of leprosy, and of the need to take into account the emotional needs of the sick. The former text refers to 'gravioribus' ['the more gravely ill'] among the leprous women, and states: 'priorisse, que adeo sit discreta, quod sciat et velit compati infirmitatibus aliarum' ['the prioress should be discreet, so that she recognises and shows pity towards the infirmities of the sisters'].[51] The Amiens *leprosarium* statutes describe the arrangements for those who are so sick that they cannot get out of bed:

47 Damien Jeanne, 'Le Groupe des lépreux à Saint-Lazare de Falaise aux XIVe et XVe siècles', in *Lépreux et sociabilité du Moyen Âge aux temps modernes*, ed. Bruno Tabuteau ([Rouen], 2000), pp. 39–61 (p. 52); Rawcliffe, *Leprosy*, p. 241.

48 See Carole Rawcliffe, *Urban Bodies: Communal Health in Late Medieval English Towns and Cities* (Woodbridge, 2013), pp. 30–2.

49 Rawcliffe, *Leprosy*, p. 213.

50 *Regestrum*, p. 101; *Register*, p. 116.

51 *Regestrum*, p. 102; *Register*, p. 117.

they are to be taken out of the dormitory of the sick and put to one side.[52] At the leper house at Sherburn, the very sick were to be given everything they needed, including a fire and a candle, ensuring that they had the reassurance of warmth and light.[53] An ordinance for the *leprosarium* at Meaux (north-east of Paris), drawn up almost certainly in Latin in the late twelfth century and surviving in a French translation in a fourteenth-century cartulary, instructs that 'aux malades les quielx ne se puent lever de leur lit senz ayde, que on leur face misericorde et que on praingne pitié et compassion' ['one should be merciful and compassionate to, and take pity upon, those sick who cannot get out of their beds without help'].[54]

These provisions indicate an awareness of the need to provide emotional support to lepers within the *leprosarium*, particularly as their condition worsened. Such support would naturally have intersected with spiritual care, upon which great emphasis was placed. At Amiens, for example, the residents were required to make frequent confession to their priest, and it was also possible for them to confess to another priest elsewhere, presumably temporarily leaving the *leprosarium* for this purpose.[55] Confession might well have been the occasion for the sick to discuss their anxieties and physical suffering with a priest, and to receive reassurance and sympathy from him, as well as spiritual guidance and preparation for what was to come. The requirement to attend regular divine service within the *leprosarium*'s chapel, as specified in, for example, the Sherburn statutes and an ordinance for the leper house of St Mary Magdalene, Exeter, recorded in the early fifteenth century, also ensured that the community assembled regularly as a body, which in ideal circumstances would have promoted a collective sense of solidarity and support.[56]

CONCLUSION

Although leprosy had mixed associations in the Middle Ages, provoking concern about sexual misconduct and, particularly from the fourteenth century, anxiety regarding contagion, medical and religious responses to the disease in northern France and England nonetheless reveal a dedication to meeting the long-term bodily and spiritual needs of sufferers. Medical practitioners took seriously the necessity of diagnosing suspected cases of leprosy, and medical theory to some extent shaped the palliative care provided within

52 'Statuts de la léproserie d'Amiens', p. 227.

53 'Constitutiones Hospitalis domus leprosorum de Shirburne', p. 126.

54 'Statuts de la léproserie de Meaux', in *Statuts d'Hôtels-Dieu et de léproseries*, ed. Le Grand, pp. 184–90 (p. 186).

55 'Statuts de la léproserie d'Amiens', p. 226.

56 'Constitutiones Hospitalis domus leprosorum de Shirburne', p. 125; 'Regulations of the Leper Hospital of St Mary Magdalene, Exeter, as Restated Early in the Fifteenth Century', in Richards, *Medieval Leper*, pp. 140–1, especially p. 140.

leprosaria. While the emphasis on chastity and religious observance in these communities paints a picture of a strictly regulated and controlled existence, this way of life ensured the future salvation of lepers' souls, considered to be of primary importance, especially since they were believed to have been specially selected by God to be saved. At the same time, life within a *leprosarium* could be somewhat comfortable – as indicated by the arrangements made for Jehan Duquesnoy at Pontoise in 1412 – and granted to lepers essential facilities that were not available to those that did not gain entry to a *leprosarium*. Itinerant, begging lepers were a recognisable social category by the later Middle Ages; yet they too could benefit from the distribution of alms and occasional medical attention.[57] They were also sometimes temporarily accommodated at *leprosaria*, as revealed by a clause in the Les Andelys statutes regarding provision for 'lez povres malades trespassans' ['the poor passing sick'].[58] Both within and outside institutions, responses to leprosy were complex and varied, reflecting stigma and fear, but also compassion and a sense of duty towards the chronically ill. While *leprosaria* did not usually employ high-status medical practitioners, they provided arguably the best overall environment within which lepers could live with their disease.

57 At Nuremberg, Germany, there was an annual medical examination of vagrant lepers in Holy Week: see Demaitre, *Leprosy*, pp. 45–6.

58 'Statuts de la léproserie des Andelys', p. 249.

AFTERWORD

Denis Renevey

Medical information and knowledge, however complex they may be, pervade our lives through the large number of media that are available to us nowadays. A simple look at *The Guardian* of 22 March 2014 is suggestive of the ways in which medical lore makes the headlines. The first front-page article conveys information about a debate triggered by a response to a study that questions the validity of prescribing a specific drug as a preventative for people who have a 20% risk of heart attack or stroke. The article continues in the 'Health' section of the broadsheet, and more information in the form of a second article, with diagrams and pictures, addresses the question of whether the product does more good than harm as a preventative drug. Continuing further into the newspaper, the 'Saturday Features, Comments & Reviews' section headlines discussion about the celebrity doctor Christian Jessen, who has reached popularity through his television series *Embarrassing Bodies*, *Supersize vs. Superskinny* and *The Ugly Face of Beauty*, shows that have generated controversies about the potentially negative impact some episodes may have on some viewers. The Saturday interview is triggered by a recent and equally controversial television programme, *Cure Me, I'm Gay*, which featured Dr Christian Jessen, who is gay, going undercover as a patient seeking a cure for what many people still consider to be a disease. Dr Jessen's documentary shows the kind of abuse 'patients' undergo as a result of gross misconceptions about homosexuality.[1] A click on my computer allows me to investigate further the information about Dr Jessen's medical and television performances, gaining access to some parts of the television programme, some of his books, and even a free downloadable signed copy of his photo! These brief references to the newspaper articles and electronic devices show the extent to which medicine, besides its therapeutic function, has a social and cultural role in contemporary society that is further exacerbated by the new media and the globalisation of the circulation of information. The cult of celebrity and strong

1 See *The Guardian, Weekend Edition* (London and Manchester, Saturday 22 March 2014), 1, 16–17, 27, 30–1.

sense of self-centredness displayed by many in the field contribute further to the high status and visibility given to the medical profession and its sphere of knowledge.

Things differed in the medieval period in degree rather than in kind. As this collection of essays demonstrates, medicine contributes significantly to medieval culture, but according to a different set of paradigms. As a result of the medieval period's holistic approach to human nature, medical and religious cultures were in constant dialogue with one another, as is evidenced by a large number of Latinate and vernacular medieval codices in which religious and medical knowledge are bound together. This volume gives particular emphasis to the literariness of medical knowledge, and to the 'medicality' of religious literature, exploring, for instance, the way in which medical metaphors and medical roles are used to define particular characters from sacred history, such as Christ and the Virgin Mary. The book also assesses the way in which some medical texts became bestsellers in their own time. Following the devastating and scientifically unexplained advent of the plague in the fourteenth century, the genre of the *regimen sanitatis*, or guide for health, was produced on a large scale for the use of the general public.

While several of the essays in this book focus on the literariness of medical knowledge, emphasis is also placed on the material conditions enabling the practice of medicine as a therapeutic art. Recent studies on charitable institutions and welfare, as well as archaeological studies on medieval hospitals, provide useful evidence for medieval medical practice and care for the privileged few who were allowed access to such institutions.[2] The space which medical practitioners and patients used for treatment was also defined by gender restrictions and specificities, based on beliefs about the link between deficient moral conduct, especially of a sexual nature, and disease. Male/female segregation for both medical practitioners and patients was the norm in the medieval hospital.

Gender issues are at the heart of several chapters in this book. They are part of Brenner's chapter dealing with medical and religious responses to leprosy, which will be discussed later. They inform much of the chapters written by Watt and Magnani. On the basis of the well-known theme of Christ the physician, which is also discussed in Yoshikawa's chapter, Watt explores the ways in which healing powers are associated with the Virgin Mary, who becomes the *Maria medica* and the model for several female authors. The

2 See for instance Tiffany A. Ziegler, 'The Hospital of Saint John: Exploring Charitable Distribution in High Medieval Brussels', *Eä: Journal of Medical Humanities & Social Studies of Science and Technology* 3 (2011), 1–32; available online at http://issuu.com/eajournal/docs/hospital-saint-john-charity-brussels (last accessed 24 March 2014); see also Carole Rawcliffe, *Leprosy in Medieval England* (Woodbridge, 2009); and *Medicine for the Soul: The Life, Death and Resurrection of an English Medieval Hospital, St Giles, Norwich c. 1249-1550* (Stroud, 1999).

existence of such a powerful model demonstrates increasingly authoritative medical stances on the part of women. Despite limitations in receiving formal medical education, the female acquisition of medical knowledge is nevertheless attested early in the medieval period, with the attribution of a guide to female health to Trotula in Salerno. Hildegard of Bingen's medical treatises are further testimony to formal female medical training. However, together with Cecilia of Oxford, also mentioned by Watt, these women were the exception rather than the rule. Watt is instead keen to explore the use of the *Maria medica* theme in the context of the household and domestic spaces, stressing the links between physical illness and sinfulness, as attested by the example of Aethelthryth of Ely provided by Bede in his *Historia ecclesiastica gentis Anglorum*. The account of two Marian healing visions in *The Life of Christina of Markyate* serves as evidence for the assignation of healing powers on the part of the Virgin Mary. In the context of Christina, the Virgin's intercession is the agent leading to her healing from illnesses, in both cases associated with anxiety about her moral standing.

Margery Kempe's recovery from a period of insanity mentioned in the early part of *The Book of Margery Kempe* is attributed to Jesus, who appears to her to offer solace and comfort. Yet her full recovery, including her inclusion back into the community and the right to enter sacred space, is made possible following the rite of purification that takes place in her parish church, and which echoes the liturgical event of the purification of the Blessed Virgin celebrated on 2 February. Kempe's ability to endorse and perform the roles given to specific characters of sacred history, which is well attested in *The Book of Margery Kempe*, takes additional power in the episode of her healing a woman suffering from a post-partum depression similar to hers in the early part of *The Book*. Margery Kempe becomes the *Maria medica* and as such she provides useful evidence for the wide reception of the role of the Virgin Mary as physician.

The way in which the Paston women construe healing in both medical and devotional terms further supports the point about women's imitation of Mary the physician as an empowering phenomenon. In the case of Margaret Paston, for instance, there is plenty of evidence showing her medical expertise as well as her belief in the healing power of devotional acts linked to the Virgin Mary, such as the pilgrimage to the Shrine of the Virgin Mary at Walsingham.

Magnani's own take on the role played by the Virgin Mary is one that she considers to be marked by assistive agency, which she understands to be an archetypal feminine quality. Thomas Hoccleve built Chaucer's fifteenth-century moral and literary reputation on his Marian output, with a transfer of the assistive function from the Virgin Mary to Virginia, who is no less than Mary's secular counterpart in 'The Physician's Tale'. Both figures are regarded as textual 'envelopes' serving to disseminate orthodox feminine Christianity. The character of the Physician, who narrates Virginia's secular martyrdom, stands as an authority in the rhetoric rather than the practice of medicine, and as such the tale is able to explore tensions between patriarchal power and female agency in general, and the tensions created by the practice of the medical profession in the medieval period in particular.

The following two essays show the extent to which medical discourse contributes to the construction of a metaphorical language making meaning of the visionary experiences of two female mystics, Mechtild of Hackeborn and Julian of Norwich. Yoshikawa's fine exposition of the textual tradition of *The Booke of Gostlye Grace* is followed by an extensive investigation of the medical language used by Mechtild in her text. The convergence between medical and devotional discourses in this text is remarkable, the more so as Yoshikawa demonstrates the breadth of the sphere of medieval medical knowledge, including the curative properties of music and smells.[3] Mechtild's personal experience with disease and her role as chantress of her community inform her use of medical metaphors. Improper handling of emotions such as anger, fear and joy, for instance, could cause imbalance to the soul and disrupt humours within the body, thus leading to illness. Boethius' *De institutione musica* made a case for the classical belief in liturgical music's power in restoring humoral balance, thus healing and soothing both body and soul. Moreover, Mechtild's understanding of the power of music reaches beyond its therapeutic functions. Music is indeed medicine, but it also allows direct access to God.[4] *Musica humana*'s main function is to provide access to heavenly music, which stands apart from cosmic music (*musica mundana*), human music (*musica humana*) and instrumental music (*musica instrumentalis*). The acute blurring of the semantic fields of devotional and medical discourses, and the way in which each of these fields permeate one another, make a strong case for the way in which experts in the fields of medieval medicine and religion need to rethink categories. Therapeutic metaphors grow out from the storehouse of medical knowledge contained in treatises such as the *regimen sanitatis*, in which Galenic material on the six non-naturals features prominently. Because of the belief in the therapeutic qualities of sweet smells, Mechtild also explores a set of terms associated to them in the description of her heavenly visions. Mechtild's *Booke of Gostlye Grace* may represent the most sustained convergence of medical and devotional discourses in one single text. That this is so is due to the way in which Mechtild negotiates her own experience with disease with a broader application of medical knowledge as part of her narrative of mystical encounter with the divine.

3 For an initial investigation of the convergence between devotional and medical discourses, see *Poetica* 72, Special Issue, *Convergence/Divergence: The Politics of Late Medieval English Devotional and Medical Discourses*, ed. Denis Renevey and Naoë Kukita Yoshikawa (Tokyo, 2009).

4 For an in-depth consideration of heavenly music and its representation, see Katherine Zieman, 'The Perils of *Canor*: Mystical Authority, Alliteration, and Extragrammatical Meaning in Rolle, the *Cloud*-author, and Hilton', *Yearbook of Langland Studies* 22 (2008), 131–63.

Although addressing different issues, McAvoy's chapter makes another strong case for the contextualisation of experiential knowledge in dialogue with the broader issues of medicinal therapeutics. Julian asked for a sickness from God as part of her journey of discovery with the divine. Her experience is strongly linked to the female abject body, which Julian describes as part of her narrative in the Long Text. In order for Julian to make sense of her experience, her suffering needs to be understood as part of a redemptive scheme scripted in medicinal terms. Literature from antecedent centuries, and more particularly from the anchoritic tradition, offers evidence for a practice that resonates with feminine constructions of physical suffering and abjection. Grimlaicus of Metz portrays the solitary life as compounded by a trajectory of suffering and healing.[5] Perhaps even more interesting, and surprising, William Flete's *De remediis contra temptaciones*, possibly a source for Julian, portrays God both as a cruel-to-be-kind physician and a kind mother, thus providing an unexpected model of conflation of the patriarchal physician with that of the maternal figure. Further, the anchoritic tradition of which Julian's text is an offshoot promotes a form of female religious activity in which the anchoress is seduced into a partnership with Jesus based on the similarities of their phlebotomic experiences. While God the physician invites Christ to let blood as an altruistic gesture towards humankind, the female recluses for whom *Ancrene Wisse* is written undergo phlebotomy as a form of *imitatio Christi*. Julian pushes the tradition further by merging the figure of the *Christus medicus* with that of the nurturing mother, thus creating what McAvoy calls a Eucharist of the feminine.

Both Julian and Margery Kempe suffered from physical disease and thought themselves to have gone mad in the early days of their visionary experiences. Their accounts, often read as autobiographical, rather than as following a hagiographic model, have led to multiple interpretations rooted in contemporary medical, psychoanalytical and psychiatric knowledge. Vuille offers a compelling evaluation of the most influential readings analysed under this lens and shows how such readings often fail or are unable to take into consideration medieval medical, religious and social parameters as elements of their analysis. Moreover, she shows that different modern manuals of diagnostics of mental disorders differ substantially between one another. Also, comparison of content between editions of the same manual indicates changes in the classification of mental disorders reflecting new discoveries and new trends in a medical domain which relies as much on cultural paradigms as bodily manifestation for the emergence of specific illnesses. The field is hence constantly changing, its scientific veracity contested within its own sphere. While Margery's uncontrollable weeping is regarded by Lawes and Stork as

5 For a dating of Grimlaicus' *Regula solitariorum*, see Phyllis G. Jestice, *Wayward Monks and the Revolution of the Eleventh Century* (Leiden, 1997), pp. 92–3 n. 4.

evidence of epilepsy or Tourette's syndrome, Vuille opts for the influence of the continental tradition of female piety as a conventional manifestation of sanctity. It is not unlikely Margery may have been influenced by this tradition and hence that she consciously made this spiritual gift part of the representation of her mystical persona.

Audelay's idiosyncrasy, in contrast to most of the authors discussed so far who suffered from a particular illness, is that he did not seek a remedy from his blindness and from his other prolonged sickness for which there was, it seems, no cure. As a consequence of this personal attitude towards sickness, Audelay's movement from the literal to the metaphorical discourse of illness has a particular resonance. His broad understanding of purgatorial space, which includes the present earthly life if experienced as a process of penance, allows him to construct a healing continuum from the present life into Purgatory, with the certainty of coming out, which would mark the completion of the healing process. Admittance to the care of the divine surgeon, a role that is assumed interchangeably both by Jesus and Mary, gives certainty of a treatment that will provide a spiritual cure. With this vision in place, Audelay constructs his persona as that of the ghost-figure sent by a divine purpose back to earth to advise humankind about proper conduct. Spiritual healing therefore must begin in this life, but continues in Purgatory as a continual process under the direction of the divine surgeon, until the liberating completion of the cure.

The following chapter by Bishop offers a very informed account of medieval understanding of the heart's nature and function. Late medieval thought and literature, influenced by Aristotelian natural philosophy, conceives the heart as the locus for 'spirit', a material substance made of blood and air, having the same substantiality, as the soul. Spirits move throughout the body and the heart's propulsive quality is therefore central to this centrifugal movement. Within this material heart and material spirit are located will, intellect and affect. The heart is the seat of all activities that qualify as human and is therefore the material organ that may be affected most importantly, via the senses, by external particulars, be they food, thoughts or sensory perceptions. Bishop constructs a narrative in which the heart becomes the object of conquest and appropriation by vernacular theologies, an act which was regarded as politically threatening to the authorities. Pecock's tolerant attitude towards Christian matters triggered anxiety on the part of Viscount Beaumont who feared such a permissive approach towards Christian doctrine could poison men's hearts. Bishop reveals further medieval understandings of the heart by means of her reading of *The Doctrine of the Hert*, a fifteenth-century translation of the thirteenth-century *De doctrina cordis*. Her combined narratives offer a fascinating account of the heart as the seat of the passions having an impact on health. But more than that, the heart in its multiple configurations becomes the site where ideological and political thoughts are in contest and where the reading heart becomes problematic. As the heart is the target of both reading and preaching, the way one performs reading receives serious attention in the fifteenth century, as exemplified in *The Doctrine of the Hert*, which offers models of reading in imitation of the monastic and liturgical uses. Both Pecock and *The Doctrine* show trust in the apprehension of meditative reading as spiritual cure. But it seems that Pecock's belief in the ability of readers to judge their faith rationally met with the disapproval of Viscount Beaumont. Beaumont's opposition led not only to Pecock's deposition as bishop of Chichester, but also to his incapacitation as a maker of books. The suspicion expressed and put into action by Viscount Beaumont upholds the strength of the vernacular in triggering intellectual, readerly and writerly activities capable of deeply touching the human heart, the seat of the 'conscience'.

The next chapter considers further the convergence between medicine and morally sanctioned behaviour by focusing on medieval culture's attempt to understand the causes for the birth of congenitally disabled people. Medical and religious texts seem to show the same degree of gendered prejudice in explaining the causes for such abnormal births, not so much by putting the blame on women only, but rather by giving women limited agency in the act of conception. Both fields attempt to answer the question of what causes a 'wrong' child. Such a stance presupposes an inherently negative perspective on the act of procreation, which in practice, and with the authoritative voice of St Augustine, was regarded as evil throughout the medieval period. Conception occurs as part of a sinful act, and as a consequence all born creatures must undergo purification under the sacrament of baptism in order to reach a state of cleanliness. Considering the morally precarious situation of the sexual act that is prerequisite of conception, the birth of defective children was understood as a consequence of further morally improper forms of individual behaviour, which medical and moral treatises took pains to describe and vituperate against. Medical treatises agree in defining the missionary position as the only prescribed method for procreation. A couple's experiments with other positions during copulation were believed to be one of the causes for defects in children. A wandering female imagination, or an insufficiently passive female parent, could also lead to defective children, with the danger of the construction of the creative imagination imprinting itself in the physical essence of the new-born (a woman thinking about a cow during copulation could lead to the birth of child with cow-like characteristics!). Unhealthy nourishment, and more specifically alcoholic consumption could have a negative impact on the sperm or the unborn child. Such notions circulated widely in the popular medical manuals, oftentimes presenting contradictory views and understandings about defective births. The popular religious literature of the late medieval period, such as preaching manuals, also expanded upon such notions, including, for instance, warnings against sexual activity during menstruation, lactation and pregnancy. The history of the Fall generates a further bias against women and therefore directs some additional blame towards them in the case of defective births. In fact, female children were regarded as a form of deformation from the male child; then followed the severely defective child and, worst of all cases in the attempt at procreation, the absent progeny. The chapter moves on to a consideration of the way in which the medical discourse of disability is used metaphorically to discuss the care with which those newly converted to Christ should be treated by the religious authorities. The final part of the chapter tackles the question of moral pressure put on the parents of deficient children, and addresses the question of infanticide and abandonment as a result of such pressure. Congenital disability, therefore, offers another fascinating example of the way in which medical and religious discourses converge to present extraordinarily complex ways of understanding medieval culture when faced with emotionally loaded experiences for which no immediate cause could be found. Considering that medieval people understood the world in which they lived to be imperfect as a result of the original sin, the birth of an imperfect child would be understood as a further demonstration of this imperfection within the parameters of the human and social microcosm.

The following three chapters focus on medical and socio-cultural attitudes, considering facial disfigurement, blindness and responses to leprosy. Skinner's discussion of the cases of three female medieval holy women reveals the ambivalence self-inflicted disfigurement can take in medieval culture. In each of these cases, that is, those of Oda of Brabant, St Margaret of Hungary and St Margaret of Cortona, the impulse for facial disfigurement is conditioned by a strong desire for the accomplishment of a life completely devoted to Christ. Self-mutilation is motivated by the necessity of facing adversity in the strongest and most decisive manner, that is, of depriving oneself of one's own beauty to annihilate marriage as a possible prospect. Or, as in the case of Margaret of Cortona, self-mutilation is motivated by the desire to efface the cause of Margaret's early life as a sexually promiscuous woman, and in that respect this gesture differs in terms of aim from penitential fasting, which looks forwards to a possible encounter with the divine. Interestingly, the cases show that often the threat of self-mutilation would be sufficient to produce the desired effect, and cases of self-mutilation are less frequent than one could expect in a society in which violence played an important function. In the case of Oda, where the threat was followed by the actual act, without any official approval, the face-cutting episode was probably more damaging to her reputation: it was carried out secretly in a bedroom, as an act of disobedience. From the thirteenth century onwards, self-inflicted physical impairment is regarded as failure in facing temptation and showing one's own strength in the face of a carnal challenge. But facial disfigurement performed by God on female bodies is always read favourably in hagiographical literature.

Medieval culture often interpreted physical suffering and illness as divine punishments resulting from sinful activity. That perspective, although correct in many cases, is far too general and, as Hawkins's chapter shows, hides the fact of medieval society's care for the sick in general, and the blind in particular.

Also, and in contrast to the association of sickness with sin, sickness is also read as a gift given by God to test the faith of a specially chosen soul, as in the case of Julian of Norwich, for instance. So the cause of the illness decides very importantly the community's response to the sufferer. If a disproportionate diet, especially excessive alcohol consumption, was found to be the cause of blindness, as it was believed to be one of the causes for this affliction, then of course the care given to the sufferer would be handled according to his moral responsibility. However, if blindness was the result of professional exposure to risks, such as dangerous fumes for goldsmiths, or the result of old age, then the response would be much more positive and would trigger the medieval community into charitable acts that would expunge the donor from his own bank of sins. Blindness was regarded as a particularly generous divine gesture endowing its recipient with piety and wisdom. The provision of care to such a patient would allow one to perform one of the Seven Works of Mercy, which were crucial for one's spiritual health.

Social and religious responses to leprosy are as complex as responses to blindness and other physical ailments. Brenner, along with several other authors of this book, explores the intersection between bodily and spiritual spheres, and the way in which care and cure function at both levels. Leprosy within religious discourse is associated with excessive sexual activity, and finds support in the medical treatises that explain the cause of the disease as a disturbance of the humoral balance. Despite this morally condemning view, the particular physical conditions in which lepers lived, enclosed, distant from the urban centres, and with their state marked by the will of God, made them in some way exemplary individuals. Like Christ, who suffered on the cross and was marked out from his community, lepers were given the opportunity to achieve their own process of redemption, leading a quasi-religious life according to a rule. Being or not being leprous had huge social consequences, and so accusations of leprosy required careful examination. Following a protocol for leprosy examinations developed in thirteenth-century France, the accusation against Theobald of Amiens proved the accusation to be unfounded, and therefore prevented the archbishop from giving up his social identity and status. Although *leprosaria* provided mainly religious and charitable hospitality to their patients, bodily care through medical treatment based on humoral theory was provided. Evidence of the need for emotional support is also available in the records of the Amiens leprosarium.

Several of the perspectives offered in this volume signal new directions in the consideration of medieval culture's convergence between devotional and medical cultures. The groundwork that has been carried out recently in the field allows now for several innovative investigations.[6] The continuation

[6] For an up-to-date annotated bibliography on medieval medicine, with some entries that address the convergence between medical and religious discourses, see Peter Murray Jones, 'Medicine', in *Oxford Bibliographies in Medieval Studies*, ed. Paul E. Szarmach

of close examination of hermeneutic practices as performed by clerics of the late medieval period such as Arnau de Vilanova and Galvano da Levanto will yield further insights into the way medical and theological discourses fuse and feed upon one another and contribute to a dynamic exegetical practice.[7] The role played by the friars as medical practitioners in the thirteenth and fourteenth centuries, as investigated by Montford, deserves further attention.[8] As mentioned by Yoshikawa in her introduction, following the advent of the plague in 1348, anxiety and hopelessness in the face of death led to a lay interest in medical knowledge in the form of translations, adaptations and compilations of medico-spiritual treatises from the Latin clerical milieu to the European vernaculars for the use of a non-academic lay readership.[9] The exploration of this process of transference is a vast, still underexplored activity, with limited modern editions, especially in the case of Latin authors who did not attend university.[10] The study of the textual and manuscript traditions of the very popular *Secreta secretorum* and the *Regimen sanitatis Salerni*, with more than five hundred extant manuscripts for the latter, is essential for better understanding the spread of medical knowledge among non-clerical European audiences.

As studies of women's medicine have flourished in the last decades, it is now possible to carry on detailed investigation of the convergence between women's medicine and religion.[11] The model of the Virgin Mary as nurse may have been constructed on the basis of the actual role played by women in the provision of medical care in provincial England. As in the case of the Paston women discussed by Watt in this volume, and by Orlemanski elsewhere, female medical care takes precedence over professional advice in the case of Sir John Paston II taking advice from his wife based in her Norfolk house, while spending time in London, where he echoes his mother's distrust of London physicians: 'fore Goddys sake be ware what medesynys ye take of any fysissyanys of London. I schal neuer trust to hem.'[12] Monica Green's own exploration of women's medicine argues similarly for it as both therapeutic art

(New York, 2010); see especially the entry 'Religion and Medicine': http://www.oxfordbibliographies.com/view/document/obo-9780195396584/obo-9780195396584-0051.xml?rskey=uv9yvf&result=1&q=medieval+medicine#firstMatch (last accessed 9 April 2014).

7 See Joseph Ziegler, *Medicine and Religion c. 1300: The Case of Arnau de Vilanova* (Oxford, 1998).

8 See Angela Montford, *Health, Sickness, Medicine, and the Friars in the Thirteenth and Fourteenth Centuries* (Aldershot, 2004).

9 See see Yoshikawa's discussion in 'Introduction'.

10 See for instance Benvenutus Grassus, *The Wonderful Art of the Eye: A Critical Edition of the Middle English Translation of his* De probatissima arte oculorum, ed. L. M. Eldredge (East Lansing, MI, 1996).

11 See in Murray Jones, 'Medicine', the rubric 'Historiography'.

12 See Julie Orlemanski, 'Thornton's Remedies and Practices of Medical Reading', in *Robert*

and cultural phenomenon, thus pointing the way to additional case studies where female agency leads to medical and religious activity.[13] An exploration of women's medicine needs to take into account the works of abbesses, mystics and visionaries, as well as exploring medical and religious practice in the fictional female hagiographies of the late medieval period.

The hybridisation of medical texts with discourses from other spheres of knowledge shows the extent to which health was the concern not only of professional physicians but also 'of philosophers, poets, theatre (and anti-theatre) practitioners, and religious communities, all of whom sought, in their different spheres, to purge and relieve the body, soul or mind of the human sufferer'.[14] More specific to the medical and religious spheres, the way in which rhetorical strategies operate within them, with reliance on the citations of the *auctores*, and the use of the persuasive mode, will yield further interesting evidence of hermeneutic practices. However, the care of body and soul also begs the question of economic interest in spiritual healing. Reports of miraculous cases of physical healing at the shrines of saints could bring enormous economic benefits to the religious communities in charge of managing and hosting visitors wanting to pay their devotions to the shrine.[15] The cult of the saint as therapeutic alternative could be a profitable business venture, and there is a need to impose upon medical and religious discourses an economic layer that offers an account of this particular dimension. A large-scale assessment of the significance of this economic aspect in relation to miraculously performed healing could yield interesting results.

As we have seen, the (spiritual) autobiographies of Margery Kempe, Julian of Norwich and Hoccleve are often immersed in medical and religious considerations, perceived in the context of human salvation and participation in the human community. Accounts of disease and emotions about disease, as well as expressions of emotions of pain undergone through physical distress, are areas in these texts that deserve further study. They also lead us to consider the aesthetics of disease in prose texts such as spiritual autobiographies and secular accounts, and to assess the way in which the writing of poetry as such

Thornton and His Books: Essays on the London and the Lincoln Thornton Manuscripts, ed. Susannah Fein and Michael Johnston (Woodbridge, 2014), pp. 235–55 (p. 239).

13 Monica H. Green, 'Bodies, Gender, Health, Disease: Recent Work on Medieval Women's Medicine', *Studies in Medieval and Renaissance History*, 3rd series, 2 (2005), 1–46; see also Green, 'Integrative Medicine: Incorporating Medicine and Health into the Canon of Medieval European History', *History Compass* 7 (2009), 1218–45.

14 See Rachel Falconer and Denis Renevey, 'Introduction', in *Medieval and Early Modern Literature, Science and Medicine*, ed. Rachel Falconer and Denis Renevey (Tübingen, 2013), pp. 11–17 (p. 12).

15 See Christiania Whitehead, 'Spiritual Healing: Healing Miracles associated with the Twelfth-Century Northern Cult of St Cuthbert', in *Medieval and Early Modern Literature, Science and Medicine*, ed. Falconer and Renevey, pp. 167–82.

was regarded in some spheres as the only means of salvation, sanity, and cure.[16]

Advances in the medical sciences bring bodies back to health in ways that our medieval ancestors could only have dreamed of. However, despite or perhaps because of its higher fallibility, medieval medicine looked for a fruitful dialogue and interaction with other spheres of knowledge, adding to its semantic field, imitating the stance taken by other authoritative discourses, or sometimes contesting them in a self-assertive gesture. This struggle for power, acted out in the vernaculars of England in the cases under consideration in this volume, but nevertheless derived from learned pan-European medical sources, provides a captivating picture of the process by which medieval culture dynamically re-makes its constitutive discourses and ideologies.

16 See Lisana Calvi, '"Is't Lunacy to call a spade, a spade?": James Carkesse and the Forgotten Language of Madness', in *Medieval and Early Modern Literature, Science and Medicine*, ed. Falconer and Renevey, pp. 139–52.

SELECT BIBLIOGRAPHY

MANUSCRIPTS

London, Wellcome Library, MS 130 (Bernard de Gordon, *Practica medicinalis (Lilium medicinae)*, fourteenth century)

London, Wellcome Library, MS 5133/1 (agreement for Jehan Duquesnoy called 'le Bourguignon')

London, Wellcome Library, MS 5133/3 (letter from the duke of Lorraine, c. 1487)

Norwich, Norfolk Record Office, NCR, 8/F (St George's Guild Account of Receipts and Expenses, 1491-92, no foliation)

Paris, Archives nationales, S4889B, dossier 13, doc. (xxi), fols 1r–2r (Peter de Collemezzo's reforms for the *leprosarium* of Mont-aux-Malades, May 1237)

Rouen, Archives départementales de Seine-Maritime, G2134 (fifteenth-century register of the cathedral chapter of Rouen)

York, York Minster Library, D/C Reg. 1, York Diocesan Probate Registers, fol. 318v

PRIMARY SOURCES

AA.SS. vol. III, 28 January, De B. Margaritae Hungariae Virginis

AA.SS. vol. VI, 22 February, De B. Margarita Poenit. Tertii Ord. S. Francisci Cortonae in Etruria

AA.SS. vol. XI, 20 April, Vita Ven. Oda Praemonstratensis

Alberti, Leon Battista, *On the Art of Building in Ten Books*, trans. Joseph Rykwert (Cambridge, MA and London: Harvard University Press, 1988)

Albertus Magnus, *De animalibus*, Liber XV, Tractatus II ('de natura spermatis'), in *Opera Omnibus*, ed. Emile Borgnet (Paris, 1891), vol. 12

Albertus Magnus, *De animalibus*, Libri XXVI, ed. Hermann Stadler, Beiträge zur Geschichte der Philosophie des Mittelalters. Texte und Untersuchungen 16 (Münster: Aschendorff, 1920)

Albertus Magnus, *Quaestiones super De Animalibus*, in *Alberti Magni Opera Omnia*, ed. B. Geyer (Münster: Aschendorff, 1955)

Albertus Magnus, *Problemata determinata*, ed. James A. Weisheipl, in 'The Problemata determinata XLIII, Ascribed to Albertus Magnus (1271)', *Mediaeval Studies* 22 (1960), 303-54

Albertus Magnus, *De natura boni*, in *Alberti Magni Opera Omnia*, vol. XXV Pars I, ed. E. Filthaut (Münster: Aschendorff, 1974)

Albertus Magnus, *Physica*, in *Alberti Magni Opera Omnia*, vol. IV Pars I, ed. Paul Hossfeld (Münster: Aschendorff, 1987)

Albertus Magnus, *Albert the Great: Questions concerning Aristotle's On Animals*, trans. Irven M. Resnick and Kenneth F. Kitchell Jr., Fathers of the Church: Medieval Continuation 9 (Washington, DC: Catholic University of America Press, 2008)

Ancrene Wisse: A Corrected Edition of the Text in Cambridge, Corpus Christi College, MS 402 with variants from other manuscripts, ed. Bella Millett, 2 vols, EETS o.s. 325, 326 (Oxford: Oxford University Press, 2005-06)

Ancrene Wisse: A Guide for Anchoresses, ed. and trans. Bella Millett (Exeter: Exeter University Press, 2009)

The Apocryphal New Testament, trans. M. R. James (Oxford: Clarendon Press, 1924)

Audelay, John, *The Poems of John Audelay*, ed. E. K. Whiting, EETS o.s. 184 (Oxford: Oxford University Press, 1931)

Augustine, St, *On John's Gospel*, Tractatus III, PL 35, col. 1397

Augustine, St, *Enarratio in Psalmum* LV, PL 36, col. 649

Augustine, St, *De peccatorium meretis et remissione*, trans. Marcus Dodd, vol. II, *The Works of St Augustine* (Edinburgh, 1885)

Augustine, St, *Concerning the City of God Against the Pagans*, trans. Henry Bettenson (London: Penguin, 1972; repr. 2003)

Augustine, *The City of God Against the Pagans*, trans. R. W. Dyson (Cambridge: Cambridge University Press, 1998)

Augustine, St, *De Virginitate*, in *Nicene and Post-Nicene Fathers*, ed. Philip Schaff, vol. 3 (New York: Cosimo, 2007)

Avicenna, *A Treatise on the Canon of Medicine of Avicenna: Incorporating a Translation of the First Book*, ed. and trans. Oskar Cameron Gruner (London: Luzac, 1930)

The Awntyrs off Arthure, ed. Ralph Hanna, III (Manchester: University of Manchester Press, 1974)

Bacon, Roger, *Opus majus*, trans. Robert B. Burke, 2 vols (New York: Russell & Russell, 1928; repr. 1962)

Bartholomaeus Anglicus, *On the Properties of Things: John Trevisa's Translation of Bartholomaeus Anglicus De proprietatibus rerum*, ed. M. C. Seymour et al., 3 vols (Oxford: Clarendon Press, 1975-88)

Bede, *Bede's Ecclesiastical History of the English People*, ed. Bertram Colgrave and R. A. B. Mynors (Oxford: Oxford University Press, 1969)

Bede, *Ecclesiastical History of the English People*, ed. and trans. Judith McClure and Roger Collins (Oxford: Oxford University Press, 1994)

Bede, *Historiam Ecclesiasticam Gentis Anglorum.* Online edition at http://www.thelatinlibrary.com/bede.html

Benvenutus Grassus, *The Wonderful Art of the Eye: A Critical Edition of the Middle English Translation of his* De probatissima arte oculorum, ed. L. M. Eldredge (East Lansing, MI: Michigan State University Press, 1996)

Bernard de Gordon, *Practica seu Lilium medicinae* (Naples: F. del Tuppo for B. Geraldinus, 1480)
Berthold von Regensburg, *Vollständige Ausgabe Seiner Predigten*, ed. F. Pfeiffer, 2 vols (Vienna, 1862)
The Bestiary, ed. T. H. White (New York: G. P. Putnam's Sons, 1965)
Bestiary MS Bodley 764, trans. Richard Barber (Woodbridge: Boydell, 1999)
The Book of Margery Kempe, ed. Sanford Brown Meech and Hope Emily Allen, EETS o.s. 212 (Oxford: Oxford University Press, 1940)
The Book of Vices and Virtues, ed. W. Nelson Francis, EETS o.s. 217 (Oxford: Oxford University Press, 1942)
The Booke of Gostlye Grace of Mechtild of Hackeborn, ed. Theresa A. Halligan (Toronto: Pontifical Institute of Mediaeval Studies, 1979)
Caesarius von Heisterbach, *Dialogus miraculorum*, ed. J. Strange (Cologne, 1851)
Calendar of Patent Rolls, 1216–1509, 54 vols (London: HMSO, 1893–1916)
Calendar of Wills Proved and Enrolled in the Court of Hustings, London A.D. 1258–A.D. 1688, ed. R. R. Sharpe, 2 vols (London: Francis for the Corporation, 1890)
Cartulaire de la léproserie du Grand-Beaulieu et du prieuré de Notre-Dame de la Bourdinière, ed. René Merlet and Maurice Jusselin (Chartres: E. Garnier, 1909)
Cassian, John, *Conlationes*, PL 49, cols 477–1328
Cassian, John, *John Cassian: The Conferences*, ed. Boniface Ramsey (New York and Mahwah, NJ: Paulist Press, 1997)
Caterina da Genova, *Vita Mirabile / Dialogo / Trattato sul Purgatorio*, ed. Filippo Lovison (Rome: Città Nuova, 2004)
Chaucer, Geoffrey, *The Riverside Chaucer*, ed. Larry D. Benson, 3rd edn (Oxford: Oxford University Press, 1987, reissued 2008)
Cher Alme: Texts of Anglo-Norman Piety, ed. Tony Hunt (Tempe, AZ: Arizona Center for Medieval and Renaissance Studies, 2010)
The Chester Mystery Cycle, ed. R. M. Lumiansky and D. Mills, EETS n.s. 3 (Oxford: Oxford University Press, 1974)
The Chester Mystery Cycle, ed. D. Mills (East Lansing, MI: Michigan State College Press, 1992)
'Constitutiones Hospitalis domus leprosorum de Shirburne', in Peter Richards, *The Medieval Leper and his Northern Heirs* (Cambridge: D. S. Brewer, 1977; repr. Woodbridge: Boydell & Brewer, 2000), pp. 125–8
Councils and Synods with Other Documents Relating to the English Church, vol. 2, ed. F. M. Powicke and C. R. Cheney (Oxford: Clarendon, 1964)
Decrees of the Ecumenical Councils, ed. and trans. Norman P. Tanner, 2 vols (London: Sheed & Ward; Washington, DC: Georgetown University Press, 1990)
Dives and Pauper, ed. P. Heath Barnum, EETS o.s. 275 (Oxford: Oxford University Press, 1976) and 280 (1980)
The Doctrine of the Hert: A Critical Edition with Introduction and Commentary, ed. Denis Renevey, Christiania Whitehead and Anne Mouron (Exeter: Exeter University Press, 2009)

English Lawsuits from William I to Richard I, vol. 2, ed. R. C. Van Caenegem, Selden Society Publications 107 (London: Selden Society, 1991)

English Mediaeval Lapidaries, ed. Joan Evans and Mary S. Serjeantson, EETS o.s. 190 (London: Oxford University Press, 1933)

English Writings of Richard Rolle, ed. Hope Emily Allen (Oxford: Oxford University Press, 1931)

Fasciculus morum: A Fourteenth-Century Preacher's Handbook, ed. Siegfried Wenzel (University Park, PA: Pennsylvania State University Press, 1989)

Ficino, Marsilio, *The Book of Life*, trans. Charles Boer (Irving, TX: Spring Publications, 1980)

Flete, William, *The Remedy ayenst the troubles of temptacyons*, in *Richard Rolle of Hampole*, ed. C. Horstmann, 2 vols (London, 1896), vol. 2, pp. 106–23

Förster, Max, 'Kleinere Mittelenglische Texte', *Anglia* 42 (1918), 145–224

Fourth Lateran Council: 1215. Online translation, http://www.fordham.edu/halsall/basis/lateran4.asp

Froehlich, Gregory, *De motu cordis*, DeSales University Aquinas Translation Project, Internet resource, http://www4.desales.edu/~philtheo/loughlin/ATP/De_Motu_Cordis/De_Motu_Cordis.html

Fundamentals of Music: Anicius Manlius Severinus Boethius, trans. (with introduction and notes) Calvin M. Bower and ed. Claude V. Palisca (New Haven, CT and London: Yale University Press, 1989)

Gerald of Wales, *The Jewel of the Church: A Translation of Gemma Ecclesiastica by Giraldus Cambrensis*, trans. J. Hagen (Leiden: Brill, 1979)

Gesetze der Angelsachsen, ed. F. Lieberman, 3 vols (Halle: Max Niemeyer, 1903)

Grant, M., *Galen on Food and Diet* (London: Routledge, 2000)

Gregory, *Dialogorum Libri IV*, IV. 55, PL 77, cols 417A–C

Grimlaicus of Metz, *Grimlaici presbyteri regula solitariorum*, PL 103, cols 573–644

Grimlaicus of Metz, *Grimlaicus: Rule for Solitaries*, ed. and trans. Andrew Thornton (Collegeville, MN: Cistercian Publications, 2011)

Hildegard of Bingen, *Causae et curae*, ed. P. Kaiser (Leipzig: B. G. Teubner, 1903)

Hildegard of Bingen, *Saint Hildegard of Bingen, Symphonia: A Critical Edition of the* Symphonia harmonie celestium revelationum *[Symphony of the Harmony of Celestial Revelations]*, trans. Barbara Newman (Ithaca, NY and London: Cornell University Press, 1988)

Hildegard of Bingen, *Scivias*, trans. Columba Hart and Jane Bishop (New York: Paulist Press, 1990)

Hildegard of Bingen, *On Natural Philosophy and Medicine: Selections from* Cause et cure, trans. Margaret Berger (Cambridge: D. S. Brewer, 1999)

Hilton, Walter, *The Scale of Perfection*, ed. T. H. Bestul (Kalamazoo, MI: Medieval Institute Publications, 2000)

Hippocrates, *Hippocrates with an English Translation*, trans. W. H. S. Jones, 4 vols (London: Heinemann, 1948)

Hoccleve, Thomas, *The Regiment of Princes*, ed. Charles R. Blyth, TEAMS Medieval Texts Series (Rochester, NY: University of Rochester, 1999)

Hoccleve's Works, III: The Regement of Princes, A.D. 1411-12 from the Harleian MS. 4866, and fourteen of Hoccleve's minor poems from the Egerton MS. 615, ed. Frederick J. Furnivall, EETS e.s. 72 (London: Kegan Paul, Trench, Trübner, 1897)

The Holy Bible containing the Old and New Testaments in the Earliest English Versions made from the Latin Vulgate by John Wycliffe and his Followers, ed. J. Forshall and F. Madden, 4 vols (Oxford: Oxford University Press, 1850)

Horstmann, Carl (ed.), 'Lyf of Saint Katherin of Senis', *Archiv für das Studium der neueren Sprachen und Litteraturen* 76 (1886), 33–112, 265–314, 353–91

Horstmann, Carl (ed.), 'The Reuelacions of Saynt Elysabeth of Hungary', *Archiv für das Studium der neueren Sprachen und Litteraturen* 76 (1886), 392–400

John the Blind Audelay, *Poems and Carols (Oxford, Bodleian Library MS Douce 302)*, ed. Susanna Fein, TEAMS Middle English Texts Series (Kalamazoo, MI: Medieval Institute Publications, 2009)

John Mirk, *Instructions for Parish Priests*, ed. E. Peacock, EETS o.s. 31 (London: Oxford University Press, 1868)

John Mirk, *John Mirk's Festial: Edited from British Library MS Cotton Claudius A.II*, ed. Susan Powell, EETS o.s. 334 (Oxford: Oxford University Press, 2009)

Julian of Norwich, *The Writings of Julian of Norwich: A Vision Shown to a Devout Woman and A Revelation of Love*, Medieval Women: Texts and Contexts 5, ed. Nicholas Watson and Jacqueline Jenkins (Turnhout: Brepols, 2006)

Kemp, B. (ed.), 'The Miracles of the Hand of St James', *Berkshire Archaeological Journal* 65 (1970), 1–19

The Knowing of Woman's Kind in Childing: A Middle English Version of Material Derived from the Trotula and Other Sources, ed. Alexandra Barratt (Turnhout: Brepols, 2001)

Die Konstitutionen Friedrichs II für das Königsreich Sizilien, ed. Wolfgang Stürner, MGH Constitutiones et Acta Publica Imperatorum et Regum II, Supplement (Hanover: Hahn, 1996)

Langland, William, *The Vision of Piers Plowman: A Critical Edition of the B-Text*, ed. A. V. C. Schmidt (London: Dent, 1978)

A Latin Technical Phlebotomy and its Middle English Translation, ed. Linda E. Voigts and Michael R. McVaughs, *Transactions of the American Philosophical Society* 74, 2 (1984), 1–69

Leechdoms, Wortcunning and Starcraft of Early England, ed. T. O. Cockayne, 3 vols, Rolls Series (London, 1864-86)

Lennox, W. G. (trans.), 'John of Gaddesden on Epilepsy', *Annals of Medical History*, 3rd series, 1 (1939), 283-307

Lennox, W. G. (trans.), 'Bernard of Gordon on Epilepsy', *Annals of Medical History*, 3rd series, 3 (1941), 372-83

The Letters of Hildegard of Bingen, vol. 1, trans. Joseph L. Baird and Radd K. Ehrman (New York and Oxford: Oxford University Press, 1994)

The Liber Celestis of St Bridget of Sweden, ed. Roger Ellis, EETS o.s. 291 (Oxford: Oxford University Press, 1987)

The Life of Christina of Markyate, ed. Samuel Fanous and Henrietta Leyser (Oxford: Oxford University Press, 2008)

Le Livre de Seyntz Medicines: The Unpublished Devotional Treatise of Henry of Lancaster, ed. E. J. Arnould (Oxford: Basil Blackwell, 1940)

Lotario de Segni (Papst Innozenz III), *Vom Elend des menschlichen Daseins*, trans. (with introduction) Carl-Friedrich Geyer, Philosophische Texte und Studien 24 (Hildesheim: Georg Olms, 1990)

Lydgate and Burgh's 'Secrees of Old Philisoffers': A Version of the Secreta Secretorum, ed. R. Steele, EETS e.s. 66 (London: Kegan Paul, Trench & Trübner, 1894)

A Macaronic Sermon Collection from Late Medieval England: Oxford: Bodley MS 649, ed. and trans. Patrick J. Horner, Studies and Texts 153 (Toronto: Pontifical Institute of Mediaeval Studies, 2006)

A Manual of Roman Law: The Ecloga of Leo III and Constantine V of Isauria at Constantinople, AD 726, ed. E. H. Freshfield (Cambridge: Cambridge University Press, 1926)

Medieval English Prose for Women: Selections from the Katherine Group and Ancrene Wisse, ed. and trans. Bella Millett and Jocelyn Wogan-Browne (Oxford: Oxford University Press, 1990)

Medieval Medicine: A Reader, ed. Faith Wallis (Toronto: University of Toronto Press, 2010)

Medieval Writings on Secular Women, ed. Patricia Skinner and Elisabeth van Houts (London: Penguin, 2011)

Le Menagier de Paris, ed. Georgine E. Brereton and Janet M. Ferrier (Oxford: Clarendon, 1981)

Middle English Sermons, edited from British Museum MS. Royal 18 B. xxiii, ed. W. O. Ross, EETS o.s. 209 (Oxford: Oxford University Press, 1940; repr. 1960)

The Minor Poems of John Lydgate, ed. Henry Noble MacCracken, 2 parts, EETS e.s. 107, o.s.192 (London: Oxford University Press, 1911–34)

The Mirror of Justices, ed. William Joseph Whittaker, Selden Society 7 (London: B. Quaritch, 1895)

The Mission of Friar William of Rubruck, trans. Peter Jackson with notes by Peter Jackson and David Morgan, Hakluyt Society 2nd series 173 (London: Hakluyt Society, 1990)

Music in Early Christian Literature, ed. James McKinnon (Cambridge: Cambridge University Press, 1987)

Nemesius: On the Nature of Man, trans. (with introduction and notes) R. W. Sharples and P. J. van der Eijk, Translated Texts for Historians 49 (Liverpool: Liverpool University Press, 2008)

The Norwich Census of the Poor 1570, ed. J. F. Pound, Norfolk Record Society 40 (Norwich: Norfolk Record Society, 1971)

The Old English Lives of St Margaret, ed. Mary Clayton and Hugh Magennis, Cambridge Studies in Anglo-Saxon England 9 (Cambridge: Cambridge University Press, 1994)

Paré, Ambroise, *On Monsters and Marvels*, trans. Janis L. Palliser (Chicago and London: University of Chicago Press, 1983)

The Paston Letters and Papers of the Fifteenth-Century, ed. Norman Davis, 2 parts, EETS s.s. 20, 21 (Oxford: Clarendon Press, 1971, 1976)

Pastors and the Care of Souls in Medieval England, ed. John Shinners and William J. Dohar (Notre Dame, IN: University of Notre Dame Press, 1998)

Pecock, Reginald, *The Repressor of over Much Blaming of the Clergy*, ed. Babington Churchill (London: Longman, Green, Longman and Roberts, 1860)

Pecock, Reginald, *Reginald Pecock's Book of Faith: A Fifteenth Century Theological Tractate*, ed. J. L. Morison (Glasgow: J. Maclehose and Sons, 1909)

Pecock, Reginald, *The Donet*, ed. Elsie Vaughan Hitchcock, EETS o.s. 117 (Oxford: Humphrey Milford, Oxford University Press, 1921)

Pecock, Reginald, *The Folewer to the Donet*, ed. Elsie Vaughan Hitchcock, EETS o.s. 164 (Oxford: Humphrey Milford, Oxford University Press, 1924)

Pecock, Reginald, *The Reule of Crysten Religioun*, ed. Reginald Greet and William Cabell (Oxford: Humphrey Milford, Oxford University Press, 1927)

Pfolspeundt, Heinrich von, *Buch der Bündt-Ertznei (1460)*, ed. H. Haeser and A. Middeldorpf (Berlin: George Reimer, 1868)

Pliny the Elder, *Naturalis Historia*, VII, ed. W. H. S. Jones (London: Heinemann, 1956)

Podestà di Torcello, *Domenico Viglari (1290–1291)*, ed. Paolo Zolli (Venice: Il Comitato Editore, 1966)

The principal navigations, voyages, traffiques, and discoveries of the English nation, collected by Richard Hakluyt, ed. Edmund Goldsmid (Edinburgh: E. & G. Goldsmid, 1885-90), vol. 8, online at http://ebooks.adelaide.edu.au/h/hakluyt/voyages/rubruquis/

Regestrum visitationum archiepiscopi Rothomagensis: Journal des visites pastorales d'Eude Rigaud, archevêque de Rouen. MCCXLVIII–MCCLXIX, ed. Théodose Bonnin (Rouen: Le Brument, 1852)

The Register of Eudes of Rouen, ed. Jeremiah F. O'Sullivan and trans. Sidney M. Brown, Records of Civilization, Sources and Studies 72 (New York: Columbia University Press, 1964)

'Regulations of the Leper Hospital of St. Mary Magdalene, Exeter, as Restated early in the Fifteenth Century', in Peter Richards, *The Medieval Leper and his Northern Heirs* (Cambridge: D. S. Brewer, 1977; repr. 2000), pp. 140–1

Revelationes Gertrudianae ac Mechtildianae, ed. Dom Ludwig Paquelin, 2 vols (Paris: H. Oudin, 1875-77)

A Revelation of Purgatory by an Unknown Fifteenth-Century Woman Visionary, ed. and trans. Martha P. Harley (Lewiston, NY: Edwin Mellen, 1985)

The Revelations of Saint Birgitta, ed. W. P. Cumming, EETS o.s. 178 (Oxford: Oxford University Press, 1929)

Richard Morris's Prick of Conscience: A Corrected and Amplified Reading Text, ed. Ralph Hanna and Sarah Wood, EETS o.s. 342 (Oxford: Oxford University Press, 2013)

Robert of Brunne's 'Handlyng Synne', ed. F. J. Furnivall, 2 parts in 1 vol., EETS, o.s. 119, 123 (London: Kegan Paul, Trench & Trübner, 1901)

Robert of Flamborough, *Liber penitentialis*, ed. J.-J. Firth, Pontifical Institute for Mediaeval Studies, Studies and Texts 18 (Toronto: Pontifical Institute for Mediaeval Studies, 1971)

Rolle, Richard, *The Incendium Amoris of Richard Rolle of Hampole*, ed. Margaret Deanesly (Manchester: University of Manchester Press, 1915)

Sampson, Abbot, 'Opus de miraculis Sancti Ædmundi', in *Memorials of St Edmund's Abbey*, ed. T. Arnold, Rolls Series 96 (London, 1890)

Secretum secretorum: Nine English Versions, ed. M. A. Manzalaoui, EETS e.s. 276 (Oxford: Oxford University Press, 1977)

Select Pleas of the Crown, vol. I: AD 1200-1225, ed. F. W. Maitland, Selden Society Publications 1 (London: Bernard Quaritch, 1888)

Somerset Medieval Wills, 1383-1500, ed. F. W. Weaver (London: Somerset Record Society, 1901)

Soranus' Gynecology, trans. Owsei Temkin (Baltimore, MD: Johns Hopkins University Press, 1956)

A Source Book in Medieval Science, ed. Edward Grant (Cambridge, MA: Harvard University Press, 1974)

Sources for the History of Medicine in Late Medieval England, ed. and trans. Carole Rawcliffe (Kalamazoo, MI: Medieval Institute Publications, 1995)

'Statuta Hospitalis de Sancto Juliano', in Peter Richards, *The Medieval Leper and His Northern Heirs* (Cambridge: D. S. Brewer, 1977; repr., 2000), pp. 129–36

'Statuts de la léproserie d'Amiens', in *Statuts d'Hôtels-Dieu et de léproseries: recueil de textes du XIIe au XIVe siècle*, ed. Léon Le Grand (Paris: Alphonse Picard, 1901), pp. 224–30

'Statuts de la léproserie des Andelys', in *Statuts d'Hôtels-Dieu et de léproseries: recueil de textes du XIIe au XIVe siècle*, ed. Léon Le Grand (Paris: Alphonse Picard, 1901), pp. 246–52

'Statuts de la léproserie de Meaux', in *Statuts d'Hôtels-Dieu et de léproseries: recueil de textes du XIIe au XIVe siècle*, ed. Léon Le Grand (Paris: Alphonse Picard, 1901), pp. 184–90

St Patrick's Purgatory: Two Versions of Owayne Miles and the Vision of William of Stranton, Together with the Long Text of the Tractatus de Purgatorio Sancti Patricii, ed. Robert Easting, EETS o.s. 298 (Oxford: Oxford University Press, 1991)

Theodoric, *The Surgery of Theodoric, ca. A. D. 1267*, trans. Eldridge Campbell and James Colton, 2 vols (New York: Appleton-Century-Crofts, 1955)

Thietmar von Merseburg, *Chronik*, ed. Werner Trillmich, FSGA Band 9 (Darmstadt: Wissenschaftliche Buchgesellschaft, 2002)

Three Prose Versions of the Secreta secretorum, vol. 1, ed. Robert Steele, EETS e.s. 74 (London: Kegan Paul, Trench & Trübner, 1898)

Three Purgatory Poems: The Gast of Gy, Sir Owain, The Vision of Tundale, ed. Edward E. Foster (Kalamazoo, MI: Medieval Institute Publications, 2004)

Three Women of Liège, A Critical Edition of and Commentary on the Middle English Lives of Elizabeth of Spalbeek, Christina Mirabilis, and Marie d'Oignies, ed. Jennifer Brown (Turnhout: Brepols, 2008)

'A Treatise on the Elections of Times', in *Popular and Practical Science of Medieval England*, ed. Lister M. Matheson (East Lansing, MI: Colleagues Press, 1994), pp. 23-59

The Trotula: An English Translation of the Medieval Compendium of Women's Medicine, ed. and trans. Monica H. Green (Philadelphia: University of Pennsylvania Press, 2001)

The Vision of Edmund Leversedge: A Fifteenth-Century Account of a Visit to the Otherworld edited from BL MS Additional 14193, ed. Wiesje F. Nijenhuis (Nijmegen: Centrum voor Middeleeuwse Studies, Katholieke Universiteit Nijmegen, 1991)

'Les "vitae sororum" d'Unterlinden: Édition critique du manuscrit 508 de la Bibliothèque de Colmar', ed. Jeanne Ancelet-Hustache, *Archives d'histoire doctrinale et littéraire du moyen âge* 5 (1930), 317–517

de Voragine, Jacobus, *The Golden Legend*, http://www.catholic-forum.com/saints/golden145.htm

de Voragine, Jacobus, *The Golden Legend or Lives of the Saints*, trans. William Caxton, ed. F. S. Ellis, published online in Internet History Sourcebooks: http://www.fordham.edu/halsall/basis/goldenlegend/

de Voragine, Jacobus, *Legenda Aurea: Vulgo Historia Lombardica Dicta ad Optimorum Librorum Fidem*, ed. Th. Grasse. http://archive.org/details/jacobiavoragine00jacogoog

Wenzel, Siegfried, *Latin Sermon Collections from Later Medieval England: Orthodox Preaching in the Age of Wyclif* (Cambridge: Cambridge University Press, 2005)

Yorkshire Writers, ed. C. Horstmann, 2 vols (London: Swan Sonnenschein, 1895–96)

SECONDARY SOURCES

Aers, David, 'The Making of Margery Kempe: Individual and Community', in *The Book of Margery Kempe*, ed. and trans. Lynn Staley (New York and London: Norton, 2001), pp. 256–64

Albala, K., 'To Your Health: Wine as Food and Medicine in Mid-Sixteenth-Century Italy', in *Alcohol: A Social and Cultural History*, ed. Mack P. Holt (Oxford: Berg, 2006), pp. 11–24

Allers, Rudolph, 'Microcosmos: From Anaximandros to Paracelsus', *Traditio* 2 (1944), 319–407

Anderson, George Christian, 'Medieval Medicine for Sin', *Journal of Religion and Health* 2. 2 (1963), 156–65

Arbesmann, R., 'The Concept of "*Christus medicus*" in St Augustine', *Traditio* 10 (1954), 1–28

Bainbridge, V. R., *Gilds in the Countryside: Social and Religious Change in Cambridgeshire, c.1350–1558* (Woodbridge: Boydell, 1996)

Balss, H., *Albertus Magnus als Zoologe* (Munich: Münchner Drucke, 1928)

Barfield, Owen, *Saving the Appearances: A Study in Idolatry* (Middletown, CT: Wesleyan University Press, 1988)

Barratt, Alexandra, '"In the Lowest Part of Our Need": Julian and Medieval Gynecological Writing', in *Julian of Norwich: A Book of Essays*, ed. Sandra J. McEntire, Garland Medieval Casebooks 21 (New York: Garland, 1998), pp. 239–56

Barron, C. M., 'The Parish Fraternities of Medieval London', in *The Church in Pre-Reformation Society*, ed. Caroline M. Barron and Christopher Harper-Bill (Woodbridge: Boydell, 1985), pp. 13–37

Bell, Rudolph M., *Holy Anorexia* (Chicago, IL and London: University of Chicago Press, 1985)

Benedek, Thomas, 'The Roles and Images of Medieval Women in the Healing Arts', in *The Roles and Images of Women in the Middle Ages and Renaissance*, ed. Douglas Radcliffe-Umstead (Pittsburgh, PA: University of Pittsburgh Press, 1975), pp.145–59

Bennett, H. S., 'Science and Information in English Writings of the Fifteenth Century', *Modern Language Review* 39 (1944), 1–8

Bennett, Michael J., 'John Audelay: Life Records and Heaven's Ladder', in *My Wyl and My Wrytyng: Essays on John the Blind Audelay*, ed. Susanna Fein (Kalamazoo, MI: Medieval Institute Publications, 2009), pp. 30–53

Bériou, Nicole, 'Les Lépreux sous le regard des prédicateurs d'après les collections de sermons *ad status* du XIIIème siècle', in Nicole Bériou and François-Olivier Touati, *Voluntate dei leprosus: les Lépreux entre conversion et exclusion aux XIIème et XIIIème siècles*, Testi, Studi, Strumenti 4 (Spoleto: Centro italiano di studi sull'altro medioevo, 1991), pp. 33–80

Biernoff, Suzannah, *Sight and Embodiment in the Middle Ages* (Basingstoke: Palgrave Macmillan, 2002)

Biller, Peter, '"Deep Is the Heart of Man, and Inscrutable": Signs of Heresy in Medieval Languedoc', in *Text and Controversy from Wyclif to Bale: Essays in Honour of Anne Hudson*, ed. Helen Barr and Ann M. Hutchison (Turnhout: Brepols, 2005), pp. 267–80

Biller, Peter A., 'Birth-Control in the West in the Thirteenth and Early Fourteenth Centuries', *Past & Present* 94 (1982), 3–26

Biller, Peter and A. J. Minnis (eds), *Handling Sin: Confession in the Middle Ages* (York: York Medieval Press, 1998)

Biller, Peter and Joseph Ziegler (eds), *Religion and Medicine in the Middle Ages* (York: York Medieval Press, 2001)

Bishop, Louise M., *Words, Stones, Herbs: The Healing Word in Medieval and Early Modern England* (Syracuse, NY: Syracuse University Press, 2007)

Bloomfield, M. W., *The Seven Deadly Sins* (East Lansing, MI: Michigan State College Press, 1952; repr. 1967)

Boenig, Robert, 'St Augustine's *jubilus* and Richard Rolle's *canor*', in *Vox Mystica: Essays for Valerie M. Lagorio*, ed. Anne Clark Bartlett et al. (Cambridge: D. S. Brewer, 1995), pp. 75–86

Boitani, Piero, 'His desir wol fle withouten wynges: Mary and Love in Fourteenth-Century Poetry', in *Chaucer's Frame Tales*, ed. Joerg O. Fichte (Cambridge: D. S. Brewer, 1987), pp. 83–128

Bonfield, Christopher, 'The *Regimen Sanitatis* and its Dissemination in England, *c*. 1348–1550', Ph.D. thesis, University of East Anglia, 2006

Boswell, John, *The Kindness of Strangers: The Abandonment of Children in Western Europe from Late Antiquity to the Renaissance* (New York: Pantheon, 1988)

Boyle, M. O. R., 'Aquinas's Natural Heart', *Early Science and Medicine* 18, 3 (2013), 266–90

Braswell, Laurel, 'The Moon and Medicine in Chaucer's Time', *Studies in the Age of Chaucer* 8 (1986), 145–56

Brenner, Elma, 'Recent Perspectives on Leprosy in Medieval Western Europe', *History Compass* 8 (2010), 388–406

Brenner, Elma, *Leprosy and Charity in Medieval Rouen* (Woodbridge: Royal Historical Society/Boydell Press, forthcoming 2015/2016)

Brenner, Elma, Liz Herbert McAvoy and Patricia Skinner, 'Care and Cure: Diseases, Disabilities and Therapies: Conference Report', *Wellcome History* 51 (2013), 26–7

Bridges, Margaret, 'Ubi Est Thesaurus Tuus, Ibi Est Cor Tuum: Towards a History of the Displaced Heart in Medieval English', *Micrologus: Natura, Scienze e Societa Medievali/Nature, Sciences and Medieval Societies* 11 (2003), 501–19

Brinker-von der Heyde, Claudia, *Die literarische Welt des Mittelalters* (Darmstadt: Wissenschaftliche Buchgesellschaft, 2007)

Brody, Saul Nathaniel, *The Disease of the Soul: Leprosy in Medieval Literature* (Ithaca, NY and London: Cornell University Press, 1974)

Brooks, Harold F., *Chaucer's Pilgrims: The Artistic Order of the Portraits in the Prologue* (London: Methuen, 1962)

Bruce, Vicki and Andy Young, *Face Perception* (London and New York: Psychology Press, 2012)

Brundage, James A., *Law, Sex and Christian Society in Medieval Europe* (Chicago, IL: University of Chicago Press, 1987)

Buckley, Peter, 'Mystical Experience and Schizophrenia', *Schizophrenia Bulletin* 7 (1981), 516–21

Bullough, Vern L., *Sexual Variance in Society and History* (New York: John Wiley, 1976)

Bullough, Vern L. and James A. Brundage (eds), *Sexual Practices in the Medieval Church* (Buffalo, NY: Prometheus Books, 1982)

Bynum, Caroline Walker, *Holy Feast and Holy Fast: The Religious Significance of Food to Medieval Women* (Los Angles and London: University of California Press, 1987)

Bynum, Caroline Walker, *Jesus as Mother: Studies in the Spirituality of the High Middle Ages* (Berkeley, CA: University of California Press, 1992)

Bynum, Caroline Walker, *Wonderful Blood: Theology and Practice in Late Medieval Germany and Beyond* (Philadelphia: University of Pennsylvania Press, 2007)

Caballero Navas, Carmen, 'The Care of Women's Health and Beauty: an Experience Shared by Medieval Jewish and Christian Women', *Journal of Medieval History* 34 (2008), 146–63

Caciola, Nancy, *Discerning Spirits: Divine and Demonic Possession in the Middle Ages* (Ithaca, NY and London: Cornell University Press, 2003)

Cadden, Joan, *The Meanings of Sex Difference in the Middle Ages: Medicine, Science, and Culture* (Cambridge and New York: Cambridge University Press, 1993)

Calvi, Lisana, '"Is't Lunacy to call a spade, a spade?": James Carkesse and the Forgotten Language of Madness', in *Medieval and Early Modern Literature, Science and Medicine*, ed. Rachel Falconer and Denis Renevey, Swiss Papers in English Language and Literature 28 (Tübingen: Gunter Narr, 2013), pp. 139–52

Camargo, Martin, 'Defining Medieval Rhetoric', in *Rhetoric and Renewal in the Latin West 1100–1540: Essays in Honour of John O. Ward*, ed. Constant Mews, Cary Nederman and Rod M. Thomson (Turnhout: Brepols, 2003), pp. 21–34

Cameron, M. L., *Anglo-Saxon Medicine* (Cambridge: Cambridge University Press, 1993)

Carrel, Helen, 'The Ideology of Punishment in Late Medieval English Towns', *Social History* 34 (2009), 301–20

Casagrande, Carla, 'Il dolore virtuoso: per una storia medievale della pazienza', in *Piacere e Dolore: materiali per una storia delle passioni nel Medioevo*, ed. Carla Casagrande and Silvana Vecchio (Florence: Sismel-Edizione del Galluzzo, 2009), pp. 31–47

Charleston, R. J., 'Vessel Glass', in *English Medieval Industries: Craftsmen, Techniques, Products*, ed. J. Blair and N. Ramsay (London, 1991), pp. 237–64

Chewning, Susannah M. (ed.), *Intersections of Sexuality and the Divine in Medieval Culture: the Word Made Flesh* (Aldershot: Ashgate, 2005)

Citrome, Jeremy J., 'Medicine as Metaphor in the Middle English *Cleanness*', *Chaucer Review* 35 (2001), 260–80

Citrome, Jeremy J., *The Surgeon in Medieval English Literature* (New York: Palgrave Macmillan, 2006)

Claridge, Gordon, Ruth Pryor and Gwen Watkins, *Sounds from the Bell Jar: Ten Psychotic Authors* (Basingstoke: Macmillan, 1990)

Clark, Elizabeth A., 'Sane Insanity: Women and Asceticism in Late Ancient Christianity', *Medieval Encounters* 3 (1997), 211–30

Cole, Andrew, 'Heresy and Humanism', in *Oxford Twenty-First Century Approaches to Literature: Middle English*, ed. Paul Strohm (Oxford: Oxford University Press, 2007), pp. 421–3

Colledge, Edmund, 'Margery Kempe', in *Pre-Reformation English Spirituality*, ed. James Walsh (New York: Fordham University Press, 1966), pp. 210–23

Corner, George W., *Anatomical Texts of the Earlier Middle Ages: A Study in the Transmission of Culture* (Washington, DC: Carnegie Institution of Washington, 1927)

Cox Miller, Patricia, 'Visceral Seeing: the Holy Body in Late Ancient Christianity', *Journal of Early Christian Studies* 12 (2004), 391–411

Craun, Marlys S., 'Personal Accounts: The Story of Margery Kempe', *Psychiatry Services* 56 (2005), 655–6.

Crowther, J. D. W., 'Chaucer's *Physician's Tale* and its "Saint"', *English Studies in Canada* 8, 2 (1982), 125–37

Cullum, Patricia H., 'Hospitals and Charitable Provision in Medieval Yorkshire', unpublished Ph.D. thesis, University of York, 1989

Davies, M., 'The Tailors of London: Corporate Charity in the Late Medieval Town', in *Crown, Government and People in the Fifteenth Century*, ed. R. Archer (Stroud: Sutton, 1995), pp. 161–90

de Jong, Mayke, *In Samuel's Image: Child Oblation in the Early Medieval West* (Leiden: Brill, 1996)

De Pablo, Gonzales A. and N. J. R. Evans, 'The Medicine of the Soul: The Origin and Development of Thought on the Soul, Diseases of the Soul and their Treatment in Medieval and Renaissance Medicine', *History of Psychiatry* 5 (1994), 483–516

Dean, Trevor and Kate Lowe (eds), *Marriage in Italy, 1300–1650* (Cambridge: Cambridge University Press, 1998)

Delany, Sheila, 'Sexual Economics, Chaucer's Wife of Bath and *The Book of Margery Kempe*', in *Feminist Readings in Middle English Literature: The Wife of Bath and All Her Sect*, ed. Ruth Evans and Leslie Johnson (London: Routledge, 1994), pp. 72–87

Delarun, Jacques et al. (eds), *The Stigmata of Francis of Assisi: New Studies, New Perspectives* (New York: St Bonaventure, 2006)

Demaitre, Luke, *Leprosy in Premodern Medicine: A Malady of the Whole Body* (Baltimore, MD: Johns Hopkins University Press, 2007)

Diagnostic and Statistical Manual of Mental Disorders (Washington, DC: American Psychiatric Association, 2000)

Diagnostic and Statistical Manual of Mental Disorders DSM-5 (Washington, DC: American Psychiatric Association, 2013)

Dickman, Susan, 'Margery Kempe and the Continental Tradition of the Pious Woman', in *The Medieval Mystical Tradition in England*, ed. Marion Glasscoe (Cambridge: D. S. Brewer, 1984), pp. 150–68

Diepgen, Paul, 'Der Einfluß der autoritativen Theologie auf die Medizin des Mittelalters', *Akademie der Wissenschaften und der Literatur.* Abhandlungen der geistes- und sozialwissenschaftlichen Klasse, vol. 1 (Mainz: *Akademie der Wissenschaften und der Literatur*, 1958), pp. 1–20

Dols, Michael W., *Majnûn: The Madman in Medieval Islamic Society*, ed. Diana E. Immisch (Oxford: Oxford University Press, 1992)

Dondaine, H., *L'Attrition suffisante* (Paris: J. Vrin, 1943)

Douiehi, Milad, *A Perverse History of the Human Heart* (Cambridge, MA: Harvard University Press, 1997)

Driver, Martha W., 'John Audelay and the Bridgettines', in *My Wyl and My Wrytyng: Essays on John the Blind Audelay*, ed. Susanna Fein (Kalamazoo, MI: Medieval Institute Publications, 2009), pp. 191–217

Drucker, Trudi, 'The Malaise of Margery Kempe', *New York State Journal of Medicine* 72 (1972), 2911–16

Duffy, E., *The Stripping of the Altars: Traditional Religion in England c.1400–1580*, 2nd edn (New Haven, CT: Yale University Press, 2005)

Dumas, Geneviève, 'Le soin des cheveux et des poils: quelques pratiques cosmétiques (XIII–XVI siècles)', in *La chevelure dans la littérature et l'art du moyen age*, ed. Chantal Connochie-Bourgne (Aix-en-Provence: Publications de l'Université de Provence, 2004), pp. 129–41

Easting, Robert, '"Choose Yourselves Whither to Go": John Audelay's *Vision of Saint Paul*', in *My Wyl and My Wrytyng: Essays on John the Blind Audelay*, ed. Susanna Fein (Kalamazoo, MI: Medieval Institute Publications, 2009), pp. 170–90

Eberly, Susan S., 'Margery Kempe, St Mary Magdalene, and Patterns of Contemplation', *The Downside Review* 368 (1989), 209–23

Eco, Umberto, *On Beauty: The History of a Western Idea* (London: Weidenfeld, 2004)

Eco, Umberto, *On Ugliness* (London: Weidenfeld, 2007)

Economou, George D., *The Goddess Natura in Medieval Literature* (Cambridge, MA: Harvard University Press, 1972)

Elliott, Dyan, 'Women and Confession: From Empowerment to Pathology', in *Gendering the Master Narrative: Women and Power in the Middle Ages*, ed. Mary C. Erler and Maryanne Kowaleski (Ithaca, NY and London: Cornell University Press, 2003), pp. 31–51

Elliott, Dyan, *Proving Woman: Female Spirituality and Inquisitional Culture in the Later Middle Ages* (Princeton: Princeton University Press, 2004)

Enderle, A., D. Meyerhöfer and G. Unverfehrt (eds), *Kleine Menschen – Große Kunst. Kleinwuchs aus künstlerischer und medizinischer Sicht* (Hamm: Artcolor, 1992)

Erler, Mary C., *Women, Reading, and Piety in Late Medieval England* (Cambridge: Cambridge University Press, 2002)

Erler, Mary C., '"A Revelation of Purgatory" (1422): Reform and the Politics of Female Visions', *Viator* 38 (2007), 321–47

Evans, G. R., *Law and Theology in the Middle Ages* (London and New York: Routledge, 2002)

Falconer, Rachel and Denis Renevey (eds), *Medieval and Early Modern Literature, Science and Medicine*, Swiss Papers in English Language and Literature 28 (Tübingen: Gunter Narr, 2013)

Farley, Mary Hardiman, 'Her Own Creature: Religion, Feminist Criticism, and the Functional Eccentricity of Margery Kempe', *Exemplaria* 11 (1999), 1–21

Farmer, D., *The Oxford Dictionary of Saints*, 4th edn (Oxford: Oxford University Press, 1997)

Fein, Susanna, 'Good Ends in the Audelay Manuscript', *The Yearbook of English Studies* 33 (2003), 97–119

Fein, Susanna, 'Death and the Colophon in the Audelay Manuscript', in *My Wyl and My Wrytyng: Essays on John the Blind Audelay*, ed. Susanna Fein (Kalamazoo, MI: Medieval Institute Publications, 2009), pp. 294–306

Fein, Susanna, 'John Audelay and His Book: Critical Overview and Major Issues', in *My Wyl and My Wrytyng: Essays on John the Blind Audelay*, ed. Susanna Fein (Kalamazoo, MI: Medieval Institute Publications, 2009), pp. 3–29

Fein, Susanna, 'English Devotions for a Noble Household: The Long Passion in Audelay's Counsel of Conscience', in *After Arundel: Religious Writing in Fifteenth-Century England*, ed. Vincent Gillespie and Kantik Ghosh (Turnhout: Brepols, 2011), pp. 325–42

Fein, Susanna, 'Mary to Veronica: John Audelay's Sequence of Salutations to God-Bearing Women', *Speculum* 86 (2011), 964–1009

Fenster, Thelma and Daniel Lord Smail (eds), *Fama: The Politics of Talk and Reputation in Medieval Europe* (Ithaca, NY: Cornell University Press, 2003)

Fenton, Kirsten A., 'Gendering the First Crusade in William of Malmesbury's *Gesta Regum Anglorum*', in *Intersections of Gender, Religion and Ethnicity in the Middle Ages*, ed. Cordelia Beattie and Kirsten Fenton (London: Palgrave Macmillan, 2011), pp. 125–39

Finnegan, Mary Jeremy, *The Women of Helfta: Scholars and Mystics* (Athens, GA: University of Georgia Press, 1991)

Förster, M., 'Vom Fortleben antiker Sammellunare in englischen und anderen Volkssprachen', *Anglia* 67–68 (1944), 1–171

Foucault, Michel, *Discipline and Punish: The Birth of the Prison*, trans. A. Sheridan (London: Allen Lane, 1977)

Foucault, Michel, *The Will to Knowledge: History of Sexuality*, vol. 1, trans. Robert Hurley (Harmondsworth: Penguin, 1998)

Fournée, Jean, 'Les Maladreries et les vocables de leurs chapelles', *Lèpre et lépreux en Normandie, Cahiers Léopold Delisle* 46 (1997), 49–142

Frampton, Michael, *Embodiments of Will: Anatomical and Physiological Theories of Voluntary Animal Motion from Greek Antiquity to the Latin Middle Ages, 400 B.C.–A.D. 1300* (Saarbrücken: VDM Verlag Dr. Müller, 2008)

Freeman, Phyllis R., Carley R. Bogarad and Diane E. Sholomskas, 'Margery Kempe, a New Theory: The Inadequacy of Hysteria and Postpartum Psychosis as Diagnostic Categories', *History of Psychiatry* 1 (1990), 169–90

Friedman, John Block, *The Monstrous Races in Medieval Art and Thought* (Cambridge, MA: Harvard University Press, 1981)

Gasse, Rosanne, 'The Practice of Medicine in *Piers Plowman*', *The Chaucer Review* 39, 2 (2004), 177–97

Gayk, Shannon and Kathleen Tonry (eds), *Form and Reform: Reading across the Fifteenth Century* (Columbus, OH: Ohio State University Press, 2011)

Geerlings, Wilhelm, 'The Decalogue in Augustine's Theology', in *The Decalogue in Jewish and Christian Tradition*, ed. Henning Graf Reventlow and Yair Hoffman (New York: T&T Clark, 2011), pp. 106–17

Getz, Faye, *Medicine in the English Middle Ages* (Princeton: Princeton University Press, 1998)

Getz, Faye Marie, 'Charity, Translation and the Language of Medical Learning in Medieval England', *The Bulletin of the History of Medicine* 64 (1990), 1–17

Gil-Sotres, Pedro, 'Derivation and Revulsion: The Theory and Practice of Medieval Phlebotomy', in *Practical Medicine from Salerno to the Black Death*, ed. Luis Garcia-Ballester, Roger French, Jon Arrizabalaga and Andrew Cunningham (Cambridge: Cambridge University Press, 1994), pp. 110–55

Gil-Sotres, Pedro, 'The Regimens of Health', in *Western Medical Thought from Antiquity to the Middle Ages*, ed. Mirko D. Grmek (Cambridge, MA: Harvard University Press, 1998), pp. 291–318

Gillespie, Vincent, '"[S]he do the police in different voices": Pastiche, Ventriloquism and Parody in Julian of Norwich', in *A Companion to Julian of Norwich*, ed. Liz Herbert McAvoy (Cambridge: D. S. Brewer, 2008), pp. 192–207

Gillespie, Vincent, '1412–1534: Culture and History', in *The Cambridge Companion to Medieval English Mysticism*, ed. Samuel Fanous and Vincent Gillespie (Cambridge: Cambridge University Press, 2011), pp. 163–93

Gleeson, B., *Geographies of Disability* (New York: Routledge, 1999)

Goffman, Erving, *Stigma: Notes on the Management of Spoiled Identity* (Englewood Cliffs, NJ: Prentice-Hall, 1963; repr. London: Penguin, 1990)

Goldberg, P. J. P., 'Performing the Word of God: Corpus Christi Drama in the Northern Province', in *Life and Thought in the Northern Church c.1100–1700*, ed. Diana Wood, Studies in Church History, Subsidia 12 (Woodbridge: Boydell, 1999), pp. 145–70

Gonthier, Nathalie, *Le châtiment du crime au Moyen Âge (XIIe–XVIe siècles)* (Rennes: Presses Universitaires de Rennes, 1998)

Good, Byron J., *Medicine, Rationality, and Experience: An Anthropological Perspective* (Cambridge: Cambridge University Press, 1994)

Goodey, Chris, *A History of Intelligence and 'Intellectual Disability': The Shaping of Psychology in Early Modern Europe* (Farnham: Ashgate, 2011)

Goodich, Michael, *Vita Perfecta: The Ideal of Sainthood in the Thirteenth Century*, Monogr. Geschichte des Mittelalters 25 (Stuttgart: Anton Hiersemann, 1982)

Goodich, Michael, *From Birth to Old Age: The Human Life Cycle in Medieval Thought, 1250–1350* (Lanham, MD and London: University Press of America, 1989)

Graef, Hilda, 'Devotion to Our Lady', *Twentieth-Century Encyclopedia of Catholicism*, vol. 45, ed. Henri Daniel-Rops (New York: Hawthorn Books, 1963)

Graef, Hilda, *Mary: A History of Doctrine and Devotion* (New York: Sheed and Ward, 1963; repr. Notre Dame, IN: Ave Maria Press, 2009)

Green, Monica H., 'Women's Medical Practice and Health Care in Medieval Europe', *Signs* 14, 2 (1989), 434–73

Green, Monica H., 'Documenting Medieval Women's Medical Practice', in *Practical Medicine from Salerno to the Black Death*, ed. Luis Garcia-Ballester, Roger French, Jon Arrizabalaga and Andrew Cunningham (Cambridge: Cambridge University Press, 1994), pp. 322–52

Green, Monica H., 'Bodies, Gender, Health, Disease: Recent Work on Medieval Women's Medicine', *Studies in Medieval and Renaissance History*, 3rd series 2 (2005), 1–46

Green, Monica H., 'Constantine the African', in *Medical Science, Technology, and Medicine: An Encyclopedia*, ed. Thomas Glick, Steven J. Livesey and Faith Wallis (New York and Abingdon: Routledge, 2005), pp. 145–7

Green, Monica H., *Making Women's Medicine Masculine: The Rise of Male Authority in Pre-Modern Gynaecology* (Oxford: Oxford University Press, 2008)

Green, Monica H., 'Integrative Medicine: Incorporating Medicine and Health into the Canon of Medieval European History', *History Compass* 7 (2009), 1218–45

Green, Monica H., 'The Value of Historical Perspective', in *The Ashgate Research Companion to the Globalization of Health*, ed. Ted Schrecker et al. (Ashgate, forthcoming)

Green, Monica H., 'Bibliography on Medieval Women, Gender, and Medicine (1980–2009)', at http://www.sciencia.cat/biblioteca/documents/Green_Cumulative Bib_Feb2010.pdf

Green, Monica H., 'Trota and the "Trotula"', at https://independent.academia.edu/MonicaGreen1/Trota-and-the-%27Trotula%27#add

Green, Richard Firth, 'Marcolf the Fool and Blind John Audelay', in *Speaking Images: Essays in Honor of V. A. Kolve*, ed. R. F. Yeager and Charlotte C. Morse (Ashville, NC: Pegasus Press, 2001), pp. 559–76

Grisé, C. Annette, 'Continental Holy Women and the Textual Relics of Prayers in Late-Medieval England', in *The Medieval Translator*, vol. 10, ed. Jacqueline Jenkins and Olivier Bertrand (Turnhout: Brepols, 2007), pp. 165–78

Groebner, Valentin, 'Losing Face, Saving Face: Noses and Honour in the Later Medieval Town', *History Workshop Journal* 40 (1995), 1–15

Groebner, Valentin, *Defaced: the Visual Culture of Violence in the Later Middle Ages*, trans. Pamela Selwyn (New York: Zone Books, 2004)

Groebner, Valentin, *Who are You? Identification, Deception and Surveillance in Early Modern Europe*, trans. Mark Kyburz and John Peck (New York: Zone Books, 2007)

Grossel, Marie-Geneviève, 'Entre médecine et magie: les gestes de beauté (l'*Ornatus Mulierum*)', in *Le geste et les gestes au moyen age: colloque* (Aix-en-Provence: Le Centre Universitaire d'Etudes et de Recherches Médiévales d'Aix, 1998), pp. 255–72

The Guardian, Weekend Edition (London and Manchester, Saturday 22 March 2014), 1, 16–17, 27, 30–1

Hackett, Benedict, Edmund Colledge and Noel Chadwick, 'William Flete's "De Remediis contra Temptaciones" in its Latin and English Recensions: The Growth of a Text', *Mediaeval Studies* 26 (1964), 210–30

Hagen, A., *A Second Handbook of Anglo-Saxon Food and Drink: Production and Distribution* (Hockwold cum Witton, Norfolk: Anglo-Saxon Books, 1995)

Haines, Roy Martin, 'Reginald Pecock: A Tolerant Man in an Age of Intolerance', *Studies in Church History* 21 (1984), 125–37

Hamburger, Jeffrey F., *Nuns as Artists: The Visual Culture of a Medieval Convent* (Berkeley, CA: University of California Press, 1997)

Harding, Wendy, 'Medieval Women's Unwritten Discourse on Motherhood: A Reading of Two Fifteenth-Century Texts', *Women's Studies* 21 (1992), 197–209

Harington, John, Sir et al., *The School of Salernum: Regimen sanitatis Salernitanum/ The English Version by Sir John Harington; History of the School of Salernum by Francis R. Packard; and a note on the prehistory of the Regimen sanitatis by Fielding H. Garrison* (New York: A. M. Kelly, 1920; repr. 1970)

Harley, David, 'Rhetoric and the Social Construction of Sickness', *Social History of Medicine* 12 (1999), 407–35

Harvey, E. R., *The Inward Wits: Psychological Theory in the Middle Ages and Renaissance* (London: Warburg Institute, 1975)

Hasse, Dag Nikolaus, 'The Soul's Faculties', in *The Cambridge History of Medieval Philosophy*, ed. Robert Pasnau, vol. 1, 1st edn (Cambridge: Cambridge University Press, 2009), pp. 305–19

Hawkins, Joy, 'The Blind in Later Medieval England: Medical, Social and Religious Responses', unpublished Ph.D. thesis, University of East Anglia, 2011

Hawkins, Joy, 'Seeing the Light? Blindness and Sanctity in Later Medieval England', in *Saints and Sanctity*, ed. Peter Clarke and Tony Claydon, Studies in Church History 47 (Woodbridge: Boydell, 2011), pp. 148–58

Hawkins, Joy, 'Sights for Sore Eyes: Vision and Health in Medieval England', in *On Light: Aspects and Responses*, ed. K. P. Clarke and Sarah Baccianti (Oxford: Medium Aevum, 2013), pp. 137–56

Hebgin-Barnes, Penny, *The Medieval Stained Glass of the County of Lincolnshire* (Oxford: Oxford University Press, 1996)

Hecker, Justus Friedrich Karl, 'An Historical Notice by Dr Hecker', *London Medical Gazette* 15 (1834), 813

Heintel, Helmut (ed.), *Quellen zur Geschichte der Epilepsie*, Hubers Klassiker der Medizin und der Naturwissenschaften Band XIV (Berne, Stuttgart and Vienna: Hans Huber, 1975)

Henderson, John, *The Renaissance Hospital: Healing the Body and Healing the Soul* (New Haven, CT and London: Yale University Press, 2006)

Hewson, M. Anthony, *Giles of Rome and the Medieval Theory of Conception* (London: Athlone Press, 1975)

Hill, Carole, *Women and Religion in Late Medieval Norwich* (Woodbridge: Boydell for the Royal Historical Society, 2010)

Hodges, Laura F., *Chaucer and Clothing: Clerical and Academic Costume in the General Prologue to The Canterbury Tales* (Cambridge: D. S. Brewer, 2005)

Hogg, James, 'Mount Grace Charterhouse and Late Medieval English Spirituality', *Analecta Cartusiana* 82 (1980), 1–43

Holsinger, Bruce W., *Music, Body, and Desire in Medieval Culture: Hildegard of Bingen to Chaucer* (Stanford, CA: Stanford University Press, 2001)

Homer, R. F., 'Tin, Lead and Pewter', in *A History of Technology*, ed. Charles Singer et al., 5 vols (Oxford: Clarendon Press, 1954–59), vol. 3, pp. 57–80

Hope Robbins, Russell, 'The Physician's Authorities', in *Studies in Language and Literature in Honour of Margaret Schlauch* (New York: Russell & Russell, 1971), pp. 335–41

Horden, Peregrine, 'A Non-Natural Environment: Medicine without Doctors and the Medieval European Hospital', in *The Medieval Hospital and Medical Practice*, ed. Barbara S. Bowers (Aldershot: Ashgate, 2007), pp. 133–45

Hubrath, Margarete, 'The *Liber specialis gratiae* as a Collective Work of Several Nuns', *Jahrbuch der Oswald von Wolkenstein Gesellschaft* 11 (1999), 233–44

Hudson, John, 'Violence, Theft and the Making of the English Common Law', in *Crime and Punishment in the Middle Ages*, ed. T. H. Haskett (Victoria, BC: Humanities Centre of the University of Victoria, 1998), pp. 19–35

Huet, Marie-Hélène, *Monstrous Imagination* (Cambridge, MA and London: Harvard University Press, 1993)

Hughes-Edwards, Mari, *Reading the Medieval Anchoritism: Ideology and Spiritual Practices* (Cardiff: University of Wales Press, 2012)

Huizinga, Johan, *The Waning of the Middle Ages*, trans. F. Hoffman (London: Penguin, 1955)

Innes-Parker, Catherine, 'The Legacy of *Ancrene Wisse*: Translations, Adaptations, Influences and Audience, with Special Attention to Women Readers', in *A Companion to* Ancrene Wisse, ed. Yoko Wada (Cambridge: D. S. Brewer, 2003), pp. 145–73

Innes-Parker, Catherine, '*The Doctrine of the Hert* and its Manuscript Context', in *A Companion to the Doctrine of the Hert: The Middle English Translation and its Latin and European Contexts*, ed. Denis Renevey and Christiania Whitehead (Exeter: University of Exeter Press, 2010), pp. 159–81

Irigaray, Luce, *This Sex which is not One*, trans. Catherine Porter with Carolyn Burke (Ithaca, NY: Cornell University Press, 1985), pp. 170–91

Jackson, Stanley W., *Melancholia and Depression: From Hippocratic Times to Modern Times* (New Haven, CT and London: Yale University Press, 1986)

Jacquard, D. and C. Thomasset, *Sexuality and Medicine in the Middle Ages*, trans. M. Adamson (Oxford: Polity, 1998)

Jager, Eric, *The Book of the Heart* (Chicago, IL: University of Chicago Press, 2000)

Jankrift, Kai P., *Mit Gott und schwarzer Magie. Medizin im Mittelalter* (Darmstadt: Wissenschaftliche Buchgesellschaft, 2005)

Jeanne, Damien, 'Le Groupe des lépreux à Saint-Lazare de Falaise aux XIVe et XVe siècles', in *Lépreux et sociabilité du Moyen Âge aux temps modernes*, ed. Bruno Tabuteau, Cahiers du GRHIS 11 ([Rouen]: Publications de l'Université de Rouen, 2000)

Jestice, Phyllis G., *Wayward Monks and the Revolution of the Eleventh Century* (Leiden: Brill, 1997)

Jones, Anne Hudson, 'Literature and Medicine: Traditions and Innovations', in *The Body and the Text: Comparative Essays in Literature and Medicine*, ed. Bruce Clarke and Wendell Aycock (Lubbock, TX: Texas Tech University Press, 1990), pp. 11–24

Kellenberger, Edgar, *Der Schutz der Einfältigen. Menschen mit einer geistigen Behinderung in der Bibel und in weiteren Quellen* (Zurich: Theologischer Verlag Zürich, 2011)

Kempton, Daniel, '*The Physician's Tale*: the Doctor of Physic's Diplomatic "Cure"', *Chaucer Review* 19, 1 (1984), 24–38

Kieckhefer, Richard, *Unquiet Souls: Fourteenth-Century Saints and Their Religious Milieu* (Chicago, IL: University of Chicago Press, 1984)

Kline, Barbara, 'The Discourse of Heaven in Mechtild of Hackeborn's *Booke of Gostlye Grace*', in *Imagining Heaven in the Middle Ages: A Book of Essays*, ed. Jan Swango Emerson and Hugh Feiss (New York: Garland, 2000), pp. 83–99

Knowles, David, *The English Mystical Tradition* (London and New York: Harper and Brothers, 1964)

Laharie, Muriel, *La Folie au Moyen Âge: xie-xiiie siècles* (Paris: Lion d'Or, 1991)

Lane, Harlan, *The Mask of Benevolence: Disabling the Deaf Community*, 2nd edn (San Diego, CA: Dawn Sign Press, 1999)

Langum, Virginia, 'Discerning Skin: Complexion, Surgery, and Language in Medieval Confession', in *Reading Skin in Medieval Literature and Culture*, ed. Katie L. Walter (New York: Palgrave Macmillan, 2013), pp. 141–60

Laqueur, Thomas, *Making Sex: Body and Gender from the Greeks to Freud* (Cambridge, MA: Harvard University Press, 1990)

Lavin, Marilyn Aronberg, 'The Mystic Winepress in the Mérode Altarpiece', in *Studies in Late Medieval and Renaissance Painting in Honour of Millard Meiss*, ed. Irving Lavin and John Plummer, 2 vols (New York: New York University Press, 1977), vol. 1, pp. 297–301

Lawes, Richard, 'The Madness of Margery Kempe', in *The Medieval Mystical Tradition in England, Ireland and Wales*, ed. Marion Glasscoe (Cambridge: D. S. Brewer, 1999), pp. 147–68

Lawes, Richard, 'Psychological Disorder and Autobiographical Impulse in Julian of Norwich, Margery Kempe and Thomas Hoccleve', in *Writing Religious Women: Female Spiritual and Textual Practices in Late Medieval England*, ed. Denis Renevey and Christiania Whitehead (Cardiff: Wales University Press, 2000), pp. 217–43

Le Goff, Jacques, *La naissance du purgatoire* (Paris: Gallimard, 1981)

Lemay, Helen Rodnite, 'Human Sexuality in Twelfth- through Fifteenth-Century Scientific Writings', in *Sexual Practices and the Medieval Church*, ed. Vern. L. Bullough and James Brundage (Buffalo, NY: Prometheus Books, 1982), pp. 187–205

Levene, M. I. and D. Tudehope, *Essentials of Neonatal Medicine*, 2nd edn (Oxford: Oxford University Press, 1993)

Lewis, Gertrud, 'Music and Dancing in the Fourteenth-Century Sister-Books', in *Vox Mystica: Essays for Valerie M. Lagorio*, ed. Anne Clark Bartlett et al. (Cambridge: D. S. Brewer, 1995), pp. 159–69

Lewis, Gertrud, *By Women, For Women, About Women: The Sister-Books of Fourteenth-Century Germany* (Toronto: Pontifical Institute of Mediaeval Studies, 1996)

Licence, Tom, *Hermits and Recluses in English Society, 950–1200* (Oxford: Oxford University Press, 2011)

Lochrie, Karma, *Margery Kempe and Translations of Flesh* (Philadelphia: University of Pennsylvania University, 1991)

Long, Julia, 'Mysticism and Hysteria: The Histories of Margery Kempe and Anna O.', in *Feminist Readings in Middle English Literature: The Wife of Bath and All Her Sect*, ed. Ruth Evans and Leslie Johnson (New York and London: Routledge, 1994), pp. 88–111

Manly, John M., 'Chaucer and the Rhetoricians', *Proceedings of the British Academy* 12 (1926), 95–113

Manly, John M. and Edith Rickert (eds), *The Text of The Canterbury Tales Studied on the Basis of All Known Manuscripts*, vol. 3 (Chicago, IL: University of Chicago Press, 1940)

Marenbon, John, 'The Emergence of Medieval Latin Philosophy', in *The Cambridge History of Medieval Philosophy*, ed. Robert Pasnau, 1st edn, vol. 1 (Cambridge: Cambridge University Press, 2009), pp. 26–38

Marneros, Andreas, 'Psychiatry's 200th Birthday', *The British Journal of Psychiatry* 193 (2008), 1–3

Marrone, Steven P., 'The Rise of the Universities', in *The Cambridge History of Medieval Philosophy*, ed. Robert Pasnau, 1st edn, vol. 1 (Cambridge: Cambridge University Press, 2009), pp. 50–62

Martin, A. Lynn, *Alcohol, Sex, and Gender in Late Medieval and Early Modern Europe* (Basingstoke: Palgrave, 2001)

Martin, Thomas F., '*Christus Medicus*', Talk given at a retreat for the friars of the Province of Saint Thomas of Villanova (Villanova University, June 2005) http://www.augustinianfriends.com/readingroom/Christus_Medicus.pdf.

Martineau-Genieys, Christine, 'Modèles, maquillage et misogynie, à travers les textes littéraires français du moyen age', in *Les soins de beauté, moyen age–début des temps modernes*, ed. Denis Menjot (Nice: Centre d'Etudes médiévales, 2004), pp. 31–50

Matsuda, Takami, *Death and Purgatory in Middle English Didactic Poetry* (Cambridge: D. S. Brewer, 1997)

Mays, Simon, 'Human Osteology at Wharram Percy: Life and Death in a Medieval Village', http://www.english-heritage.org.uk/publications/conservation-bulletin-45/cb45p22-23.pdf

McAvoy, Liz Herbert, *Authority and the Female Body in the Writings of Julian of Norwich and Margery Kempe* (Cambridge: D. S. Brewer, 1994)

McAvoy, Liz Herbert, *The Book of Margery Kempe: An Abridged Translation*,

Translated from the Middle English with Introduction, Notes, and Interpretive Essay (Cambridge: D. S. Brewer, 2003), pp. 105–26

McAvoy, Liz Herbert, '"For we be double of God's making": Writing, Gender and the Body in Julian of Norwich', in *A Companion to Julian of Norwich*, ed. Liz Herbert McAvoy (Cambridge: D. S. Brewer, 2008), pp. 166–80

McAvoy, Liz Herbert, *Medieval Anchoritisms: Gender, Space and the Solitary Life* (Cambridge: D. S. Brewer, 2011)

McAvoy, Liz Herbert, 'Envisioning Reform: *A Revelation of Purgatory* and Anchoritic *Compassioun* in the Later Middle Ages', in *The Medieval Mystical Tradition in England*, ed. E. A. Jones (Cambridge: D. S. Brewer, 2013), pp. 141–55

McCann, Justin, 'The Book of Margery Kempe', *The Dublin Review* 200 (1937), 103–16

McCleery, Iona, 'Medical "Emplotment" and Plotting Medicine: Health and Disease in Late Medieval Portuguese Chronicles', *Social History of Medicine* 24, 1 (2011), 125–41

McClive, Cathy, 'Menstrual Knowledge and Medical Practice in Early Modern France c. 1555–1761', in *Menstruation: A Cultural History*, ed. Andrew Shail and Gillian Howie (Basingstoke: Palgrave Macmillan, 2005), pp. 76–89

McCracken, Peggy, *The Curse of Eve, the Wound of the Hero: Blood, Gender and Medieval Literature* (Philadelphia: University of Pennsylvania Press, 2003)

McGlynn, Sean, *By Sword and Fire: Cruelty and Atrocity in Medieval Warfare* (London: Weidenfeld and Nicolson, 2008)

McLaughlin, Mary M., 'Survivors and Surrogates: Children and Parents from the Ninth to the Thirteenth Centuries', in *The History of Childhood: The Untold Story of Child Abuse*, ed. Lloyd De Mause (New York: Psychohistory Press, 1974), pp. 101–81

McRee, B., 'Charity and Gild Solidarity in Late Medieval England', *Journal of British Studies* 32 (1993), 195–225

McVaugh, Michael R., 'Bedside Manners in the Middle Ages', *Bulletin of the History of Medicine* 71 (1997), 201–23

Meaney, A. L., 'Women, Witchcraft and Magic in Anglo-Saxon England', in *Superstition and Popular Medicine in Anglo-Saxon England*, ed. D. G. Scragg (Manchester: Manchester Centre for Anglo-Saxon Studies, 1989), pp. 9–40

Merback, Mitchell T., *The Thief, the Cross and the Wheel: Pain and the Spectacle of Punishment in Medieval and Renaissance Europe* (London: Reaktion Books, 1999)

Merton, T., *What Are These Wounds? The Life of a Cistercian Mystic: Saint Lutgarde of Aywières* (Dublin: Bruce Publishing, 1980)

Metzler, Irina, *Disability in Medieval Europe: Thinking about Physical Impairment during the High Middle Ages, c.1100–1400* (London and New York: Routledge, 2006)

Metzler, Irina, *A Social History of Disability in the Middle Ages: Cultural Considerations of Physical Impairment* (London and New York: Routledge, 2013)

Meyer-Lee, Robert J., 'The Vatic Penitent: John Audelay's Self-Representation', in *My Wyl and My Wrytyng: Essays on John the Blind Audelay*, ed. Susanna Fein (Kalamazoo, MI: Medieval Institute Publications, 2009), pp. 54–85

The Middle English Dictionary, in *The Middle English Compendium*, ed. Frances Ann McSparran (Ann Arbor, MI: University of Michigan, 1998), Internet resource, http://quod.lib.umich.edu/m/med/

Middleton, Anne, '*The Physician's Tale* and Love's Martyrs: "Ensamples Mo Than Ten" as a Method to the *Canterbury Tales*', *Chaucer Review* 8 (1973), 9–31

Miller, Sarah Alison, *Medieval Monstrosity and the Female Body*, Routledge Studies in Medieval Religion and Culture 8 (New York: Routledge, 2010)

Millett, Bella, *Annotated Bibliographies of Old and Middle English Literature: Ancrene Wisse, the Katherine Group, and the Wooing Group* (Cambridge: D. S. Brewer, 1996)

Minnis, Alastair, *Fallible Authors: Chaucer's Pardoner and Wife of Bath* (Philadelphia: University of Pennsylvania Press, 2008)

Molinari, Paul, *Julian of Norwich: The Teaching of a 14th Century English Mystic* (London: The Catholic Book Club, 1958)

Montford, Angela, *Health, Sickness, Medicine and the Friars in the Thirteenth and Fourteenth Centuries* (Aldershot and Burlington, VT: Ashgate, 2004)

Mooney, Linne R., 'A Middle English Text on the Seven Liberal Arts', *Speculum* 68 (1993), 1027–52

Moulinier-Brogi, Laurence, 'Esthétique et soins du corps dans les traités médicaux latins à la fin du moyen age', *Médiévales* 46 (2004), 55–71

Muessig, Carolyn, 'The Stigmata Debate in Theology and Art in the Late Middle Ages', in *The Authority of the Word: Reflecting on Image and Text in Northern Europe, 1400–1700*, ed. Celeste Brusati, Karl Enenkel and Walter Melion (Leiden: Brill, 2011), pp. 481–504

Muessig, Carolyn, George Ferzoco and Beverley Kienzle (eds), *A Companion to St Catherine of Siena* (Leiden: Brill, 2011)

Murray Jones, Peter, 'Music Therapy in the Later Middle Ages: The Case of Hugo van der Goes', in *Music as Medicine: The History of Music Therapy since Antiquity*, ed. Peregrine Horden (Aldershot: Ashgate, 2000), pp. 120–44

Murray Jones, Peter, 'John of Arderne and the Mediterranean Tradition of Scholastic Surgery', in *Practical Medicine from Salerno to the Black Death*, ed. Luis García-Ballester, Roger French, Jon Arrizabalaga and Andrew Cunningham (Cambridge: Cambridge University Press, 2010), pp. 289–321

Murray Jones, Peter, 'Medicine', in *Oxford Bibliographies in Medieval Studies*, ed. Paul E. Szarmach (New York: Oxford University Press, 2010) http://www.oxfordbibliographies.com/view/document/obo-9780195396584/obo-9780195396584-0051.xml?rskey=uv9yvf&result=1&q=medieval+medicine#firstMatch

Musacchio, Jacqueline Marie, *The Art and Ritual of Childbirth in Renaissance Italy* (New Haven, CT and London: Yale University Press, 1999)

Neugebauer, Richard, 'Treatment of the Mentally Ill in Medieval and Early

Modern England', *Journal of the History of the Behavioral Sciences* 14 (1978), 158–69

Niebryzdowski, Sue, 'Marian Literature', in *The History of British Women's Writing, 700–1500*, ed. Liz Herbert McAvoy and Diane Watt (Basingstoke: Palgrave, 2012), pp. 112–20

Noonan, J. T., *Contraception: A History of Its Treatment by the Catholic Theologians and Canonists* (Cambridge, MA: Harvard University Press, 1966)

Ober, William B., 'Margery Kempe: Hysteria and Mysticism Reconciled', *Literature and Medicine* 4 (1985), 24–40

Olson, Glending, *Literature as Recreation in the Middle Ages* (Ithaca, NY: Cornell University Press, 1982)

Orlemanski, Julie, 'Jargon and the Matter of Medicine in Middle English', *Journal of Medieval and Early Modern Studies* 42, 2 (2012), 395–420

Orlemanski, Julie, 'Thornton's Remedies and Practices of Medical Reading', in *Robert Thornton and His Books: Essays on the London and the Lincoln Thornton Manuscripts*, ed. Susanna Fein and Michael Johnston (York: York Medieval Press, 2014), pp. 235–55.

O'Tool, M. P., 'Disability and the Suppression of Historical Identity: Rediscovering the Professional Backgrounds of the Blind Residents of the Hôpital des Quinze-Vingts', in *Disability in the Middle Ages: Reconsiderations and Reverberations*, ed. Joshua R. Eyler (Farnham: Ashgate, 2010), pp. 11–24

Page, W. (ed.), *Victoria County History: Shropshire II* (London: Oxford University Press for the University of London Institute of Historical Research, 1973)

Palmer, Richard, 'In Bad Odour: Smell and its Significance in Medicine from Antiquity to the Seventeenth Century', in *Medicine and the Five Senses*, ed. W. F. Bynum and Roy Porter (Cambridge: Cambridge University Press, 1993), pp. 61–8

Paravicini-Bagliani, Agostino, *The Pope's Body*, trans. David S. Peterson (Chicago, IL and London: University of Chicago Press, 1994)

Park, Katharine, 'Medicine and Society in Medieval Europe, 500–1500', in *Medicine in Society: Historical Essays*, ed. Andrew Wear (Cambridge: Cambridge University Press, 1992), pp. 59–90

Park, Katharine, *Secrets of Women: Gender, Generation, and the Origins of Human Dissection* (New York: Zone books, 2006)

Partner, Nancy F., 'Reading the *Book of Margery Kempe*', *Exemplaria* 3 (1991), 29–66

Pelling, Margaret, 'The Women of the Family? Speculations around Early Modern British Physicians', *The Society for the Social History of Medicine* 7, 3 (1995), 383–40

Peltzer, Jörg, *Canon Law, Careers and Conquest: Episcopal Elections in Normandy and Greater Anjou, c.1140–c.1230* (Cambridge: Cambridge University Press, 2008)

Pepler, Conrad, *The English Religious Heritage* (London: Blackfriars, 1958)

Petroff, Elizabeth, *Body and Soul: Essays on Medieval Women and Mysticism* (Oxford: Oxford University Press, 1994)

Peyroux, Catherine, 'The Leper's Kiss', in *Monks and Nuns, Saints and Outcasts: Religion in Medieval Society, Essays in Honor of Lester K. Little*, ed. Sharon Farmer and Barbara H. Rosenwein (Ithaca, NY: Cornell University Press, 2000), pp. 172–88

Phillips, Helen, 'Chaucer and Deguileville: The *ABC* in Context', *Medium Aevum* 62 (1993), 1–19

Phillips, Helen (ed.), *Chaucer and Religion* (Cambridge: D. S. Brewer, 2010)

Pitcher, John A., *Chaucer's Feminine Subjects: Figures of Desire in The Canterbury Tales* (New York: Palgrave Macmillan, 2012)

Porter, Roy, *Blood and Guts: A Short History of Medicine* (London: Penguin, 2002)

Pouchelle, Marie-Christine, *The Body and Surgery in the Middle Ages*, trans. R. Morris (Oxford: Polity Press, 1990)

Powell, Susan, 'John Audelay and John Mirk: Comparisons and Contrasts', in *My Wyl and My Wrytyng: Essays on John the Blind Audelay*, ed. Susanna Fein (Kalamazoo, MI: Medieval Institute Publications, 2009), pp. 86–111

Price, B. B., 'The Physical Astronomy and Astrology of Albertus Magnus', in *Albertus Magnus and the Sciences*, ed. J. A. Weisheipl (Toronto: Pontifical Institute of Mediaeval Studies, 1980), 155–85

Rawcliffe, Carole, *Medicine and Society in Later Medieval England* (Stroud: Alan Sutton, 1995)

Rawcliffe, Carole, 'Hospital Nurses and Their Work', in *Daily Life in the Late Middle Ages*, ed. Richard Britnell (Stroud: Sutton, 1998), pp. 43–64

Rawcliffe, Carole, *Medicine for the Soul: The Life, Death and Resurrection of an English Medieval Hospital, St Giles's, Norwich, c. 1249–1550* (Stroud: Sutton, 1999)

Rawcliffe, Carole, 'Learning to Love the Leper: Aspects of Institutional Charity in Anglo-Norman England', *Anglo-Norman Studies* 23 (2000), 231–50

Rawcliffe, Carole, *Leprosy in Medieval England* (Woodbridge: Boydell, 2006)

Rawcliffe, Carole, '"Delectable Sightes and Fragrant Smelles": Gardens and Health in Late Medieval and Early Modern England', *Garden History* 36 (2008), 3–21

Rawcliffe, Carole, *Urban Bodies: Communal Health in Late Medieval English Towns and Cities* (Woodbridge: Boydell, 2013)

Reames, Sherry, 'Mary, Sanctity and Prayers to Saints: Chaucer and Late-Medieval Piety', in *Chaucer and Religion*, ed. Helen Phillips (Cambridge: D. S. Brewer, 2010), pp. 81–96

Reed, Teresa, *Shadows of Mary: Reading the Virgin Mary in Medieval Texts* (Cardiff: University of Wales Press, 2003)

Renevey, Denis, 'Margery's Performing Body: The Translation of Late Medieval Discursive Religious Practices', in *Writing Religious Women: Female Spiritual and Textual Practices in Late Medieval England*, ed. Denis Renevey and Christiania Whitehead (Cardiff: Wales University Press, 2000), pp. 197–216

Renevey, Denis and Christiania Whitehead (eds), *A Companion to* The Doctrine of the Hert*: The Middle English Translation and Its Latin and European Contexts* (Exeter: University of Exeter Press, 2010)

Renevey, Denis and Naoë Kukita Yoshikawa (eds), *Poetica* 72, Special Issue, *Convergence/ Divergence: The Politics and Late Medieval English Devotional and Medical Discourses* (Tokyo: Yushodo Press, 2009)

Reynolds, Anna Marie, 'Some Literary Influences in the *Revelations* of Julian of Norwich (c. 1342–post-1416)', *Leeds Studies in English* 7–8 (1952), 18–28

Riddle, J. M., 'Oral Contraceptives and Early-Term Abortifacients during Classical Antiquity and the Middle Ages', *Past & Present* 132 (1991), 3–32

Roberts, C. and M. Cox, *Health and Disease in Britain: From Prehistory to the Present Day* (Stroud: Sutton, 2003)

Roberts, Marie Mulvey and Roy Porter (eds), *Literature and Medicine during the Eighteenth Century* (London and New York: Routledge, 1993)

Robertson, Elizabeth A., 'The Corporeality of Sanctity in the Life of St Margaret', in *Images of Sainthood in Medieval Europe*, ed. Renate Blumenfeld-Kosinski and Timea Szell (Ithaca, NY: Cornell University Press, 1991), pp. 268–87

Robertson, Elizabeth, 'Medieval Medical Views of Women and Female Spirituality in the *Ancrene Wisse* and Julian of Norwich's *Showings*', in *Feminist Approaches to the Body in Medieval Literature*, ed. Linda Lomperis and Sarah Stanbury (Philadelphia: University of Pennsylvania Press, 1993), pp. 142–67

Robinson, Duncan, *Lectio Divina: The Medieval Experience of Reading*, Cistercian Studies 238 (Collegeville, MN: Liturgical Press, 2011)

Rosenthal, Joel T., *Margaret Paston's Piety* (New York: Palgrave Macmillan, 2010)

Rosser, G., 'Communities of Parish and Guild in the Late Middle Ages', in *Parish, Church and People: Local Studies in Lay Religion 1350–1750*, ed. S. J. Wright (London: Harper-Collins, 1988), pp. 29–55

Rousseau, George S., *Enlightenment Borders: Pre- and Post-modern Discourses: Medical, Scientific* (Manchester and New York: Manchester University Press, 1991)

Rousseau, George S., 'Bridges of Light: The Domains of Literature and Medicine', *The Aberdeen University Review* 56 (1995), 1–22

Rubin, Miri, *Mother of God: A History of the Virgin Mary* (London: Penguin, 2009)

Safilios-Rothschild, C., *The Sociology and Social Psychology of Disability and Rehabilitation* (New York: Random House, 1970)

Savage, Anne, 'From Anchorhold to Cell of Self-Knowledge: Points along a History of the Human Body', in *Rhetoric of the Anchorhold: Space, Place and Body within the Discourses of Enclosure*, ed. Liz Herbert McAvoy (Cardiff: University of Wales Press, 2005), pp. 157–72

Scase, Wendy, 'Reginald Pecock', in *English Writers of the Middle Ages*, ed. M. C. Seymour, Authors of the Middle Ages 3 (Aldershot: Variorum, 1996), pp. 69–146

Scheerenberger, R. C., *A History of Mental Retardation* (Baltimore, MD and London: Brookes, 1983)

Schelberg, Antje M., 'The Beauty and the Beast? Medieval Ideas on Physical Appearance and Their Psychological Meaning with regard to Leprosy Sufferers', in *The Myths of Medieval Leprosy: A Collection of Essays*, ed. Antje M. Schelberg (Göttingen: Tempus, 2006), pp. 35–50

Schroder-Sheket, Therese, 'The Alchemical Harp of Mechthild of Hackeborn', *Vox Benedictina* 6, 1 (1989), 40–55

Scully, Terence, *The Art of Cookery in the Middle Ages* (Woodbridge: Boydell, 1995)

Sedgwick, Peter, *Psycho Politics* (London: Pluto Press, 1982)

Shahar, Shulamith, *Childhood in the Middle Ages* (London and New York: Routledge, 1990)

Shahar, Shulamith, *Growing Old in the Middle Ages: 'Winter Clothes Us in Shadow and Pain'* (London and New York: Routledge, 1997)

Shoham, S. Giora, *The Mark of Cain: the Stigma Theory of Crime and Social Deviation* (Jerusalem: Israel Universities Press, 1970)

Simpson, James, 'Saving Satire after Arundel's Constitutions: John Audelay's "Marcol and Solomon"', in *Text and Controversy from Wyclif to Bale: Essays in Honour of Anne Hudson*, ed. Helen Barr and Ann M. Hutchison (Turnhout: Brepols, 2005), pp. 387–404

Siraisi, Nancy G., 'The Music of the Pulse in the Writings of Italian Academic Physician (Fourteenth and Fifteenth Centuries)', *Speculum* 50 (1975), 689–710

Siraisi, Nancy, *Medieval and Early Renaissance Medicine: An Introduction to Knowledge and Practice* (Chicago, IL: University of Chicago Press, 1990)

Skerpan, Elizabeth P., 'Chaucer's Physicians: Their Texts, Contents, and the *Canterbury Tales*', *Journal of the Rocky Mountain Medieval and Renaissance Association* 5 (1984), 41–56

Skinner, Patricia, *Health and Medicine in Early Medieval Southern Italy* (Leiden: Brill, 1997)

Skinner, Patricia, 'Forum: The Gendered Nose and Its Lack: "Medieval" Nose-cutting and Its Modern Manifestations', *Journal of Women's History* 26, 1 (2014)

Slack, Paul, 'Mirrors of Health and Treasures of Poor Men: The Uses of the Vernacular Medical Literature of Tudor England', in *Health, Medicine and Mortality in the Sixteenth Century*, ed. Charles Webster (Cambridge: Cambridge University Press, 1979), pp. 237–73

Smith, Lesley, 'William of Auvergne and Confession', in *Handling Sin: Confession in the Middle Ages*, ed. Peter Biller and A. J. Minnis (York: York Medieval Press, 1998), pp. 95–107

Solórzana Telechea, Jesús Ángel, 'Fama publica, Infamy and Defamation: Judicial Violence and Social Control of Crimes against Sexual Morals in Medieval Castile', *Journal of Medieval History* 33 (2007), 398–413

St-Jacques, Raymond, 'Langland's Christus Medicus Image and the Structure of *Piers Plowman*', *Yearbook of Langland Studies* 5 (1991), 111–27

Stiker, H.-J., *A History of Disability*, trans. William Sayer (Ann Arbor, MI: University of Michigan Press, 1999)

Stork, Nancy P., 'Did Margery Kempe Suffer from Tourette's Syndrome?', *Mediaeval Studies* 59 (1997), 261–300

Sture, Judi, 'Congenital and Developmental Conditions', in *'Lepers outside the*

Gate': Excavations at the Cemetery of the Hospital of St James and St Mary Magdalene, Chichester, 1986–87 and 1993, ed. John Magilton, Frances Lee and Anthea Bolston, Chichester Excavations vol. 10, CBA Research Report 158 (York: Council for British Archaeology, 2008), pp. 157–63

Swanson, R. N., *Religion and Devotion in Europe, c.1215–c.1515* (Cambridge: Cambridge University Press, 1995)

Swanson, Robert N., 'Praying for Pardon: Devotional Indulgences in Late Medieval England', in *Promissory Notes on the Treasury of Merits: Indulgences in Late Medieval Europe*, ed. Robert N. Swanson (Leiden: Brill, 2006), pp. 215–40

Swanson, Robert N., *Indulgences in Late Medieval England: Passport to Paradise?* (Cambridge: Cambridge University Press, 2007)

Tabbagh, Vincent, *Fasti ecclesiae gallicanae: répertoire prosopographique des éveques, dignitaires et chanoines de France de 1200 à 1500. Tome II: diocèse de Rouen* (Turnhout: Brepols, 1998)

Tanner, N. P., *The Church in Medieval Norwich* (Toronto: Pontifical Institute of Mediaeval Studies, 1984)

Temkin, Owsei, *The Falling Sickness: A History of Epilepsy from the Greeks to the Beginnings of Modern Neurology*, 2nd edn (Baltimore, MD: Johns Hopkins University Press, 1971)

Thorndike, Lynn, *A History of Magic and Experimental Science*, vol. 1 (New York and London: Columbia University Press, 1923)

Thouless, Robert H., *The Lady Julian: A Psychological Study* (London: Society for Promoting Christian Knowledge, 1924)

Tibbetts Schulenberg, Jane, 'The Heroics of Virginity: Brides of Christ and Sacrificial Mutilation', in *Women in the Middle Ages and Renaissance: Literary and Historical Perspectives*, ed. Mary Beth Rose (Syracuse, NY: Syracuse University Press, 1986), pp. 29–72

Tobin, Thomas J., '"He made his confession and told all his misdeeds": The Rise of the Internal Consciousness between 1100 and 1500', *Janus Head* (Summer 1998), Internet resource, http://www.janushead.org/JHSummer98/ThomasTobin.cfm

Torn, Alison, 'Margery Kempe: Madwoman or Mystic – A Narrative Approach to the Representation of Madness and Mysticism in Medieval England', in *Narratives and Fiction: An Interdisciplinary Approach*, ed. David Robinson et al. (Huddersfield: University of Huddersfield Press, 2008), pp. 79–89

Torn, Alison, 'Madness and Mysticism: Can a Mediaeval Narrative Inform our Understanding of Psychosis?', *History and Philosophy of Psychology* 13 (2011), 1–14

Torn, Alison, 'Looking Back: Medieval Mysticism or Psychosis?', *The Psychologist* 24 (2011), 788–90

Touati, François-Olivier, 'Les Léproseries aux XIIème et XIIIème siècles, lieux de conversion?', in Nicole Bériou and François-Olivier Touati, *Voluntate dei leprosus: les Lépreux entre conversion et exclusion aux XIIème et XIIIème siècles,*

Testi, Studi, Strumenti 4 (Spoleto: Centro italiano di studi sull'altro medioevo, 1991), pp. 1–32

Touati, François-Olivier, *Maladie et société au Moyen Âge: la lèpre, les lépreux et les léproseries dans la province ecclésiastique de Sens jusqu'au milieu du XIVe siècle*, Bibliothèque du Moyen Âge 11 (Brussels: De Boeck Université, 1998)

Tucker, M. J., 'The Child as Beginning and End: Fifteenth and Sixteenth Century English Childhood', in *The History of Childhood: The Untold Story of Child Abuse*, ed. Lloyd De Mause (New York: Psychohistory Press, 1974), pp. 229–58

Tyrrell, George S. J., 'Julian of Norwich', *The Faith of the Millions* (London: Longman, Green, 1901), Internet resource, http://www.gutenberg.org/files/10139/10139.txt

Udry, Susan, 'Robert de Blois and Geoffroy de la Tour Landry on Feminine Beauty: Two Late-Medieval French Conduct Books', *Essays in Medieval Studies* 19 (2002), 70–89

Ussery, Huling E., *Chaucer's Physician: Medicine and Literature in Fourteenth-Century England*, Tulane Studies in English 19 (New Orleans, LA: Department of English, Tulane University, 1971)

Vale, Malcolm, 'Aristocratic Violence: Trial by Battle in the Later Middle Ages', in *Violence in Medieval Society*, ed. Richard W. Kaeuper (Woodbridge: Boydell, 2000), pp. 159–81

Vincent, Nicholas, *Holy Blood: King Henry III and the Westminster Blood Relic* (Cambridge: Cambridge University Press, 2001)

Voaden, Rosalynn, 'The Company She Keeps: Mechtild of Hackeborn in Late-Medieval Devotional Compilations', in *Prophets Abroad: The Reception of Continental Holy Women in Late-Medieval England*, ed. Rosalynn Voaden (Cambridge: D. S. Brewer, 1996), pp. 51–69

Voaden, Rosalynn, *God's Words, Women's Voices: The Discernment of Spirits in the Writing of Late-Medieval Women Visionaries* (York: York Medieval Press, 1999)

Voaden, Rosalynn, 'Mechtild of Hackeborn', in *Medieval Holy Women in the Christian Tradition, c. 1100–c. 1500*, ed. Alastair Minnis and Rosalynn Voaden (Turnhout: Brepols, 2010), pp. 431–51

Vuille, Juliette, '"I wolde I wer as worthy to ben sekyr of thy lofe as Mary Mawdelyn was": The Magdalene as an Authorizing Tool in the *Book of Margery Kempe*', in *Mary Magdalene in Medieval Culture: Conflicted Roles*, ed. Peter Loewen and Robin Waugh (London: Routledge, 2014), pp. 208–25

Wack, Mary, *Lovesickness in the Middle Ages: The Viaticum and Its Commentaries* (Philadelphia: University of Pennsylvania Press, 1990)

Walter, Katie, 'Discourses of the Human: Mouths in Late Medieval Religious Literature', unpublished doctoral thesis, University of Cambridge, 2007

Warner, Marina, *Alone of All Her Sex: The Myth and the Cult of the Virgin Mary* (London: Picador, 1985)

Watson, Nicholas, 'The Composition of Julian of Norwich's Revelation of Love', *Speculum* 68 (1993), 637–83

Watson, Nicholas, 'Censorship and Cultural Change in Late-Medieval England: Vernacular Theology, the Oxford Translation Debate, and Arundel's Constitutions of 1409', *Speculum* 70 (1995), 822–64

Watson, Nicholas, '"Yf women be double naturally": Remaking "Woman" in Julian of Norwich's *Revelation of Love*', *Exemplaria* 8, 1 (1996), 1–34

Watt, Diane, *Secretaries of God: Women Prophets in Late Medieval and Early Modern England* (Cambridge: D. S. Brewer, 1997)

Webb, Heather, 'Cardiosensory Impulses in Late Medieval Spirituality', in *Rethinking the Medieval Senses: Heritage, Fascinations, Frames*, ed. Stephen G. Nichols, Andreas Kablitz and Alison Calhoun (Baltimore, MD: Johns Hopkins University Press, 2008), pp. 265–85

Webb, Heather, *The Medieval Heart* (New Haven, CT: Yale University Press, 2010)

Weiss-Adamson, Melitta, '*Regimen sanitatis*', in *Medieval Science, Technology, and Medicine: An Encyclopedia*, ed. Thomas Glick, Steven J. Livesey and Faith Wallis (New York and Abingdon: Routledge, 2005), pp. 438–9

Weissman, Hope P., 'Margery Kempe in Jerusalem: *Hysterica Compassio* in the Late Middle Ages', in *Acts of Interpretation: The Text in Context, 700–1600*, ed. Mary J. Carruthers and Elizabeth D. Kirk (Norman, OK: Pilgrim Books, 1982)

Westlake, H. F., *The Parish Gilds of Mediaeval England* (London: Society for Promoting Christian Knowledge, 1919)

Wheatley, Edward, *Stumbling Blocks before the Blind: Medieval Constructions of a Disability* (Ann Arbor, MI: Michigan University Press, 2010)

Whitaker, Elaine E., 'Reading the Pastons Medically', *English Language Notes* 31 (1993), 19–27

Whitehead, Christiania, 'Spiritual Healing: Healing Miracles associated with the Twelfth-Century Northern Cult of St Cuthbert', in *Medieval and Early Modern Literature, Science and Medicine*, ed. Rachel Falconer and Denis Renevey, Swiss Papers in English Language and Literature 28 (Tübingen: Gunter Narr, 2013), pp. 167–82

Wickham, Chris, 'Gossip and Resistance among the Medieval Peasantry', *Past & Present* 160 (1998), 3–20

Wiethaus, Ulrike, 'Sexuality, Gender and the Body in Late Medieval Women's Spirituality: Cases from Germany and the Netherlands', *Journal of Feminist Studies in Religion* 7 (1991), 35–52

Wilmart, A., 'La légende de Ste Édith en prose et vers par le moine Goscelin', *Analecta Bollandiana* 56 (1938), 265–307

Winzer, M. A., 'Disability and Society before the Eighteenth Century: Dread and Despair', in *The Disability Studies Reader*, ed. L. J. Davis (New York: Routledge 1997), pp. 75–109

Wogan-Browne, Jocelyn and Ian R. Johnson (eds), *The Idea of the Vernacular: An Anthology of Middle English Literary Theory, 1280–1520* (University Park, PA: Pennsylvania State University Press, 1999)

Wood, Charles C., 'The Doctor's Dilemma: Sin, Salvation and the Menstrual Cycle in Medieval Thought', *Speculum* 56, 4 (1981), 710–27

Woolgar, C. M., *The Senses in Late Medieval England* (New Haven, CT: Yale University Press, 2006)

World Health Organization, *ICD 10: International Statistical Classification of Diseases and Related Health Problems: Classification of Mental and Behavioural Disorders* (Geneva: WHO, 1992–94)

World Health Organisation, WHO Fact sheet no. 370, October 2012, http://www.who.int/mediacentre/factsheets/fs370/en/

Wormald, Patrick, *The Making of English Law: King Alfred to the Twelfth Century*, I (Oxford: Blackwell, 1999)

Yearl, Mary K. K. H., 'Medieval Monastic Customaries on *Minuti* and *Infirmi*', in *The Medieval Hospital and Medical Practice*, ed. Barbara S. Bowers, AVISTA Studies in the History of Medieval Technology, Science and Art 3 (Aldershot: Ashgate, 2007), pp. 175–94

Yoshikawa, Naoë Kukita, *Margery Kempe's Meditations: The Context of Medieval Devotional Literature, Liturgy and Iconography* (Cardiff: University of Wales Press, 2007)

Yoshikawa, Naoë Kukita, 'Holy Medicine and Diseases of the Soul: Henry of Lancaster and *Le Livre de Seyntz Medicines*', *Medical History* 53, 3 (2009), 397–414

Yoshikawa, Naoë Kukita, 'Mysticism and Medicine: Holy Communion in the *Vita of Marie d'Oignies* and *The Book of Margery Kempe*', *Poetica* 72, Special Issue, *Convergence/Divergence: The Politics and Late Medieval English Devotional and Medical Discourses*, ed. Denis Renevey and Naoë Kukita Yoshikawa (Tokyo: Yushodo Press, 2009), pp. 109–22

Yoshikawa, Naoë Kukita, 'The Translation of the *Regimen Sanitatis* into a Handbook for the Devout Laity: a New Look at the *Kalender of Shepherds* and its Context', in *Medieval Translator XV: In Principio Fuit Interpres*, ed. Alessandra Petrina (Turnhout: Brepols, 2013), pp. 303–15

Ziegler, Joseph, 'Medical Similes in Religious Discourse: The Case of Giovanni di San Gimignano OP (ca.1250–ca.1333)', *Sciences in Context* 8 (1995), 103–31

Ziegler, Joseph, *Medicine and Religion c. 1300: The Case of Arnau de Vilanova* (Oxford: Clarendon, 1998)

Ziegler, Joseph, 'Medicine and Immortality in Terrestrial Paradise', in *Religion and Medicine in the Middle Ages*, ed. Joseph Ziegler and Peter Biller (York: York Medieval Press, 2001), pp. 201–42

Ziegler, Tiffany A., 'The Hospital of Saint John: Exploring Charitable Distribution in High Medieval Brussels', *Eä: Journal of Medical Humanities & Social Studies of Science and Technology* 3 (2011), 1–32, at http://issuu.com/eajournal/docs/hospital-saint-john-charity-brussels

Zieman, Katherine, 'The Perils of *Canor*: Mystical Authority, Alliteration, and Extragrammatical Meaning in Rolle, the *Cloud*-author, and Hilton', *Yearbook of Langland Studies* 22 (2008), 131–63

INDEX

GENDER IN THE MIDDLE AGES

I *Gender and Medieval Drama,* Katie Normington, 2004

II *Gender and Petty Crime in Late Medieval England: The Local Courts in Kent, 1460–1560,* Karen Jones, 2006

III *The Pastoral Care of Women in Late Medieval England,* Beth Allison Barr, 2008

IV *Gender, Nation and Conquest in the Works of William of Malmesbury,* Kirsten A. Fenton, 2008

V *Monsters, Gender and Sexuality in Medieval English Literature,* Dana M. Oswald, 2010

VI *Medieval Anchoritisms: Gender, Space and the Solitary Life,* Liz Herbert McAvoy, 2011

VII *Middle-Aged Women in the Middle Ages,* edited by Sue Niebrzydowski, 2011

VIII *Married Women and the Law in Premodern Northwest Europe,* edited by Cordelia Beattie and Matthew Frank Stevens, 2013

IX *Religious Men and Masculine Identity in the Middle Ages,* edited by P. H. Cullum and Katherine J. Lewis, 2013

X *Reconsidering Gender, Time and Memory in Medieval Culture,* edited by Elizabeth Cox, Liz Herbert McAvoy and Roberta Magnani, 2015

Lightning Source UK Ltd.
Milton Keynes UK
UKOW06n0004120416

272055UK00019B/543/P